ACP | MKSAP® 18

Medical Knowledge Self-Assessment Program®

Cardiovascular Medicine

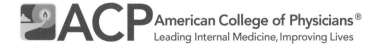

American College of Physicians®
Leading Internal Medicine, Improving Lives

Welcome to the Cardiovascular Medicine Section of MKSAP 18!

In these pages, you will find updated information on risk assessment in cardiovascular disease, diagnostic testing, coronary artery disease, heart failure, arrhythmias, valvular heart disease, myocardial and pericardial disease, peripheral artery disease, and other clinical challenges. All of these topics are uniquely focused on the needs of generalists and subspecialists *outside* of cardiovascular medicine.

The core content of MKSAP 18 has been developed as in previous editions—all essential information that is newly researched and written in 11 topic areas of internal medicine—created by dozens of leading generalists and subspecialists and guided by certification and recertification requirements, emerging knowledge in the field, and user feedback. MKSAP 18 also contains 1200 all-new peer-reviewed, psychometrically validated, multiple-choice questions (MCQs) for self-assessment and study, including 120 in Cardiovascular Medicine. MKSAP 18 continues to include *High Value Care* (HVC) recommendations, based on the concept of balancing clinical benefit with costs and harms, with associated MCQs illustrating these principles and HVC Key Points called out in the text. Internists practicing in the hospital setting can easily find comprehensive *Hospitalist*-focused content and MCQs, specially designated in blue and with the 🄷 symbol.

If you purchased MKSAP 18 Complete, you also have access to MKSAP 18 Digital, with additional tools allowing you to customize your learning experience. MKSAP Digital includes regular text updates with new, practice-changing information, 200 new self-assessment questions, and enhanced custom-quiz options. MKSAP Complete also includes more than 1200 electronic, adaptive learning–enhanced flashcards for quick review of important concepts, as well as an updated and enhanced version of Virtual Dx, MKSAP's image-based self-assessment tool. As before, MKSAP 18 Digital is optimized for use on your mobile devices, with iOS- and Android-based apps allowing you to sync between your apps and online account and submit for CME credits and MOC points online.

Please visit us at the MKSAP Resource Site (mksap.acponline.org) to find out how we can help you study, earn CME credit and MOC points, and stay up to date.

On behalf of the many internists who have offered their time and expertise to create the content for MKSAP 18 and the editorial staff who work to bring this material to you in the best possible way, we are honored that you have chosen to use MKSAP 18 and appreciate any feedback about the program you may have. Please feel free to send any comments to mksap_editors@acponline.org.

Sincerely,

Patrick C. Alguire, MD, FACP
Editor-in-Chief
Senior Vice President Emeritus
Medical Education Division
American College of Physicians

Cardiovascular Medicine

Committee

Andrew Wang, MD, Section Editor[2]
Professor of Medicine
Director, Cardiovascular Disease Fellowship Program
Division of Cardiology
Duke University Health System
Durham, North Carolina

R. Michael Benitez, MD[1]
Professor of Medicine
Associate Chief (Clinical)
Division of Cardiovascular Medicine
Department of Medicine
University of Maryland School of Medicine
Baltimore, Maryland

Heidi M. Connolly, MD[1]
Professor of Medicine
Mayo Clinic College of Medicine
Rochester, Minnesota

W. Schuyler Jones, MD[2]
Associate Professor of Medicine
Director, Adult Cardiac Catheterization Laboratory
Division of Cardiology
Duke University Health System
Durham, North Carolina

Jonathan P. Piccini, MD, MHS[2]
Associate Professor of Medicine
Director, Duke Center for Atrial Fibrillation
Duke University Health System
Duke Clinical Research Institute
Durham, North Carolina

Donna Polk, MD, MPH[2]
Director, Cardiovascular Fellowship Program
Brigham and Women's Hospital
Boston, Massachusetts

Stuart D. Russell, MD, FACP[2]
Temporary Instructor of Medicine
Duke University Health System
Durham, North Carolina

Paul Sorajja, MD[1]
Roger L. and Lynn C. Headrick Family Chair
Valve Science Center
Minneapolis Heart Institute Foundation
Director, Center for Valve and Structural Heart Disease
Abbott Northwestern Hospital
Minneapolis, Minnesota

Aslan Turer, MD, MHS, MBA[2]
Associate Professor
Director, Clinical Heart Center
Division of Cardiology
Department of Internal Medicine
UT Southwestern Medical Center
Dallas, Texas

Consultant

Kevin Curl, MD[1]
Cardiology Fellow
Division of Cardiology
Department of Internal Medicine
Thomas Jefferson University
Philadelphia, Pennsylvania

Editor-in-Chief

Patrick C. Alguire, MD, FACP[2]
Senior Vice President Emeritus, Medical Education
American College of Physicians
Philadelphia, Pennsylvania

Deputy Editor

Denise M. Dupras, MD, PhD, FACP[1]
Associate Program Director
Department of Internal Medicine
Associate Professor of Medicine
Mayo Clinic College of Medicine
Rochester, Minnesota

Cardiovascular Medicine Reviewers

Yousaf Ali, MD, FACP[1]
Muhammad W. Amir, MD, FACP[1]
Nandini Anandu, MD, FACP[1]
Rebecca A. Andrews, MD, FACP[1]
Sivakumar Ardhanari, MD, FACP[1]
David Barcay, MD, FACP[1]
Abdallah Kamouh, MD, FACP[1]
Robert M. Monger, MD, FACP[1]
Rinah I. Shopnick, DO, FACP[1]
Sung K. Yang, MD, FACP[1]

Hospital Medicine Cardiovascular Medicine Reviewers

David H. Chong, MD, FACP[1]
Catharine Malmsten, MD, FACP[1]
Tony I. Oliver, MD, FACP[1]

Cardiovascular Medicine ACP Editorial Staff

Jackie Twomey[1], Staff Editor, Self-Assessment and Educational Programs
Linnea Donnarumma[1], Staff Editor, Self-Assessment and Educational Programs
Margaret Wells[1], Director, Self-Assessment and Educational Programs
Becky Krumm[1], Managing Editor, Self-Assessment and Educational Programs

ACP Principal Staff

Davoren Chick, MD, FACP[2]
Senior Vice President, Medical Education

Patrick C. Alguire, MD, FACP[2]
Senior Vice President Emeritus, Medical Education

Sean McKinney[1]
Vice President, Medical Education

Margaret Wells[1]
Director, Self-Assessment and Educational Programs

Becky Krumm[1]
Managing Editor

Valerie Dangovetsky[1]
Administrator

Ellen McDonald, PhD[1]
Senior Staff Editor

Megan Zborowski[1]
Senior Staff Editor

Randy Hendrickson[1]
Production Administrator/Editor

Julia Nawrocki[1]
Digital Content Associate/Editor

Linnea Donnarumma[1]
Staff Editor

Chuck Emig[1]
Staff Editor

Jackie Twomey[1]
Staff Editor

Joysa Winter[1]
Staff Editor

Kimberly Kerns[1]
Administrative Coordinator

---

1. Has no relationships with any entity producing, marketing, reselling, or distributing health care goods or services consumed by, or used on, patients.

2. Has disclosed relationship(s) with any entity producing, marketing, reselling, or distributing health care goods or services consumed by, or used on, patients.

Disclosure of relationships with any entity producing, marketing, reselling, or distributing health care goods or services consumed by, or used on, patients.

Patrick C. Alguire, MD, FACP
Royalties
UpToDate

Davoren Chick, MD, FACP
Royalties
Wolters Kluwer Publishing
Consultantship
EBSCO Health's DynaMed Plus
Other: Owner and sole proprietor of Coding 101 LLC; research consultant (spouse) for Vedanta Biosciences Inc.

W. Schuyler Jones, MD
Research Grants/Contracts
AstraZeneca, Bristol-Myers Squibb Co., Doris Duke Charitable Foundation, Patient-Centered Outcomes Research Institute
Consultantship
Pfizer Inc.
Other
American Physician Institute (Maintenance of Certification lectures on peripheral artery disease); Daiichi Sankyo Inc. (clinical adjudication program)

Jonathan P. Piccini, MD, MHS
Research Grants/Contracts
Abbott Medical, ARCA biopharma Inc., Boston Scientific Corp., GE Healthcare, Janssen Pharmaceutical, ResMed
Consultantship
Forest Laboratories Inc., GlaxoSmithKline plc., Johnson & Johnson, Laguna Pharmaceuticals, Medtronic plc., Pfizer Inc./Bristol-Meyers Squibb Co., Spectranetics Corp.

Donna Polk, MD, MPH
Honoraria
American College of Cardiology
Board Member
American Society of Nuclear Cardiology

Stuart D. Russell, MD, FACP
Consultantship
Abbott Laboratories, Amgen
Honoraria
American College of Cardiology
Research Grants/Contracts
SQ Pharmaceuticals

Aslan Turer, MD, MHS, MBA
Consultantship
MyoKardia Inc.

Andrew Wang, MD
Research Grants/Contracts
Abbott Vascular Inc., Gilead Sciences Inc., MyoKardia Inc.
Other: MyoKardia Inc. (educational grant)

Acknowledgments

The American College of Physicians (ACP) gratefully acknowledges the special contributions to the development and production of the 18th edition of the Medical Knowledge Self-Assessment Program® (MKSAP® 18) made by the following people:

Graphic Design: Barry Moshinski (Director, Graphic Services), Michael Ripca (Graphics Technical Administrator), and Jennifer Gropper (Graphic Designer).

Production/Systems: Dan Hoffmann (Director, Information Technology), Scott Hurd (Manager, Content Systems), Neil Kohl (Senior Architect), and Chris Patterson (Senior Architect).

MKSAP 18 Digital: Under the direction of Steven Spadt (Senior Vice President, Technology), the digital version of MKSAP 18 was developed within the ACP's Digital Products and Services Department, led by Brian Sweigard (Director, Digital Products and Services). Other members of the team included Dan Barron (Senior Web Application Developer/ Architect), Chris Forrest (Senior Software Developer/Design Lead), Kathleen Hoover (Senior Web Developer), Kara Regis (Manager, User Interface Design and Development), Brad Lord (Senior Web Application Developer), and John McKnight (Senior Web Developer).

The College also wishes to acknowledge that many other persons, too numerous to mention, have contributed to the production of this program. Without their dedicated efforts, this program would not have been possible.

MKSAP Resource Site (mksap.acponline.org)

The MKSAP Resource Site (mksap.acponline.org) is a continually updated site that provides links to MKSAP 18 online answer sheets for print subscribers; access to MKSAP 18 Digital; Board Basics® e-book access instructions; information on Continuing Medical Education (CME), Maintenance of Certification (MOC), and international Continuing Professional Development (CPD) and MOC; errata; and other new information.

International MOC/CPD

For information and instructions on submission of international MOC/CPD, please go to the MKSAP Resource Site (mksap.acponline.org).

Continuing Medical Education

The American College of Physicians is accredited by the Accreditation Council for Continuing Medical Education (ACCME) to provide continuing medical education for physicians.

The American College of Physicians designates this enduring material, MKSAP 18, for a maximum of 275 *AMA PRA Category 1 Credits*™. Physicians should claim only the credit commensurate with the extent of their participation in the activity.

Up to 30 *AMA PRA Category 1 Credits*™ are available from July 31, 2018, to July 31, 2021, for the MKSAP 18 Cardiovascular Medicine section.

Learning Objectives

The learning objectives of MKSAP 18 are to:

- Close gaps between actual care in your practice and preferred standards of care, based on best evidence
- Diagnose disease states that are less common and sometimes overlooked and confusing
- Improve management of comorbid conditions that can complicate patient care
- Determine when to refer patients for surgery or care by subspecialists
- Pass the ABIM Certification Examination
- Pass the ABIM Maintenance of Certification Examination

Target Audience

- General internists and primary care physicians
- Subspecialists who need to remain up to date in internal medicine
- Residents preparing for the certifying examination in internal medicine
- Physicians preparing for maintenance of certification in internal medicine (recertification)

ABIM Maintenance of Certification

Check the MKSAP Resource Site (mksap.acponline.org) for the latest information on how MKSAP tests can be used to apply to the American Board of Internal Medicine (ABIM) for Maintenance of Certification (MOC) points following completion of the CME activity.

Successful completion of the CME activity, which includes participation in the evaluation component, enables the participant to earn up to 275 medical knowledge MOC points in the ABIM's MOC program. It is the CME activity provider's responsibility to submit participant completion information to ACCME for the purpose of granting MOC credit.

Earn Instantaneous CME Credits or MOC Points Online

Print subscribers can enter their answers online to earn instantaneous CME credits or MOC points. You can submit your answers using online answer sheets that are provided at mksap.acponline.org, where a record of your MKSAP 18 credits will be available. To earn CME credits or to apply for MOC points, you need to answer all of the questions in a test and earn a score of at least 50% correct (number of correct answers divided by the total number of questions). Please note that if you are applying for MOC points, you must also enter your birth date and ABIM candidate number.

Take either of the following approaches:

1. Use the printed answer sheet at the back of this book to record your answers. Go to mksap.acponline.org, access the appropriate online answer sheet, transcribe your answers, and submit your test for instantaneous CME credits or MOC points. There is no additional fee for this service.
2. Go to mksap.acponline.org, access the appropriate online answer sheet, directly enter your answers, and submit your test for instantaneous CME credits or MOC points. There is no additional fee for this service.

Earn CME Credits or MOC Points by Mail or Fax

Pay a $20 processing fee per answer sheet and submit the printed answer sheet at the back of this book by mail or fax, as instructed on the answer sheet. Make sure you calculate your score and enter your birth date and ABIM candidate number, and fax the answer sheet to 215-351-2799 or mail the answer sheet to Member and Customer Service, American College of Physicians, 190 N. Independence Mall West, Philadelphia, PA 19106-1572, using the courtesy envelope provided in your MKSAP 18 slipcase. You will need your 10-digit order number and

8-digit ACP ID number, which are printed on your packing slip. Please allow 4 to 6 weeks for your score report to be emailed back to you. Be sure to include your email address for a response.

If you do not have a 10-digit order number and 8-digit ACP ID number, or if you need help creating a username and password to access the MKSAP 18 online answer sheets, go to mksap.acponline.org or email custserv@acponline.org.

Disclosure Policy

It is the policy of the American College of Physicians (ACP) to ensure balance, independence, objectivity, and scientific rigor in all of its educational activities. To this end, and consistent with the policies of the ACP and the Accreditation Council for Continuing Medical Education (ACCME), contributors to all ACP continuing medical education activities are required to disclose all relevant financial relationships with any entity producing, marketing, re-selling, or distributing health care goods or services consumed by, or used on, patients. Contributors are required to use generic names in the discussion of therapeutic options and are required to identify any unapproved, off-label, or investigative use of commercial products or devices. Where a trade name is used, all available trade names for the same product type are also included. If trade-name products manufactured by companies with whom contributors have relationships are discussed, contributors are asked to provide evidence-based citations in support of the discussion. The information is reviewed by the committee responsible for producing this text. If necessary, adjustments to topics or contributors' roles in content development are made to balance the discussion. Further, all readers of this text are asked to evaluate the content for evidence of commercial bias and send any relevant comments to mksap_editors@acponline.org so that future decisions about content and contributors can be made in light of this information.

Resolution of Conflicts

To resolve all conflicts of interest and influences of vested interests, ACP's content planners used best evidence and updated clinical care guidelines in developing content, when such evidence and guidelines were available. All content underwent review by peer reviewers not on the committee to ensure that the material was balanced and unbiased. Contributors' disclosure information can be found with the list of contributors' names and those of ACP principal staff listed in the beginning of this book.

Hospital-Based Medicine

For the convenience of subscribers who provide care in hospital settings, content that is specific to the hospital setting has been highlighted in blue. Hospital icons (H) highlight where the hospital-only content begins, continues over more than one page, and ends.

High Value Care Key Points

Key Points in the text that relate to High Value Care concepts (that is, concepts that discuss balancing clinical benefit with costs and harms) are designated by the HVC icon [HVC].

Educational Disclaimer

The editors and publisher of MKSAP 18 recognize that the development of new material offers many opportunities for error. Despite our best efforts, some errors may persist in print. Drug dosage schedules are, we believe, accurate and in accordance with current standards. Readers are advised, however, to ensure that the recommended dosages in MKSAP 18 concur with the information provided in the product information material. This is especially important in cases of new, infrequently used, or highly toxic drugs. Application of the information in MKSAP 18 remains the professional responsibility of the practitioner.

The primary purpose of MKSAP 18 is educational. Information presented, as well as publications, technologies, products, and/or services discussed, is intended to inform subscribers about the knowledge, techniques, and experiences of the contributors. A diversity of professional opinion exists, and the views of the contributors are their own and not those of the ACP. Inclusion of any material in the program does not constitute endorsement or recommendation by the ACP. The ACP does not warrant the safety, reliability, accuracy, completeness, or usefulness of and disclaims any and all liability for damages and claims that may result from the use of information, publications, technologies, products, and/or services discussed in this program.

Publisher's Information

Disclaimer Regarding Direct Purchases from Online Retailers

CME and/or MOC for MKSAP 18 is available only if you purchase the program directly from ACP. CME credits and MOC points cannot be awarded to those purchasers who have purchased the program from non-authorized sellers such as Amazon, eBay, or any other such online retailer.

Unauthorized Use of This Book Is Against the Law

MKSAP 18 ISBN: 978-1-938245-47-3
Cardiovascular Medicine ISBN: 978-1-938245-48-0

Printed in the United States of America.

For order information in the U.S. or Canada call 800-ACP-1915. All other countries call 215-351-2600 (Monday to Friday, 9 AM – 5 PM ET). Fax inquiries to 215-351-2799 or email to custserv@acponline.org.

Errata

Errata for MKSAP 18 will be available through the MKSAP Resource Site at mksap.acponline.org as new information becomes known to the editors.

Table of Contents

Cardiovascular Medicine High Value Care Recommendations

The American College of Physicians, in collaboration with multiple other organizations, is engaged in a worldwide initiative to promote the practice of High Value Care (HVC). The goals of the HVC initiative are to improve health care outcomes by providing care of proven benefit and reducing costs by avoiding unnecessary and even harmful interventions. The initiative comprises several programs that integrate the important concept of health care value (balancing clinical benefit with costs and harms) for a given intervention into a broad range of educational materials to address the needs of trainees, practicing physicians, and patients.

HVC content has been integrated into MKSAP 18 in several important ways. MKSAP 18 includes HVC-identified key points in the text, HVC-focused multiple choice questions, and, for subscribers to MKSAP Digital, an HVC custom quiz. From the text and questions, we have generated the following list of HVC recommendations that meet the definition below of high value care and bring us closer to our goal of improving patient outcomes while conserving finite resources.

High Value Care Recommendation: A recommendation to choose diagnostic and management strategies for patients in specific clinical situations that balance clinical benefit with cost and harms with the goal of improving patient outcomes.

Below are the High Value Care Recommendations for the Cardiovascular Medicine section of MKSAP 18.

- Exercise electrocardiography is the initial stress test in patients who can exercise and have normal findings on a baseline electrocardiogram (see Item 27).
- Stress testing is not routinely recommended in asymptomatic patients with diabetes mellitus to detect subclinical coronary artery disease.
- Coronary artery calcification assessment in asymptomatic patients should be limited to those at intermediate risk in whom reclassification of risk will influence primary prevention therapy.
- Percutaneous coronary intervention in chronic stable angina is reserved for patients with refractory symptoms, high-risk features, or an inability to tolerate medical therapy (see Item 79).
- An ischemia-guided approach is appropriate for low-risk non–ST-elevation acute coronary syndrome (see Item 96).
- Do not use thrombolytic therapy for treatment of non–ST-elevation acute coronary syndromes.

- Do not use statin therapy for secondary prevention of cardiovascular disease in patients on hemodialysis.
- Do not use serial B-type natriuretic peptide measurements to guide heart failure therapy.
- Office follow-up within 1 week of discharge reduces early readmission for heart failure (see Item 83).
- Guideline-directed medical therapy for heart failure with reduced ejection fraction reduces cardiovascular mortality (see Item 114).
- Guideline-directed medical therapy precedes consideration of device therapy for symptomatic heart failure (see Item 28).
- Do not routinely use pulmonary artery catheterization to guide heart failure therapy.
- Low-risk premature ventricular contractions require no intervention.
- Pacemaker implantation is not indicated for asymptomatic first-degree atrioventricular block with bifascicular block (see Item 113).
- Do not perform genetic testing for hypertrophic cardiomyopathy in the absence of an identified mutation in the proband.
- No treatment or follow-up is needed for an asymptomatic patent foramen ovale.
- Treatment of iron deficiency in patients with congenital cyanotic heart disease improves exercise capacity and quality of life (see Item 22).
- Manage uncomplicated ventricular septal defect with periodic clinical follow-up and imaging (see Item 67).
- Do not screen for peripheral artery disease with ankle-brachial index testing in asymptomatic patients without risk factors.
- Primary therapy for asymptomatic peripheral artery disease is risk factor modification (see Item 39).
- Obtain a toe-brachial index in patients with an ankle-brachial index greater than 1.40 to diagnose peripheral artery disease (see Item 24).
- Primary treatment for intermittent claudication is exercise training (see Item 15).
- Benign asymptomatic murmurs do not require investigation (see Item 50).
- Transthoracic echocardiography is indicated for systolic murmurs grade 3/6 or higher, late or holosystolic murmurs, diastolic or continuous murmurs, and murmurs with symptoms (see Item 110).
- Transthoracic echocardiography is the initial imaging modality for suspected infective endocarditis (see Item 95).

Cardiovascular Medicine

Epidemiology and Risk Factors

Overview

Cardiovascular disease (CVD) encompasses many conditions, including coronary artery disease (CAD), heart failure, valvular heart disease, stroke, congenital heart defects, heart rhythm disorders, and sudden cardiac arrest. CVD is the leading cause of death in the United States; however, from 2004 to 2014, the mortality rate attributable to CVD fell approximately 25%, likely as a result of improved primary and secondary prevention. Despite this improvement, CVD was responsible for nearly 31% of all deaths in the United States in 2014 (roughly 800,000 people). Globally, CVD resulted in more than 17.3 million deaths in 2013, representing 31% of all deaths.

More than one in three U.S. adults currently have some form of CVD. Prevalence increases with age, and more than 70% of persons aged 60 to 79 years have CVD. The American Heart Association projects that 44% of the U.S. population will have some form of CVD by 2030. Lifetime risk for CVD is estimated to be one in three for women and two in three for men according to data from the Framingham Heart Study.

Hospitalizations for cardiovascular-related diseases continue to increase. In 2011, heart failure and heart rhythm problems were among the top 10 diagnoses associated with hospital admission in the United States, accounting for approximately 1.7 million hospital stays. The number of inpatient cardiovascular operations and procedures increased 28% to more than 7.5 million from 2000 to 2010. CVD, including stroke, was associated with a cost of $316.6 billion in 2011.

An estimated 5.7 million U.S. adults older than 20 years have a diagnosis of heart failure, a final common pathway for many cardiovascular conditions. The prevalence of heart failure is projected to increase by 46% between 2012 and 2030, and the current annual incidence is 1 in 1000 persons in those older than 65 years. Most patients with heart failure (75%) have a history of hypertension. The overall mortality rate after the diagnosis of heart failure is roughly 50% at 5 years, with about half of those deaths due to cardiovascular causes.

Risk Factors for Cardiovascular Disease

Lifestyle

Cardiovascular risk can be mostly attributed to modifiable risk factors. Very few persons meet the seven metrics of cardiovascular health: optimal lipid, blood pressure, and glucose levels; healthy diet; appropriate energy intake; physical activity; and avoidance of tobacco. Elevated cholesterol levels impart the highest risk for myocardial infarction (MI), followed by current smoking, diabetes mellitus, hypertension, abdominal obesity, no alcohol intake, inadequate exercise, and suboptimal consumption of fruits and vegetables.

Elevations in serum cholesterol levels are associated with increased cardiovascular risk, and reductions in cholesterol levels can reduce overall risk. Thirteen percent of adults older than age 20 years, or 31 million persons, have total cholesterol levels greater than 240 mg/dL (6.22 mmol/L), and 6% of adults are estimated to have undiagnosed hypercholesterolemia. Elevated LDL cholesterol and low HDL cholesterol levels are also independently associated with increased risk for CVD. A 1% reduction in LDL cholesterol level decreases risk for CAD by 1%. Risk for CAD decreases 2% to 3% for every 1% increase in HDL cholesterol level; however, pharmacologic therapies that increase HDL cholesterol levels in patients with acceptable LDL cholesterol levels do not reduce cardiovascular events. Current cholesterol treatment guidelines are based on cardiovascular risk rather than absolute lipid levels. For primary prevention of cardiovascular events, the treatment goal is at least a 50% reduction in LDL cholesterol level in high-risk patients and a 30% to 50% reduction in moderate-risk patients (see MKSAP 18 General Internal Medicine).

Tobacco exposure is a significant risk factor for CVD, including CAD, stroke, and peripheral vascular disease. In 2010, smoking was the second leading risk factor for death in the United States, exceeded only by dietary risks. The prevalence of tobacco use continues to decline; 18.8% of men and 15.1% of women were current smokers in 2014. The percentage of adolescents who smoke tobacco daily has also decreased significantly, from 15.2% in 2003 to 7.8% in 2013. In patients who smoke, overall mortality is increased two to three times, and risk for stroke is increased two to four times. The use of tobacco increases the risk for CAD by 25% in women. Secondhand smoke increases the risk for CVD by 25% to 30%. Smoking cessation substantially reduces cardiovascular risk within 2 years, with risk returning to the level of a nonsmoker after approximately 10 years. Smokers who quit extend their life expectancy by several years. Smoking status should be assessed at every visit, and cessation counseling should be offered to active smokers (see MKSAP 18 General Internal Medicine).

Psychosocial stressors, including depression, anger, and anxiety, are associated with worse cardiovascular outcomes. Depression has been linked with higher risk for cardiovascular events, and psychosocial stressors also affect the course of treatment and adherence to healthy lifestyles after an event.

Sedentary lifestyle, poor diet, and obesity contribute to increased cardiovascular risk and increase the risk for diabetes. According to the Centers for Disease Control and Prevention, 23.7% of adults report no leisure time physical activity, and only 20.2% of adults meet aerobic and strengthening recommendations. Average fruit and vegetable consumption in the United States is less than 1 cup of fruit daily (recommended is 1.5-2 cups daily) and less than 1.5 cups of vegetables daily (recommended is 2-3 cups daily). On the basis of adherence to 2010 U.S. dietary guidelines, average diet quality is worse in men than in women, in younger adults than in older adults, and in smokers than in nonsmokers. The National Diabetes Prevention Program found that in persons at high risk for diabetes, interventions such as changes in diet, exercise, and moderate weight loss of 5% to 7% reduced the risk for developing diabetes by 58% but did not reduce CVD events.

Genetics

Although CVD risk is mainly attributable to traditional risk factors, additional risk may be caused by other factors, including genetic predisposition. A history of premature CAD (male younger than 55 years, female younger than 65 years) in parents doubles risk for MI in men and increases risk in women by 70%. CVD in a sibling increases risk for CVD by 45%, and stroke in a first-degree relative increases risk for stroke by 50%. A parental history of atrial fibrillation increases odds of this condition by 80%. In addition to genetics, the shared environment (that is, lifestyle) may contribute to increased risk in family members.

Ethnicity

There are significant racial and ethnic differences in the risk and prevalence for CVD in the United States. The prevalence of heart disease, including MI, chest pain, heart failure, and stroke, is highest among Hawaiians and Pacific Islanders (19.1%), followed by American Indians and Alaska Natives (13.7%), non-Hispanic whites (11.1%), blacks (10.3%), Hispanics and Latinos (7.8%), and Asians (6.0%).

Risk factor prevalence varies by ethnicity, location, income, and education level. Prevalence of hypertension (blood pressure ≥130/80 mm Hg) is highest among non-Hispanic black men (59%) and non-Hispanic black women (56%) and lowest among Hispanic men (44%) and non-Hispanic Asian women (36%). In contrast, the risk for diabetes is highest among American Indians and Alaska Natives (15.9%), followed by non-Hispanic blacks (13.2%) and Hispanics (12.8%). Tobacco use is highest among non-Hispanic blacks (19.9%) and lowest among Asian men (13.8%) and Hispanics (13.8%).

Globally, the prevalence of cardiovascular risk factors and subsequent CVD is increasing as a result of changes in eating habits, tobacco use, and lifestyle factors.

KEY POINT

- Risk for cardiovascular disease is mostly attributed to modifiable risk factors, including dyslipidemia, smoking, diabetes mellitus, hypertension, obesity, inadequate exercise, and diet.

Calculating Cardiovascular Risk

Cardiovascular risk scores and calculators can be used to assess a patient's future risk for major cardiovascular events and to identify which interventions are most effective for prevention. Traditionally, the Framingham risk score, which includes age, systolic blood pressure, total cholesterol level, HDL cholesterol level, smoking status, and presence of diabetes, was used to estimate the 10-year risk for a major coronary heart disease event (MI or coronary death). The Framingham risk score classifies a 10-year risk for coronary heart disease of less than 10% as low risk, 10% to 20% as intermediate risk, and greater than 20% as high risk (considered a CVD risk equivalent). A limitation of the Framingham risk score is its underestimation of risk in women and minority populations. The Reynolds risk score, which was developed in an effort to create a more accurate risk assessment tool, is a sex-specific score for both men and women that includes family history and high-sensitivity C-reactive protein level.

The American College of Cardiology/American Heart Association (ACC/AHA) Pooled Cohort Equations are a risk assessment instrument derived from several community-based cohorts that included large minority populations in addition to the cohort included in the Framingham Heart Study. The Pooled Cohort Equations include the cardiovascular endpoints of MI, angina, ischemic or hemorrhagic stroke, transient ischemic attack, claudication, and heart failure. The ACC/AHA CVD risk calculator based on the Pooled Cohort Equations (available at http://tools.acc.org/ASCVD-Risk-Estimator/) may be used to identify persons at risk for the development of CVD who would benefit from preventive measures, including statin therapy. The risk calculator can also be used to risk-stratify patients with diabetes to determine the appropriate intensity of statin therapy. However, there are concerns that the Pooled Cohort Equations overestimate risk in certain populations, including women and some minorities.

The ACC/AHA and U.S. Preventive Services Task Force do not recommend routinely using several previously considered cardiovascular risk factors, including a history of premature cardiovascular disease in a first-degree relative, elevated lifetime ASCVD risk, and LDL cholesterol level of 160 mg/dL (4.14 mmol/L) or higher, for cardiovascular risk calculation. Other nontraditional risk factors, such as high-sensitivity C-reactive protein level of 2 mg/L or greater, coronary artery calcium score of 300 or higher or in the 75th percentile or greater, and ankle-brachial index below 0.90, have been associated with an increased risk of cardiovascular events; however, the value of these measurements, and whether they should affect treatment decisions, is unclear.

> **KEY POINT**
>
> - The American College of Cardiology/American Heart Association Pooled Cohort Equations are used to identify persons at risk for the development of cardiovascular disease who would benefit from preventive measures, including statin therapy.

Specific Risk Groups

Hypertension

Hypertension, defined as a blood pressure of 130/80 mm Hg or higher, affects approximately 46% of individuals aged 20 years and older. Before age 45 years, the prevalence of hypertension is higher in men than in women; however, after age 65 years, the prevalence is higher in women than in men. The population attributable risk of hypertension for first MI is 18%. Among the modifiable risk factors, hypertension is the leading cause of death in women. Treatment of hypertension reduces risk for stroke, heart failure, and kidney disease.

Women

Although mortality from CVD has decreased in the past decade, the death rate remains higher in women than in men. CVD remains the leading cause of death in women, resulting in more deaths than caused by cancer, diabetes, and kidney disease combined. In 2013, heart disease caused 398,086, or 1 in 3.2, deaths in women. Mortality within the first year after first MI is higher in women (26%) than in men (19%), and younger women are particularly at risk for death. Within 5 years of MI, nearly 50% of women will die, develop heart failure, or have a stroke, compared with 36% of men. Women have a higher risk for stroke than men throughout their lifetime as well.

The prevalence of and risk for CVD are higher in nonwhite women than in white women. Prevalence of acute MI and mortality are highest among black women. Black women also have a higher prevalence of heart disease (7.0%) compared with Hispanic women (5.9%) and white women (4.6%). Hispanic women develop heart disease nearly 10 years earlier than white women. In the past decade, heart disease mortality has increased in Asian Indian women.

Hyperlipidemia, type 2 diabetes, obesity, and tobacco use confer greater risk for CAD in women compared with men. Additional factors associated with increased risk for CVD include depression; preterm labor; and less aggressive management of recognized CVD risk factors, such as hypertension.

Significant anatomic obstruction in coronary arteries is less predictive of clinical CAD in women than in men.

Approximately two thirds of women who die of MI have no previous symptoms or have symptoms that were unrecognized as cardiac in origin. Many women have symptoms described as chest discomfort, indigestion, shortness of breath, or unusual fatigue, but less than 50% of women seek medical attention for these symptoms. Because of the atypical presentation of angina, diagnosis and treatment in women are delayed when compared with men.

Treatments and outcomes also differ between men and women. After an acute coronary syndrome, women undergo fewer interventions, have more complications, and have higher unadjusted mortality. Women with non–ST-elevation MI have worse outcomes, with higher rates of bleeding, heart failure, shock, kidney failure, stroke, and reinfarction.

Obesity and Metabolic Syndrome

In the United States, 33.1% of adults older than 20 years are overweight (BMI, 25-29.9), 35.7% are obese (BMI >30), and 6.3% are extremely obese (BMI >40). Rates are increased in nonwhite adults. Obesity may increase the risk for CVD events, even in the absence of metabolic risk factors.

Metabolic syndrome is characterized by the presence of at least three of the following conditions: elevated glucose level, central obesity, low HDL cholesterol level, elevated triglyceride level, and elevated blood pressure. The hallmark feature of metabolic syndrome is glucose intolerance. Approximately 23% of adults older than 20 years meet the criteria for metabolic syndrome, but the prevalence varies considerably among different ethnicities. The highest prevalence is among Mexican American men (35%) and lowest among non–Mexican American black men (19%). Metabolic syndrome is associated with increased risk for CVD, with risk increasing as the number of component conditions increases. The cardiovascular risk associated with metabolic syndrome also appears to be higher among women.

Diabetes Mellitus

Diabetes has been diagnosed in approximately 23.4 million U.S. adults, and an estimated 7.6 million U.S. adults have undiagnosed diabetes. The prevalence of diabetes and prediabetes is increasing among adolescents aged 12 to 19 years and in those older than 65 years. Additionally, diabetes prevalence is disproportionately higher in nonwhite ethnic groups, including African Americans and Hispanics/Latinos.

Diabetes increases cardiovascular risk, especially in women, and is considered a CVD risk equivalent. Persons with diabetes have a two to four times increased risk for CVD; 68% of those with diabetes eventually die of heart disease, and 16% die of stroke. In persons with diabetes, the risk for stroke is increased 1.8- to 6-fold. Additionally, CAD is more extensive in persons with diabetes, and the incidence of multivessel disease is increased. Patients with diabetes are more likely to have undiagnosed CAD and have worse outcomes when hospitalized for other CVDs, such as heart failure. Undiagnosed diabetes may be recognized at the time of an acute event, such as MI.

Aggressive treatment of cardiovascular risk factors, such as elevated cholesterol levels, is associated with reduced cardiovascular risk in patients with diabetes. Early recognition and treatment are important in reducing the burden of CVD and the morbidity and mortality associated with diabetes.

Systemic Inflammatory Conditions

The prevalence of atherosclerosis is increased and the risk for CVD is higher in patients with systemic inflammatory conditions, such as systemic lupus erythematosus and rheumatoid arthritis. The risk for CAD is nearly 60% higher in patients with rheumatoid arthritis and is doubled in patients with systemic lupus erythematosus. Patients with systemic lupus erythematosus and antiphospholipid antibodies have a higher prevalence of CAD and MI; the relative risk for MI is higher in younger patients with systemic lupus erythematosus than in age-matched controls. The risk for CVD in patients with rheumatoid arthritis increases from twofold at baseline to threefold over 10 years when compared with the general population. The increased risk is likely a result of the inflammatory process, including a prothrombic state, in addition to traditional cardiovascular risk factors.

Chronic Kidney Disease

Chronic kidney disease, defined as reduced estimated glomerular filtration rate, is associated with higher incidence of CVD and worse cardiovascular outcomes. Beyond the risk attributable to traditional risk factors, the risk for cardiovascular events is higher in patients with kidney dysfunction. CVD is the leading cause of death in patients with end-stage kidney disease, and the risk for CVD-related death is 5 to 30 times higher in patients undergoing dialysis than in those with similar risk factors and preserved kidney function. The presence of moderately increased albuminuria (microalbuminuria) independently increases the risk for cardiovascular events.

Despite excessive cardiovascular risk, there is evidence that patients with chronic kidney disease do not receive appropriate preventive therapies, such as statins. Data indicate that patients undergoing hemodialysis do not benefit from secondary prevention with statins.

HIV

Increased survival of patients infected with HIV due to effective antiretroviral therapy has resulted in the increased development of non–AIDS-related complications, including CVD. Patients with HIV have a 1.5 times increased risk for CVD, and cardiovascular mortality is increasing in the HIV-infected population. The increased risk is likely multifactorial, related to antiretroviral therapy–associated dyslipidemia, insulin resistance,

medications associated with CVD events (such as protease inhibitors), viral load, and disease-related increases in risk factors (dyslipidemia, diabetes).

KEY POINTS

- Hyperlipidemia, type 2 diabetes mellitus, obesity, and tobacco use confer greater risk for coronary artery disease in women than in men.
- Delayed diagnosis of coronary artery disease in women is often due to the presentation of atypical chest pain.
- Cardiovascular disease risk is increased in patients with diabetes mellitus, systemic inflammatory conditions, HIV, and chronic kidney disease.
- Statin therapy should not be used for secondary prevention of cardiovascular disease in patients on hemodialysis.

HVC

Diagnostic Testing in Cardiology

Clinical History and Physical Examination

The clinical history and physical examination are cornerstones in the diagnosis of cardiovascular disease. A careful history that includes symptom characteristics, timing, and duration; factors that exacerbate or relieve symptoms; and functional capacity is critical to ensure a focused and appropriate diagnostic evaluation. Abnormal findings on the cardiovascular examination may also raise suspicion for specific cardiac conditions and guide the selection of tests.

Cardiovascular testing provides both diagnostic and prognostic information, and its use should be guided by symptoms, the pretest likelihood of heart disease, and whether testing results will alter patient management.

Diagnostic Testing for Atherosclerotic Coronary Artery Disease

Diagnostic testing for coronary artery disease (CAD) can be categorized as providing functional and/or anatomic information regarding atherosclerotic disease burden. Functional studies reveal the presence of ischemia (exercise electrocardiography [ECG], single-photon emission CT [SPECT], PET), the extent and severity of ischemia (SPECT, PET), information on coronary blood flow (PET, fractional flow reserve (FFR)–CT), and development of wall motion abnormalities (echocardiography, cardiac magnetic resonance [CMR] imaging). Anatomic information is obtained from invasive angiography, coronary CT angiography (CTA), and coronary artery calcium (CAC) scoring. Cardiac diagnostic testing modalities are summarized in **Table 1**.

TABLE 1. Diagnostic Testing for Coronary Artery Disease

Diagnostic Test	Utility	Advantages	Limitations
Exercise Stress Testing			
Exercise ECG	Initial diagnostic test in most patients suspected of having CAD	Data acquired on exercise capacity, blood pressure and heart rate response, and provoked symptoms	Not useful when baseline ECG is abnormal (LVH, LBBB, paced rhythm, preexcitation, >1-mm ST-segment depression)
Stress echocardiography	Recommended when baseline ECG findings are abnormal or when information on a particular area of myocardium at risk is needed	Exercise data acquired along with imaging for wall motion abnormalities to indicate ischemia Allows evaluation of valve function and pulmonary pressures Relatively portable and less costly than nuclear protocols Entire study is completed in <1 h	Image quality is suboptimal in some patients but can be improved with microbubble transpulmonary contrast Image interpretation is difficult when baseline wall motion abnormalities are present Diagnostic accuracy decreases with single-vessel disease or delayed stress image acquisition
Nuclear SPECT perfusion	Recommended when baseline ECG findings are abnormal or when information on a particular area of myocardium at risk is needed With LBBB, conduction delay in the septum may cause false-positive abnormalities; vasodilator stress can improve the accuracy of perfusion imaging	Gating (image acquisition coordinated with the cardiac cycle); use of higher-energy agents, such as technetium; and techniques used to correct for attenuation provide improved specificity Late reperfusion imaging allows evaluation of myocardial viability if thallium is used	Attenuation artifacts can be caused by breast tissue or diaphragm interference; attenuation correction and software programs can improve image interpretation Radiation exposure
Pharmacologic Stress Testing			
Dobutamine echocardiography	Recommended in patients who cannot exercise or when information on an area of myocardium at risk is needed	Because the patient is supine, images are acquired continuously, allowing the test to be stopped as soon as ischemia is evident	Contraindications are severe baseline hypertension, unstable angina, severe tachyarrhythmias, hypertrophic cardiomyopathy, severe aortic stenosis, and large aortic aneurysm
Vasodilator nuclear perfusion (adenosine, dipyridamole, regadenoson)	Recommended in patients who cannot exercise Minimizes septal abnormalities frequently seen with nuclear perfusion scanning in patients with LBBB	Vasodilator stress testing may minimize effect of β-blockade on perfusion defect size Imaging can be performed sooner after myocardial infarction with vasodilator stress	Contraindications are active bronchospastic airway disease, theophylline use, sick sinus syndrome, hypotension, and high-degree AV block Caffeine must be withheld 12-24 h before the test Adenosine or dipyridamole may cause chest pain, dyspnea, or flushing Radiation exposure
Dobutamine nuclear perfusion	Recommended in patients who cannot exercise and have contraindications to vasodilator stress Recommended when information on an area of myocardium at risk is needed	Has sensitivity and specificity similar to those of exercise or vasodilator perfusion imaging for diagnosis of myocardial ischemia	Contraindications are severe baseline hypertension, unstable angina, severe tachyarrhythmias, hypertrophic cardiomyopathy, severe aortic stenosis, and large aortic aneurysm Radiation exposure
PET/CT	Provides best perfusion images in larger patients Provides data on myocardial perfusion, function, and viability	Study duration is shorter and radiation dose is lower than with conventional nuclear perfusion imaging Absolute myocardial blood flow can be measured Can be combined with CAC scoring	Not widely available More expensive than other imaging modalities Used with pharmacologic stress only (no exercise protocol) Radiation exposure

(Continued on the next page)

TABLE 1. Diagnostic Testing for Coronary Artery Disease *(Continued)*

Diagnostic Test	Utility	Advantages	Limitations
Dobutamine or adenosine CMR imaging	Provides excellent spatial resolution for wall motion abnormalities during dobutamine infusion Identifies perfusion abnormalities during adenosine infusion with gadolinium as contrast agent Provides data on infarction and viability using gadolinium contrast Identifies anomalous coronary artery origin	Accurate test for myocardial ischemia or viability	Some patients experience claustrophobia May be contraindicated in patients with pacemaker, ICD, or other implanted device Gadolinium is contraindicated in patients with kidney failure Sinus rhythm and a slower heart rate are needed for improved image quality Limited availability and expertise
Other Tests			
Coronary angiography	Provides anatomic diagnosis of the presence and severity of CAD	Percutaneous revascularization can be performed after diagnostic study	Invasive Risks of vascular access and radiocontrast exposure (kidney dysfunction, allergy, bleeding) Radiation exposure
CAC scoring	May inform treatment decisions for patients with intermediate 10-year risk for cardiovascular events	CAC scores are predictive of cardiovascular risk in selected patients	Does not provide data on coronary luminal narrowing Radiation exposure
Coronary CT angiography	Identifies anomalous coronary arteries Useful for selected patients with intermediate risk for CAD	Coronary artery vessel lumen and atherosclerotic lesions can be visualized in detail	Requires high-resolution (64-slice) CT instruments Does not provide detailed images of distal vessel anatomy Catheterization will be needed if intervention is planned Ability to quantify lesion severity can be limited by significant calcification Radiation and radiocontrast exposure

AV = atrioventricular; CAC = coronary artery calcium; CAD = coronary artery disease; CMR = cardiac magnetic resonance; ECG = electrocardiography; ICD = implantable cardioverter-defibrillator; LBBB = left bundle branch block; LVH = left ventricular hypertrophy; SPECT = single-photon emission CT.

Cardiac Stress Testing

Cardiac stress testing is commonly performed to diagnose CAD. Appropriate, cost-effective stress testing is based on the history, physical examination, and pretest probability of CAD, which takes into account age, sex, symptoms, and prevalence of disease. Cardiac stress testing is most effectively used in patients with an intermediate pretest probability of CAD, in whom a positive test result significantly increases disease likelihood and a negative test result significantly decreases likelihood (see Coronary Artery Disease). Performing stress testing in persons with a low likelihood of disease (such as young patients with atypical symptoms) yields a high incidence of false-positive test results, potentially resulting in unnecessary testing, inaccurate diagnoses, and harms. In patients with a high pretest probability of disease, invasive angiography rather than stress testing is appropriate.

Assessment of the patient's functional capacity and ability to exercise is important in determining the most appropriate stress testing. Exercise ECG is recommended as the initial test of choice in patients with normal findings on baseline ECG. If there are baseline ECG abnormalities (such as ST-segment depression >1 mm, left bundle branch block, left ventricular hypertrophy, paced rhythm, or preexcitation), ST-segment changes with exercise cannot be used to evaluate for the presence of obstructive CAD; these abnormalities will result in a nondiagnostic ECG stress test. Functional testing with imaging (with exercise or pharmacologic stress) or anatomic assessment with coronary CTA is indicated in these instances.

Stress testing may also be used for risk assessment in patients known or suspected to have CAD. The ability to exercise and, more important, exercise capacity are strong predictors of cardiovascular events. ECG changes, hemodynamic response to exercise (blood pressure and heart rate recovery), and other measures (such as the Duke Treadmill Score) also provide prognostic information. Stress imaging studies provide information on the extent and severity of disease, which is helpful for risk assessment.

The decision of whether to withhold cardiac medications, such as nitrates and β-blockers, before stress testing should be individualized. In patients who are undergoing exercise stress testing to diagnose CAD, cardiac medications that impair heart rate response (β-blockers) should be withheld for at least 24 hours before testing because these agents may lead to an inadequate peak heart rate. If the stress test is being performed to evaluate symptoms or determine prognosis in a patient with known CAD, patients should continue their cardioactive medication regimen.

Exercise Electrocardiography

Stress testing should always be performed with exercise, unless exercise is contraindicated or the patient is unable to exercise. Exercise stress testing protocols use treadmill or stationary bicycle ergometry, and each protocol should increase workload in a stepwise manner over a period of 6 to 12 minutes to allow adequate time for development of maximal metabolic demand. A standard Bruce protocol increases the speed and grade of the treadmill every 3 minutes. Achieving 85% of the age-predicted maximal heart rate adequately rules out obstructive CAD; however, patients should exercise until limited by symptoms. Because heart rate and blood pressure are the major determinants of myocardial oxygen demand, achieving a rate pressure product (heart rate × systolic blood pressure) of at least 25,000 is considered an adequate workload and reflects overall left ventricular myocardial performance. Stress testing should be terminated when the patient has

exerted maximal effort, requests to stop, or experiences significant angina or other physical symptoms. The test should also be stopped for exertional hypotension, significant hypertension (>200/110 mm Hg), ST-segment elevation or significant ST-segment depression, or ventricular or supraventricular arrhythmias.

Ischemia is defined by the development of horizontal or downsloping ST-segment depression of at least 1 mm occurring 80 milliseconds after the J point on exercise ECG, although ST-segment depression cannot localize ischemia (**Figure 1**). The development of hypotension or lack of blood pressure augmentation during exercise can indicate the presence of significant obstructive disease. Heart rate recovery after cessation of exercise provides incremental prognostic information. A heart rate drop of less than 12/min in the first minute after exercise termination is associated with higher mortality. Functional capacity is also a powerful predictor of outcomes; individuals unable to achieve 5 metabolic equivalents, or the first stage of a Bruce protocol, have higher all-cause mortality. Information obtained from exercise stress testing can be combined with clinical information in risk prediction models. The Duke Treadmill Score incorporates duration of exercise, development of symptoms, and degree of ST-segment depression to calculate 5-year all-cause mortality in patients without CAD.

Stress Testing with Adjunctive Imaging

In patients with obstructive CAD, reduced blood flow and myocardial ischemia lead to a progression of myocardial abnormalities, termed the ischemic cascade. Initially, ischemia induces changes in perfusion, followed by diastolic and (at a later stage) systolic dysfunction, ECG changes, and eventually angina. The addition of imaging studies to ECG stress testing

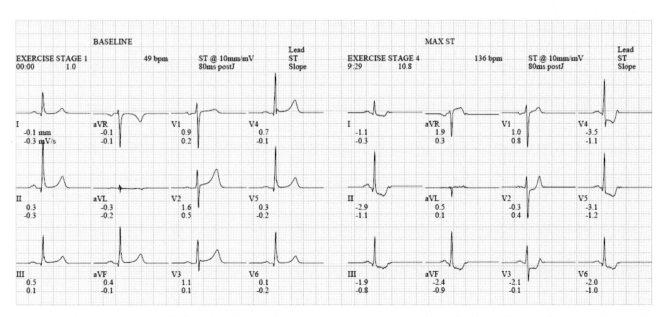

FIGURE 1. Electrocardiogram recorded before (*left*) and during (*right*) exercise stress testing. The presence of 2-mm downsloping ST-segment depressions in leads I, II, III, and aVF, and leads V$_3$ through V$_6$, during exercise indicates ischemia.

CONT.

increases diagnostic sensitivity by detecting earlier signs of ischemia.

Stress testing with imaging is indicated in patients with an inability to exercise, contraindications to exercise, baseline ECG abnormalities that would preclude interpretation of the exercise ECG, or indeterminate findings on the exercise ECG. Imaging with SPECT, PET, or CMR can be used to detect reduced myocardial perfusion as early evidence of ischemia. Systolic dysfunction, indicated by wall motion abnormalities during stress, can be detected by echocardiography or CMR imaging. Overall, imaging choice should consider characteristics of the patient and modality as well as local availability and expertise (see Table 1).

Stress testing with adjunctive imaging compares wall motion, perfusion, and/or metabolism at baseline and after stress, depending on the modality used (**Table 2**). Exercise is the stress modality of choice. Patients should undergo pharmacologic stress if they are unable to exercise or have contraindications to exercise. Dobutamine, like exercise, increases myocardial oxygen demand and elicits ischemia because of insufficient perfusion to the affected myocardium. Vasodilators, such as dipyridamole, regadenoson, and adenosine, produce hyperemia and a flow disparity between myocardium supplied by unobstructed vessels and myocardium supplied by the stenotic vessel because of the inability of the distal vasculature to dilate. In patients with left bundle branch block undergoing nuclear stress testing, vasodilator-induced stress is preferred to exercise or dobutamine because of the potential for false-positive septal perfusion abnormalities.

Stress Echocardiography

Exercise stress echocardiography provides information on ischemia, hemodynamic significance of valvular abnormalities, and pulmonary pressures during exercise. Exercise is performed with supine or upright bicycle ergometry, which allows for continuous imaging, or with a treadmill protocol, which requires acquisition of post-stress images within 90 seconds. The development of new wall motion abnormalities indicates ischemia in the visualized territory. Resting wall motion abnormalities that do not change at peak exercise may indicate infarcted or hibernating myocardium (chronic but potentially reversible ischemic dysfunction).

With pharmacologic stress echocardiography, dobutamine is progressively infused (up to 40 μg/kg/min) to achieve 85% of age-predicted maximal heart rate. Atropine is administered if the target heart rate is not achieved. The development of new wall motion abnormalities indicates myocardial ischemia. Dobutamine infusion may also be used in patients with low-gradient aortic stenosis to help differentiate between severe aortic stenosis and pseudostenosis. Patients with reduced systolic function who are able to augment their stroke volume in the setting of severe aortic stenosis may benefit from aortic valve replacement.

Interpretation of stress echocardiography findings is more subjective than with other tests, and the sensitivity of stress echocardiography may be reduced in the setting of baseline wall motion abnormalities, systolic dysfunction, or single-vessel disease.

Nuclear Stress Testing

Nuclear stress testing compares blood flow in the myocardium to diagnose ischemia. In SPECT myocardial perfusion imaging, a radiotracer is injected at rest and at peak exercise/vasodilation, and the radiotracer is taken up by the myocardium relative to blood flow. Rest images are compared with those obtained after exercise or pharmacologic stress. Perfusion defects observed on images obtained after stress indicate flow-limiting CAD (**Figure 2**). Regions with fixed defects can indicate infarcted or hibernating myocardium, and viability assessment can help distinguish between the two. Gated images can provide an assessment of left ventricular systolic function.

SPECT imaging can also quantify the extent and severity of disease, providing additional prognostic information. High-risk features, such as several regions of hypoperfusion, a lack of augmentation or a reduction in post-stress ejection fraction, transient cavity dilatation, and wall motion abnormalities, are associated with a worse prognosis.

Technetium-based myocardial perfusion imaging has higher sensitivity and specificity than thallium-based studies and also provides better image quality. Technetium-based

TABLE 2. Interpretation of Stress Testing with Imaging Results		
Stress SPECT		
At Rest	**After Stressor**	**Interpretation**
Normal	Normal	Normal
Normal	Perfusion defect	Stress-induced myocardial ischemia
Perfusion defect	Perfusion defect	Infarct
Normal	LV dilation	Small or no distinct zone of ischemia, possible balanced ischemia or multivessel CAD
Stress Echocardiography		
At Rest	**After Stressor**	**Interpretation**
Normal	Normal	Normal
Normal	Wall motion abnormality	Stress-induced myocardial ischemia
Regional wall motion abnormalities	Regional wall motion abnormalities	Infarct
Normal	LV dilation	Small or no distinct zone of ischemia, possible balanced ischemia or multivessel CAD

CAD = coronary artery disease; LV = left ventricular; SPECT = single-photon emission CT.

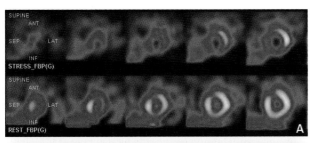

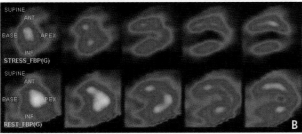

FIGURE 2. Selected images from a nuclear perfusion single-photon emission CT (SPECT) stress study. Short-axis views (*panel A*) of the heart with stress (*top row*) and at rest (*bottom row*) show a radiotracer defect in the septum and inferior wall that is filled on the rest images. Long-axis views (*panel B*) demonstrate an apical filling defect with stress (*top row*) that is perfused on rest images (*bottom row*).

agents are taken up with blood flow and are bound to the mitochondria, allowing for delayed imaging. In contrast, uptake of thallium requires active metabolism, which can be useful to assess myocardial viability (**Table 3**).

TABLE 3. Interpretation of Myocardial Viability Study Results		
SPECT Viability Testing		
Initial Study (at Rest)	**Rest Study Repeated After 4-24 h (with Thallium)**	**Interpretation**
Perfusion defect	Perfusion defect	Fixed defect: infarct, no viability
Perfusion defect	Reperfusion of area	Viable myocardium
PET Viability Testing		
Baseline	**Metabolism**	**Interpretation**
Perfusion defect	Metabolically active	Viable myocardium
Echocardiographic Viability Testing		
Baseline	**Response to Dobutamine**	**Interpretation**
Wall motion abnormality	Low dose: improvement of function Higher dose: worsening of function	Biphasic response indicates viable myocardium
SPECT = single-photon emission CT.		

Cardiac PET provides excellent diagnostic and prognostic information for patients known or suspected to have CAD. PET provides better temporal and spatial resolution than does SPECT imaging, which is helpful in patients who are obese or who have nondiagnostic SPECT results. CT may be used with PET to provide information on the presence of coronary artery calcification. PET radiotracers have a short half-life, resulting in lower radiation exposure and necessitating the use of vasodilators. Vasodilator stress allows for assessment of peak stress ejection fraction, quantification of absolute myocardial blood flow, and evaluation of myocardial metabolism. The utility of PET imaging in cardiac patients is limited by availability of the technology.

Cardiovascular Magnetic Resonance Imaging
CMR imaging is used with dobutamine to assess development of wall motion abnormalities or with vasodilators to assess perfusion. Right and left systolic function can be assessed with gated imaging. CMR imaging is commonly used to evaluate inflammatory or infiltrative diseases, pericardial diseases, and the extent and severity of infarction. Viability can be determined by evaluating the extent of myocardial fibrosis (nonviable myocardium) within the left ventricular region. CMR imaging is limited by operator expertise, length of time for image acquisition, and availability. ◧

KEY POINTS

- Cardiac stress testing is best used in patients with an intermediate pretest probability of coronary artery disease.

- In patients undergoing cardiac stress testing, exercise is the preferred stressor because it provides additional prognostic information, including functional capacity and hemodynamic response.

- Stress testing with imaging is indicated in patients with an inability to exercise, contraindications to exercise, baseline electrocardiographic (ECG) abnormalities that would preclude interpretation of exercise ECG results, or indeterminate findings on exercise ECG.

Visualization of the Coronary Anatomy

Anatomic assessment of the coronary arteries can be performed with noninvasive coronary CTA or invasive angiography. Both tests require administration of contrast agents and expose the patient to radiation. CTA interpretation can be limited in cases of extensive calcification and with assessment of distal arteries.

In symptomatic patients with an intermediate risk for CAD, CTA may be helpful in ruling out CAD. In the PROMISE trial, 10,000 symptomatic patients suspected of having CAD were evaluated with an initial strategy of anatomic testing with CTA or functional testing. In patients with an intermediate pretest probability of CAD, the composite cardiovascular event rate was low (<1% per year) in both groups, and outcomes (death, myocardial infarction, hospitalization for unstable angina, or major procedural complication) at 2 years did not differ between groups.

Coronary CTA may also play a role in the evaluation of acute chest pain in the emergency department. CTA is appropriate in patients suspected of having an acute aortic syndrome or a coronary embolism. Coronary CTA may be helpful in patients with low or intermediate likelihood of non–ST-elevation acute coronary syndrome who have a low TIMI risk score, negative troponin level, or nonischemic ECG. It may also be useful in patients with an equivocal diagnosis of non–ST-elevation acute coronary syndrome who have an equivocal initial troponin level or single troponin elevation without further symptoms of acute coronary syndrome, or in patients who have ischemic symptoms that resolved hours before undergoing testing. Careful consideration of patient factors and selection of appropriate testing are essential to avoid additional unnecessary testing and the associated costs and potential harms.

Coronary angiography during a cardiac catheterization procedure is an invasive test in which nonionic contrast material is injected into the coronary arteries (or bypass grafts) by using long, thin (<2-mm) catheters. Arterial access is obtained by using the femoral or radial artery, and radiation exposure is required. This test should be considered in patients who have a high pretest probability of obstructive CAD, including symptomatic patients with abnormal findings on noninvasive functional or anatomic testing or with an acute coronary syndrome.

The addition of FFR to invasive angiography and CTA can provide additional functional information, including the hemodynamic significance of a lesion and need for intervention. FFR is the ratio of blood flow distal to the stenosis to blood flow proximal to the stenosis at maximal flow. It is typically measured during cardiac catheterization by placing a pressure wire across the stenosis and inducing conditions of maximal hyperemia, usually with adenosine. FFR-CT is an FDA-approved diagnostic test that provides both anatomic and functional data; it has higher specificity for the diagnosis of obstructive CAD than does CTA alone. Performance of FFR-CT is similar to performance of invasive FFR during angiography. The availability of this test and its delayed interpretation may limit its use in patients with acute symptoms. **H**

KEY POINT

- Coronary angiography and CT angiography (CTA) provide anatomic information regarding the extent and severity of coronary artery disease; however, the diagnostic value of CTA may be limited in cases of extensive calcification.

Coronary Artery Calcium Scoring

Coronary artery calcification indicates atherosclerosis and may be quantified with electron-beam or multidetector CT. Although CAC scoring provides information regarding the burden of disease, it cannot determine the degree of obstruction.

CAC measurement has been used for diagnosis and risk assessment in both symptomatic and asymptomatic patients; however, assessment of CAC in asymptomatic patients should be limited to those at intermediate risk (according to the Framingham score) in whom risk reclassification will influence primary prevention therapy.

CAC scores are categorized as follows: 0, no disease; 1 to 99, mild disease; 100 to 399, moderate disease; and above 400, severe disease. These scores should be interpreted in the setting of age, ethnicity, and sex. Specific nomograms and risk calculators, such as the MESA risk calculator (www.mesa-nhlbi.org/MESACHDRisk/MesaRiskScore/RiskScore.aspx), can be used for risk prediction. The absence of CAC is associated with a low risk for cardiovascular events.

KEY POINT

- Assessment of coronary artery calcification in asymptomatic patients should be limited to those at intermediate risk in whom reclassification of risk will influence primary prevention therapy.

Risks of Diagnostic Testing for Coronary Artery Disease

Cardiac diagnostic testing carries risks related to exercise; exposure to pharmacologic stress testing agents, radiation, or contrast agents; and vascular access for invasive procedures. Additionally, inappropriate initial testing may lead to unnecessary downstream testing with added physical and financial costs.

There is a very small risk for myocardial infarction or death (1/2500 patients) in patients undergoing exercise stress testing. Absolute contraindications to exercise include unstable angina or acute myocardial infarction, uncontrolled arrhythmias, decompensated heart failure, acute pulmonary embolism or deep venous thrombosis, acute pericarditis or myocarditis, acute aortic dissection, and severe symptomatic aortic stenosis. Relative contraindications are left main coronary artery stenosis, hypertrophic cardiomyopathy with severe obstruction, electrolyte abnormalities, high-degree atrioventricular block, and significant arrhythmias.

Vasodilator stress agents (most commonly adenosine) are associated with the side effects of chest pain, headache, and flushing. Atrioventricular block and bronchospasm may also occur. Theophylline may be given after the test to reverse these effects. Vasodilator stress testing is contraindicated in patients with reactive airways disease with active wheezing, systolic blood pressure of less than 90 mm Hg, sick sinus syndrome, or high-degree atrioventricular block.

Nuclear stress testing with SPECT and PET, CAC scoring, coronary CTA, and coronary angiography all expose the patient to radiation; however, advances in techniques have resulted in reduction of overall radiation exposure. The level of radiation exposure depends on the procedure, equipment, radiopharmaceutical agent, operator technique, and patient characteristics (such as body size).

HVC

Contrast agents used in invasive angiography, coronary CTA, CMR imaging, and echocardiography also pose a risk to the patient. CMR imaging that requires gadolinium contrast may rarely cause nephrogenic systemic fibrosis, particularly in patients with underlying kidney disease. Iodinated contrast material used in CT may result in acute kidney injury. Microbubble contrast agents are used to enhance the endocardial borders in echocardiography and can cause hypersensitivity reactions in rare instances.

Coronary angiography can be complicated by vascular access problems; bleeding complications; coronary artery dissection; aortic dissection; and plaque disruption or thrombus leading to peripheral emboli, stroke, or myocardial infarction. Femoral artery access can be complicated by retroperitoneal hemorrhage, which should be suspected in patients with hypotension, back or flank pain, and/or a drop in hemoglobin level. Pseudoaneurysms at the arterial puncture sites occur more commonly with femoral artery access and may manifest as a large hematoma or new bruit at the access site.

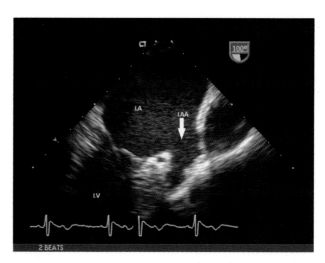

FIGURE 3. Transesophageal echocardiogram. The transducer is posterior to the heart, and the left atrium (LA) and left atrial appendage (LAA, *arrow*) are more easily seen than with transthoracic echocardiography, showing an absence of thrombus in the appendage. LV = left ventricle.

Diagnostic Testing for Structural Heart Disease

Diagnostic testing for structural heart disease should be considered in patients with a suggestive history and physical examination, such as those with a systolic murmur that is grade 3/6 or higher, a late or holosystolic murmur, a diastolic or continuous murmur, or a murmur with accompanying symptoms. Routine imaging of known structural disease is unnecessary unless there is a change in the clinical presentation or examination. A change in functional status in patients with known underlying structural disease warrants evaluation. Imaging modalities to evaluate for structural heart disease are listed in **Table 4**.

The mainstay of noninvasive cardiovascular imaging for structural abnormalities is transthoracic echocardiography (TTE). TTE evaluates right and left ventricular size, thickness, and function, including wall motion abnormalities. It can also be used to obtain information on valvular function (including regurgitation or stenosis), diastolic function, filling pressures, and the pericardium. The presence of an intracardiac shunt can be evaluated with the use of agitated saline contrast. Initial assessment for endocarditis can also be performed with TTE.

Transesophageal echocardiography (TEE) is commonly used to evaluate for the diagnosis of infective endocarditis in patients with a high pretest probability and to assess for complications of endocarditis (such as abscess). TEE may also be used to better visualize valvular pathology, particularly when surgical repair or percutaneous intervention is planned; to evaluate specific structures that cannot be well visualized on TTE (such as prosthetic heart valves) or patients with poor transthoracic imaging; to evaluate acute aortic abnormalities; and to rule out left atrial thrombus before cardioversion (**Figure 3**). TEE requires moderate sedation and placement of

the TEE probe in the distal esophagus and stomach. Contraindications include esophageal strictures or active esophageal varices. Esophageal injury, including perforation and bleeding, are potential complications of TEE.

> **KEY POINTS**
>
> - Transthoracic echocardiography is used to evaluate patients with valvular abnormalities, congenital heart disease, pericardial disease, or left or right ventricular dysfunction.
> - Transesophageal echocardiography is the most accurate test to evaluate endocarditis, prosthetic valves, and left atrial thrombus.

Diagnostic Testing for Cardiac Arrhythmias

The initial study in patients with a history of palpitations, presyncope, or syncope when an arrhythmia is suspected should be 12-lead resting ECG. The ECG may show evidence of preexcitation, ectopic rhythms, atrioventricular block, or intraventricular conduction delay, providing insight into the cause of the symptoms. Echocardiography should be performed in patients suspected of having structural heart disease.

The intermittent and fleeting nature of arrhythmias can make diagnosis difficult. Diagnostic studies are selected on the basis of the presence and frequency of symptoms and the duration and timing of the recording (**Table 5**). If symptoms occur daily, a 24- or 48-hour ambulatory ECG monitor (Holter monitor) may be used. Infrequent symptomatic events may be captured with an external patient-triggered event recorder if the event lasts long enough for the patient to trigger the device. A looping event recorder captures several seconds of the ECG

TABLE 4. Diagnostic Testing for Structural Heart Disease

Diagnostic Test	Major Indications	Advantages	Limitations
Transthoracic echocardiography	Heart failure Cardiomyopathy Valve disease Congenital heart disease Pulmonary hypertension Aortic disease Pericardial disease	Accurate diagnosis of presence and severity of structural heart disease Quantitation of LV size and function, pulmonary pressures, valve function, and intracardiac shunts Widely available, portable, fast	Operator-dependent data acquisition; interpretation requires expertise Variability in instrumentation Image quality limits diagnosis in some patients (COPD, large body habitus) May require microbubble contrast agents
Transesophageal echocardiography	Endocarditis Prosthetic valve dysfunction Aortic disease Left atrial thrombus	High-quality images, especially of posterior cardiac structures Most accurate test for evaluation of endocarditis, prosthetic valves, and left atrial thrombus	Requires esophageal intubation, typically with conscious sedation
Three-dimensional echocardiography	Mitral valve disease ASD (percutaneous ASD closure)	Improved tomographic imaging Used during cardiac procedures for device placement Improved assessment of LV global/regional systolic function	Adjunct to two-dimensional imaging Limited by availability and expertise
Radionuclide angiography (MUGA)	Evaluation of LV systolic function	Quantitative EF measurements Accurate for serial LVEF measurements (e.g., to evaluate for cardiotoxicity from chemotherapy)	Radiation exposure Provides no data on other cardiac structures
Cardiac catheterization (left and right)	Congenital heart disease Coronary artery disease Valve assessment Shunt assessment	Direct measurement of intracardiac pressures, gradients, and shunts Contrast angiography provides visualization of complex cardiac anatomy Allows percutaneous intervention for structural heart disease	Invasive Radiation and radiocontrast exposure Images not tomographic, limiting evaluation of complex three-dimensional anatomy
Coronary CT angiography	Coronary artery disease Congenital heart disease	Visualization of complex cardiac anatomy High-resolution tomographic images	Invasive Radiation and radiocontrast exposure Image acquisition improved with sinus rhythm and slower heart rate
CMR imaging	Congenital heart disease Aortic disease Myocardial disease (infiltrative disease, myocarditis, hypertrophic cardiomyopathy) RV cardiomyopathy (ARVC) Quantitation of LV mass and function	High-resolution tomographic imaging and blood-flow data Quantitative RV volumes and EF No ionizing radiation or contrast material Enables three-dimensional reconstruction of aortic and coronary anatomy	Limited by availability and expertise Patient claustrophobia May be contraindicated in patients with pacemaker, ICD, or other implanted devices Gadolinium is contraindicated in patients with kidney failure Sinus rhythm and slower heart rate are needed for improved image quality
Chest CT with contrast	Aortic disease Coronary artery disease Cardiac masses Pericardial disease	High-resolution tomographic images Enables three-dimensional reconstruction of vascular structures	Radiation and radiocontrast exposure

ARVC = arrhythmogenic right ventricular cardiomyopathy; ASD = atrial septal defect; CMR = cardiac magnetic resonance; EF = ejection fraction; ICD = implantable cardioverter-defibrillator; LV = left ventricular; LVEF = left ventricular ejection fraction; MUGA = multigated acquisition; RV = right ventricular.

TABLE 5. Diagnostic Testing for Suspected or Known Cardiac Arrhythmias

Diagnostic Test or Device	Indications	Advantages	Limitations
Resting ECG	Initial diagnostic test in all patients	12-lead ECG recorded during the arrhythmia often identifies the specific arrhythmia	Most arrhythmias are intermittent and not recorded on resting ECG
Ambulatory ECG (Holter monitor)	Frequent (at least daily) asymptomatic or symptomatic arrhythmias	Records every heart beat during a 24- or 48-h period for later analysis Patient log allows correlation with symptoms	Not helpful when arrhythmia occurs less frequently ECG leads limit patient activities
Long-term external ECG monitor	Infrequent asymptomatic or symptomatic arrhythmias	Provides continuous rhythm recording for up to 30 days	Adhesive attachment to chest Detection of rhythm abnormalities that are asymptomatic or not clinically significant
Exercise ECG	Arrhythmias provoked by exercise	Allows diagnosis of exercise-related arrhythmias Allows assessment of impact of arrhythmia on blood pressure	Physician supervision needed during testing Most arrhythmias are not exercise related
Patient-triggered event recorder	Infrequent symptomatic arrhythmias that last more than 1-2 min	Small, pocket-sized recorder is held to the chest when symptoms are present Recorded data are transmitted to central monitoring service	Symptomatic arrhythmias must last long enough for patient to activate the device Arrhythmia onset is not recorded Not useful for syncope or extremely brief arrhythmias
Looping event recorder (wearable)	Infrequent, symptomatic, brief arrhythmias Syncope	Continuous ECG signal is recorded (with the previous 30 s to 2 min saved) when the patient activates the recording mode Arrhythmia onset is recorded	ECG leads limit patient activities Device records only when activated by patient
Implantable loop recorder	Very infrequent asymptomatic or symptomatic arrhythmias	Long-term continuous ECG monitoring with patient-triggered or heart rate–triggered episode storage Specific heart rate or QRS parameters can be set to initiate recording of data	Invasive procedure with minor risks Device must be explanted later
Mobile cardiac outpatient telemetry	Continuous outpatient ECG recording for precise quantification or capture of rare arrhythmia	Auto-triggered and patient-triggered capture of arrhythmic events Up to 96 h of retrievable memory	ECG leads limit patient activities Resource intensive
Electrophysiology study	Used for inducing, identifying, and clarifying the mechanism of arrhythmia as well as potential treatment (catheter ablation)	Origin and mechanism of an arrhythmia can be precisely defined	Invasive procedure with some risk Some arrhythmias may not be inducible, particularly if the patient is sedated

ECG = electrocardiography.

signal before the device is triggered; it is useful for syncope or presyncope associated with arrhythmias. A longer-term external ECG monitor or an implanted loop recorder may be warranted in patients with very infrequent events.

Exercise stress testing is also frequently used in patients suspected of having or known to have arrhythmia. Treadmill stress testing is an important tool for evaluating chronotropic response, ischemia, and exercise-induced or adrenergically induced arrhythmia.

Most patients do not require diagnostic electrophysiology testing. Electrophysiology testing may be indicated in patients in whom the diagnosis remains indeterminate or in settings in which catheter-based interventions may be needed to treat refractory arrhythmias.

Coronary Artery Disease

Stable Angina Pectoris

Diagnosis and Evaluation

Stable angina pectoris is defined as reproducible angina symptoms (chest pain or pressure) of at least 2 months' duration that are precipitated by exertion or emotional stress and have not appreciably worsened. In contrast, unstable angina is defined by new-onset angina or angina occurring at a relatively low level of exertion, occurring at rest, or accelerating in frequency or severity. Unstable angina is associated with increased short-term risk for acute myocardial infarction (MI). As such, the evaluation of patients with angina should include a focused history, eliciting the duration of symptoms, aggravating and relieving factors, and whether symptoms have worsened. Although angina is classically described as tightness, heaviness, or gripping in the chest, it is important to recognize that classic symptoms may be absent, and some demographic groups (women and patients with diabetes mellitus) may have atypical symptoms, including exertional dyspnea.

The physical examination should include an evaluation of the cardiovascular system and a search for findings suggesting conditions that mimic angina, including heart failure, pulmonary hypertension, valvular heart disease (particularly aortic stenosis), and hypertrophic cardiomyopathy. The first step in diagnostic testing is to determine the pretest probability (or likelihood) of coronary artery disease (CAD) (**Table 6**). Baseline resting electrocardiography (ECG) is required to rule out ongoing ischemia and to guide the choice of stress test

(**Figure 4**). The selection of tests for evaluating chest pain is discussed in Diagnostic Testing in Cardiology. Stress testing is most useful in patients with an intermediate probability of CAD; however, when the pretest probability of CAD is high, testing may provide prognostic information. Other diagnoses should be pursued in patients with normal findings on stress testing. If the stress test yields abnormal results, additional evaluation should be considered.

General Approach to Treatment of Stable Angina Pectoris

All patients with angina should receive guideline-directed medical therapy consisting of risk factor modification, cardioprotective medications, and antianginal medications (**Figure 5**). Lifestyle modifications, including regular physical activity, weight loss, tobacco cessation, and dietary changes, should be strongly encouraged, and blood pressure control (with a goal of <130/80 mm Hg) and diabetes management should be emphasized. Cardioprotective medications are indicated in patients with CAD to prevent thrombosis and halt further progression of atherosclerotic plaque. Antianginal medications reduce cardiac workload or increase myocardial oxygen delivery, resulting in decreased angina and improved functional capacity.

Cardioprotective Medications

Aspirin reduces the risk for MI and cardiovascular death in patients with stable angina. Guidelines recommend low-dose aspirin (75-162 mg/d) because it is as effective in preventing MI as high-dose aspirin (325 mg/d) and confers a lower bleeding risk. In aspirin-intolerant patients, clopidogrel, a platelet $P2Y_{12}$ receptor inhibitor, is an acceptable alternative. Neither prasugrel nor ticagrelor has been studied in the context of stable angina, and their role in managing this condition remains to be established.

Lipid-lowering therapy, targeting LDL cholesterol in particular, is indicated to reduce the risk for vascular events and

TABLE 6. Pretest Likelihood of Coronary Artery Disease in Symptomatic Patients According to Age and Sex[a]

Age (y)	Nonanginal Chest Pain[b]		Atypical Angina[c]		Typical Angina[d]	
	Men	Women	Men	Women	Men	Women
30-39	4	2	34	12	76	26
40-49	13	3	51	22	87	55
50-59	20	7	65	31	93	73
60-69	27	14	72	51	94	86

[a]Each value represents the percentage with significant coronary artery disease on catheterization.

[b]Nonanginal chest pain has one or none of the components for typical angina.

[c]Atypical angina has two of the three components for typical angina.

[d]Typical angina has three components: (1) substernal chest pain or discomfort that is (2) provoked by exertion or emotional stress and (3) relieved by rest and/or nitroglycerin.

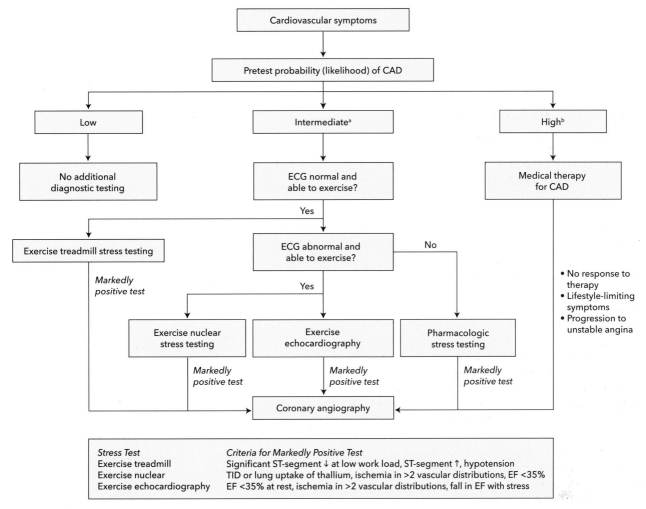

FIGURE 4. Diagnosis of coronary artery disease. CAD = coronary artery disease; ECG = electrocardiography; EF = ejection fraction; TID = transient ischemic dilation.

[a]Intermediate pretest probability (likelihood) is variably defined as between 10% and 90% or between 25% and 75%.

[b]Stress testing in patients with high pretest probability can be used to obtain prognostic information, but the results should not affect the initiation of optimal medical therapy.

progression of underlying CAD. Statin therapy remains the cornerstone of lipid management for secondary prevention, as it has been shown to reduce the risk for MI, death, and stroke. High-intensity statin therapy (atorvastatin, 40-80 mg/d, or rosuvastatin, 20-40 mg/d) decreases LDL cholesterol levels by 50% or more and is preferred to moderate-intensity therapy in patients with no contraindications to its use. In patients who are intolerant of statins (such as those who develop significant myalgia) or who do not achieve adequate LDL cholesterol reduction with statin therapy, it is reasonable to address LDL cholesterol levels with nonstatin medications, including ezetimibe, bile acid sequestrants, fibrates, and proprotein convertase subtilisin/kexin type 9 inhibitors. Management of statin therapy and nonstatin cholesterol-lowering therapy is discussed in MKSAP 18 General Internal Medicine.

ACE inhibitor therapy is indicated in patients with stable angina if there is concomitant diabetes, chronic kidney disease, left ventricular dysfunction (ejection fraction ≤40%),

heart failure, or a history of MI. In these populations, ACE inhibitors have additional benefits that are unrelated to CAD, such as preservation of kidney function and improvement in left ventricular function. Angiotensin receptor blockers (ARBs) may be used as an alternative to ACE inhibitors in these same patient populations.

Chelation therapy involves a series of intravenous infusions of ethylene diamine tetra-acetic acid or similar compounds to bind cations (such as calcium) and increase their excretion from the body. There has been no convincing evidence of any benefit with chelation therapy, and it is not recommended for treatment of CAD.

Antianginal Medications

β-Blockers are recommended as first-line agents in patients with stable angina. β-Blockers simultaneously lower heart rate and blood pressure to reduce myocardial oxygen consumption. All β-blockers are equally efficacious in reducing angina, and dosage should be titrated to achieve a resting heart rate

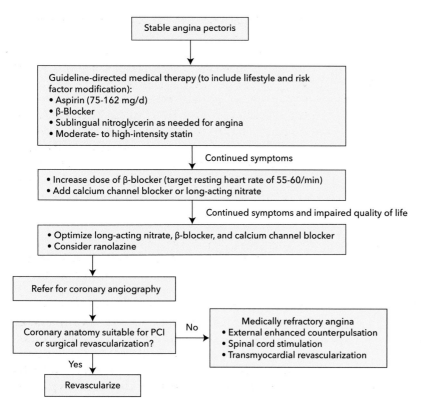

FIGURE 5. Management of stable angina pectoris. PCI = percutaneous coronary intervention.

Recommendations based on Qaseem A, Fihn SD, Dallas P, Williams S, Owens DK, Shekelle P; Clinical Guidelines Committee of the American College of Physicians. Management of stable ischemic heart disease: summary of a clinical practice guideline from the American College of Physicians/American College of Cardiology Foundation/American Heart Association/American Association for Thoracic Surgery/Preventive Cardiovascular Nurses Association/Society of Thoracic Surgeons. Ann Intern Med. 2012;157:735-43. [PMID: 23165665] doi:10.7326/0003-4819-157-10-201211200-00011

between 55/min and 60/min. The choice of β-blocker may depend on other medical conditions, such as concomitant left ventricular dysfunction, kidney dysfunction, lung disease, and significant hypertension. β-Blockers should be used with caution in patients taking nondihydropyridine calcium channel blockers (verapamil, diltiazem) because of additive negative inotropic and chronotropic actions. Caution should also be exercised with these agents in the setting of significant conduction disease on ECG or left ventricular dysfunction. β_1-Selective β-blockers, such as metoprolol, should be used in patients with significant lung disease to avoid worsening respiratory function. Reported side effects include fatigue, lethargy, sleep disturbances, and impotence.

Calcium channel blockers can be useful in patients with symptoms despite β-blocker therapy or in patients intolerant of β-blockers. All calcium channel blockers improve myocardial oxygen delivery by causing coronary vasodilation and reduction in coronary vascular resistance. Additionally, calcium channel blockers can decrease myocardial oxygen consumption through their antihypertensive and negative inotropic effects. The nondihydropyridine calcium channel blockers have negative chronotropic effects and lower heart rate, which can worsen heart failure and increase mortality; therefore, they should not be used in patients with left ventricular dysfunction. Short-acting dihydropyridine formulations, such as short-acting nifedipine, should be avoided because they can paradoxically worsen angina by causing an acute drop in blood pressure, resulting in reflex tachycardia and increased myocardial oxygen demand.

Nitrates cause coronary vasodilation, thereby improving myocardial oxygen delivery. These agents also decrease oxygen consumption by reducing preload, which reduces ventricular wall stress. The beneficial effects may be offset by reflex tachycardia unless β-blockers or calcium channel blockers are used. Short-acting sublingual nitrates should be prescribed to patients with CAD for acute relief of angina. Long-acting nitrates, including isosorbide mononitrate or dinitrate and nitroglycerin patch formulations, provide a constant level of vasodilation throughout the day. A nitrate-free interval of about 12 hours, generally during sleep hours, is needed to avoid development of nitrate tolerance. Side effects include headache, flushing, and hypotension, particularly with rapid-acting formulations. Concomitant use of nitrates and phosphodiesterase 5 inhibitors, such as sildenafil, should be avoided because of the risk for significant hypotension.

Ranolazine decreases angina and modestly increases exercise times in patients with stable angina. It inhibits the late sodium current, which in turn reduces sodium-dependent calcium currents, resulting in reduced wall tension and myocardial oxygen consumption. Ranolazine also has a modest QT-prolonging effect, but no proarrhythmic effect has been directly attributed to ranolazine. The QT interval should be monitored carefully when other QT-prolonging drugs are coadministered. The typical dosage is 1000 mg twice daily; however, the dosage should be reduced to 500 mg twice daily in patients receiving moderate inhibitors of cytochrome P-450 3A4 (verapamil, diltiazem). Ranolazine should not be used in patients receiving strong inhibitors of cytochrome P-450 3A4 (clarithromycin, itraconazole, ketoconazole, several HIV medications) because serum levels of ranolazine will significantly increase.

KEY POINTS

- Stable angina is characterized by reproducible angina symptoms (chest pain or pressure) that are present for more than 2 months without appreciable worsening and are precipitated by exertion or emotional stress.

- Initial evaluation of a patient with angina should include a focused history, eliciting duration of symptoms, aggravating and relieving factors, and whether symptoms have worsened.

- All patients with coronary artery disease should be counseled on lifestyle modifications, blood pressure control, and management of diabetes mellitus.

- First-line therapy in patients with stable angina includes aspirin (or clopidogrel in aspirin-intolerant patients), statin therapy, and β-blocker therapy.

- ACE inhibitor therapy is indicated in patients with stable angina if there is concomitant left ventricular dysfunction, heart failure, diabetes mellitus, chronic kidney disease, or history of myocardial infarction.

Coronary Revascularization
Decision to Revascularize

Patients with progressive angina symptoms refractory to medical therapy or markedly abnormal stress testing results should be considered for coronary angiography. Before angiography, the risks, benefits, and alternatives to the procedure should be discussed with the patient. It is also important to discuss possible findings and the therapeutic options available after angiography. The goals of revascularization are to improve symptoms of angina and quality of life, prevent future CAD events, and improve survival.

Coronary angiography with fractional flow reserve testing can provide information on the functional significance of angiographically indeterminate lesions (see Diagnostic Testing in Cardiology). Determining the hemodynamic significance of lesions reduces both unnecessary stenting and the need for urgent revascularization. Abnormal fractional flow reserve measures (values <0.80) suggest that a lesion is hemodynamically significant.

Percutaneous Coronary Intervention

Percutaneous coronary intervention (PCI) encompasses several different catheter-based techniques to improve coronary blood flow by relieving coronary obstruction. Initially, PCI was most commonly performed with balloon angioplasty; however, this technique was replaced in the 1990s with bare metal stenting. Currently, most PCI procedures involve drug-eluting stent implantation, which has reduced the risk for in-stent restenosis (the process by which neointimal proliferation

within or adjacent to the treated section of coronary artery renarrows the vessel lumen).

Despite advancements in PCI technology, there is no evidence that PCI is superior to guideline-directed medical therapy in the treatment of stable CAD. Specifically, neither the COURAGE trial of patients with stable angina nor the BARI-2D trial of patients with concomitant CAD and diabetes showed any difference in mortality or incidence of MI between treatment strategies. PCI is indicated for the treatment of patients with medically refractory angina, those who are unable to tolerate optimal medical therapy owing to side effects, or those with high-risk features on noninvasive exercise and imaging tests.

Coronary Artery Bypass Graft Surgery

Coronary artery bypass grafting (CABG) is generally recommended for patients with extensive CAD and in certain subsets of patients for whom studies have shown CABG to be superior to PCI or medical therapy. In patients with multivessel CAD, revascularization with CABG results in decreased recurrence of angina, lower rates of MI, and fewer repeat revascularization procedures compared with PCI. Unlike PCI, CABG improves survival in patients with left main or three-vessel CAD and is recommended to reduce mortality in these high-risk patients. Additionally, CABG has an established role in revascularization of patients with diabetes and in those with left ventricular dysfunction. Long-term (10-year) follow-up of the STICH trial demonstrated a survival advantage with CABG compared with medical therapy alone among patients with multivessel CAD and severe left ventricular dysfunction.

After Revascularization

Patients should continue receiving guideline-directed medical therapy following surgical or percutaneous revascularization, although some antianginal therapies may be reduced or discontinued. Aspirin is recommended indefinitely after revascularization. The addition of a P2Y$_{12}$ inhibitor to aspirin therapy, known as dual antiplatelet therapy (DAPT), is also indicated; the recommended duration of DAPT depends on many clinical considerations. Clopidogrel is the only antiplatelet drug that has been studied in combination with aspirin after revascularization of patients with stable CAD. The role of newer antiplatelet agents is unclear at this time.

In patients treated with bare metal stent placement, guidelines recommend a minimum of 1 month of DAPT. Studies of the optimal duration of DAPT after drug-eluting stent implantation have suggested safety and benefits with both shorter (6-month) and longer (30-month) treatment courses. Current guidelines recommend treating patients with stable angina with DAPT for at least 6 months after drug-eluting stent placement, with the option to continue therapy for a longer duration in those with a high risk for thrombosis-related complications (such as depressed left ventricular function, saphenous vein graft stenting, and diabetes) and a favorable bleeding profile. Although guidelines define minimum DAPT duration, the optimal duration should be individualized according to the patient's risks for thrombotic and bleeding complications.

In patients undergoing CABG for stable CAD, DAPT for 12 months may be reasonable to improve the patency of vein grafts.

KEY POINTS

- Percutaneous coronary intervention may alleviate angina symptoms but does not decrease mortality or risk for myocardial infarction in patients with stable angina.

- Coronary artery bypass graft revascularization is associated with improved survival in patients with multivessel coronary artery disease, diabetes mellitus, or severe left ventricular dysfunction.

- In patients with stable angina who undergo percutaneous coronary intervention, dual antiplatelet therapy should be continued for at least 1 month after bare metal stent implantation and at least 6 months after drug-eluting stent implantation.

Acute Coronary Syndromes

General Considerations

An acute coronary syndrome (ACS) results from acute or subacute disruption in coronary blood flow. Patients present with acute-onset chest pain or an angina equivalent that occurs without a clear precipitant. Unlike stable angina, which involves a gradual narrowing in the coronary artery, an ACS is caused by acute plaque rupture or erosion, often in sections of the coronary artery with mild or moderate stenosis. The presentation depends on the degree of coronary flow impairment.

ACS is classified as ST-elevation myocardial infarction (STEMI) or non–ST-elevation acute coronary syndrome (NSTE-ACS) based on findings on ECG (**Figure 6**). The hall-

mark ECG features of STEMI are ST-segment elevation of 1 mm or more in two or more contiguous limb or chest leads, excepting leads V_2 and V_3. STEMI is defined as ST-segment elevation of 2 mm or greater in men and 1.5 mm or greater in women in leads V_2 and V_3. Posterior MI typically manifests as ST-segment depression greater than 2 mm in the anterior leads (V_1 through V_4), often with ST-segment elevation in the inferior or lateral leads. New left bundle branch block is considered a STEMI equivalent and potentially reflects an acute left anterior descending artery occlusion.

NSTE-ACS is further categorized according to the presence of biomarkers of cardiac injury (troponin T or I) in the serum. Non–ST-elevation myocardial infarction (NSTEMI) is defined as a biomarker-positive presentation that does not meet criteria for STEMI. Unstable angina is characterized by new or worsening angina, with or without ECG changes, and without detectable levels of cardiac injury markers. The use of troponin assays has resulted in increased diagnosis of NSTEMI. New high-sensitivity troponin assays can detect cardiac injury with even greater sensitivity and earlier in the setting of ACS than previous tests. Their clinical use may expedite risk stratification in patients with chest pain but may increase detection of non-ACS events and consequent downstream testing.

ST-Elevation Myocardial Infarction
Recognition

The pathogenesis of STEMI typically involves plaque rupture within a coronary artery. The rupture causes platelet adhesion, activation, and aggregation, resulting in a thrombosed coronary artery and acute vessel occlusion. The sudden loss of coronary blood flow leads to transmural ischemia of the myocardium and the ECG manifestation of ST-segment elevation. Because oxygen delivery to the affected artery is acutely and completely obstructed, prompt recognition and initiation of reperfusion therapy are vital (**Figure 7**).

Although the presentation of STEMI is often dramatic and clear, several diagnoses can mimic STEMI. These disease entities need to be distinguished from STEMI to minimize patient harm. Acute pericarditis presents with acute chest pain, albeit pain with a pleuritic and positional nature, and ST-segment elevation. The ST-segment elevation of pericarditis tends to be diffuse and concave; however, it can be easily misinterpreted for STEMI on ECG (**Figure 8**). Pericarditis can also be localized and present with regional ST-segment elevation, such as in the inferior leads. Myopericarditis resulting from viral infections or autoimmune conditions can cause cardiac enzyme release, further confusing the clinical picture. A thorough history and physical examination combined with review of the ECG findings may help differentiate the conditions.

Left ventricular hypertrophy–induced ECG changes may also look similar to ST-segment elevation injury currents; however, these changes are typically concave in appearance. Comparison with previous ECG results is helpful in assessing for acute changes.

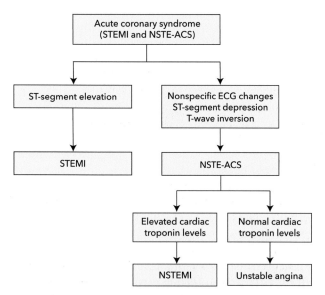

FIGURE 6. Diagnosis of acute coronary syndromes. ECG = electrocardiographic; NSTE-ACS = non–ST-elevation acute coronary syndrome; NSTEMI = non–ST-elevation myocardial infarction; STEMI = ST-elevation myocardial infarction.

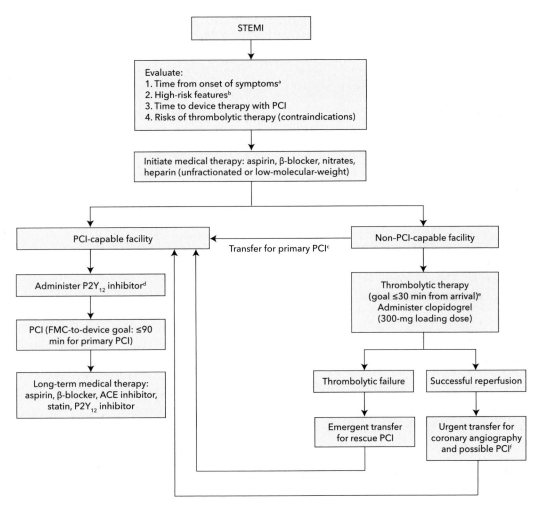

FIGURE 7. Management of ST-elevation myocardial infarction. FMC = first medical contact; PCI = percutaneous coronary intervention; STEMI = ST-elevation myocardial infarction.

[a]If 4 or more hours have elapsed since symptom onset, PCI is preferred.

[b]High-risk features, such as cardiogenic shock and heart failure, favor PCI.

[c]FMC-to-device ("door-to-balloon") goal for patients being transferred for primary PCI is as soon as possible and ≤120 minutes.

[d]P2Y$_{12}$ inhibitors: clopidogrel, prasugrel, ticagrelor.

[e]Patients with STEMI presenting to a hospital without PCI capabilities and who cannot be transferred to a PCI-capable center and undergo PCI within 120 minutes of FMC ("door-to-balloon time") should be treated with thrombolytic therapy within 30 minutes of hospital presentation ("door-to-needle time") as a systems goal unless thrombolytic therapy is contraindicated.

[f]In patients with successful reperfusion after thrombolytic therapy, it is reasonable to transfer these patients to a PCI-capable center for subsequent coronary angiography. Angiography should not be performed within 2 to 3 hours after thrombolytic administration but is ideally performed within 24 hours.

Recommendations based on O'Gara PT, Kushner FG, Ascheim DD, Casey DE Jr, Chung MK, de Lemos JA, et al; American College of Cardiology Foundation/American Heart Association Task Force on Practice Guidelines. 2013 ACCF/AHA guideline for the management of ST-elevation myocardial infarction: a report of the American College of Cardiology Foundation/American Heart Association Task Force on Practice Guidelines. Circulation. 2013;127:e362-425. [PMID: 23247304] doi:10.1161/CIR.0b013e3182742cf6

Aortic dissection can cause ST-segment elevation if the dissection involves the left or right coronary artery. In these cases, the ST-segment elevation is due to transmural myocardial ischemia. Aortic dissection is a surgical emergency and must be recognized early because treatment paradigms are drastically different. Diagnostic clues that help differentiate the two conditions include differential blood pressures in the upper extremities and mediastinal widening on chest radiograph with aortic dissection.

Severe hypercalcemia may result in ST-segment elevation that mimics ACS; however, other findings include a short QT interval and flattened T waves.

Reperfusion

Upon STEMI recognition, reperfusion with thrombolytic agents or primary PCI (PPCI) is necessary. PPCI is the preferred method of reperfusion in most cases.

Thrombolytic Therapy

Thrombolytic therapy is recommended for patients with STEMI when symptom onset is within 12 hours and PPCI is not available within 120 minutes of first medical contact. If symptoms began 12 to 24 hours before presentation and there is evidence of hemodynamic instability or significant myocardium at risk

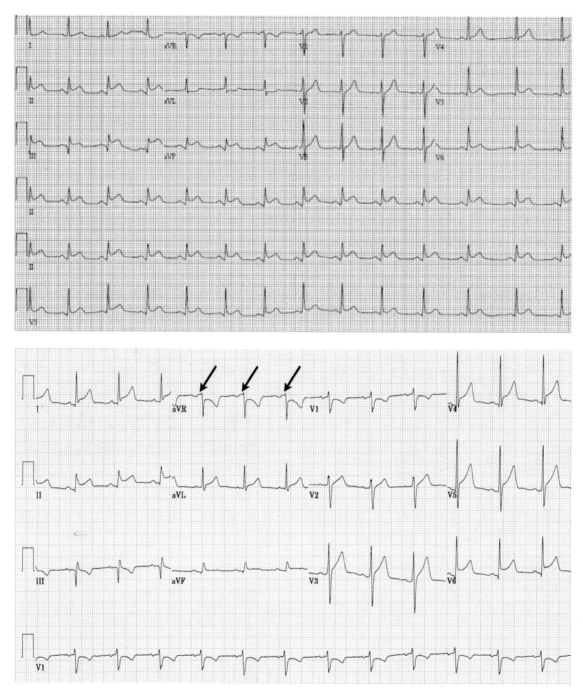

FIGURE 8. *Top panel:* Electrocardiogram showing findings consistent with an acute inferior ST-elevation myocardial infarction. Note the ST-segment elevation isolated to the inferior and lateral precordial leads, which is consistent with a single coronary vascular distribution (that is, the right coronary artery in this case). *Bottom panel:* Electrocardiogram demonstrating acute pericarditis with diffuse ST-segment elevation and slight PR-segment depression (see lead I) and reciprocal PR-segment elevation ("knuckle sign") in lead aVR (*arrows*).

(such as with anterior MI), thrombolytic therapy should be considered. Characteristics of the various thrombolytic agents are presented in **Table 7**.

In addition to thrombolytic therapy, all patients without a specific contraindication should receive a loading dose of aspirin (162–325 mg) as well as intravenous heparin, enoxaparin, or fondaparinux. Clopidogrel loading has been demonstrated to increase rates of vessel patency and is also recommended in this setting.

After thrombolytic therapy is administered, the ECG should be monitored at 60 minutes and 90 minutes to confirm at least 50% improvement in maximal ST-segment

TABLE 7. Characteristics of Thrombolytic Agents Commonly Used in the Treatment of ST-Elevation Myocardial Infarction

Characteristic	Streptokinase	Alteplase	Reteplase	Tenecteplase
Dose	1.5 megaunits over 30-60 min	Up to 100 mg in 90 min (based on weight)[a]	10 units × 2 (30 min apart), each over 2 min	30-50 mg based on weight[b]
Bolus administration	No	No	Yes	Yes
Antigenic	Yes	No	No	No
Allergic reactions (hypotension most common)	Yes	No	No	No
Systemic fibrinogen depletion	Marked	Mild	Moderate	Minimal
TIMI flow grade 3	~30%	~50%	~60%	~60%
TIMI flow grade 2/3	~55%	~75%	~83%	~83%
Rate of intracerebral hemorrhage	~0.4%	~0.4%-0.7% (100-mg dose)	~0.8%	~0.9%
Fibrin specificity	None	++	+	+++
Fibrin affinity	None	+++	+	++++
Cost per recommended MI dose (U.S.)[c]	$562.50	$3404.78	$2872.50	$2917.48 for 50 mg

[a]Bolus 15 mg, infusion 0.75 mg/kg × 30 min (maximum 50 mg), then 0.5 mg/kg not to exceed 35 mg over the next 60 min to an overall maximum of 100 mg.

[b]30 mg for weight <60 kg (132 lb), 35 mg for 60-69 kg (132-152 lb), 40 mg for 70-79 kg (154-174 lb), 45 mg for 80-89 kg (176-196 lb), and 50 mg for 90 kg (198 lb) or more.

[c]Department of Health and Human Services, Office of Inspector General. Red Book, 2005. Available at https://oig.hhs.gov/publications/docs/redbook/Red%20Book%202005.pdf.

Reproduced with permission from Boden WE, Eagle K, Granger CB. Reperfusion strategies in acute ST-segment elevation myocardial infarction: a comprehensive review of contemporary management options. J Am Coll Cardiol. 2007;50:917-29. [PMID: 17765117] Copyright 2007, Elsevier.

elevation. ~~One quarter to one third of patients do not achieve reperfusion, particularly if time from symptom onset to receipt of thrombolytic therapy is delayed.~~ Owing to the potential for thrombolytic failure, patients with STEMI treated with thrombolytic therapy should be subsequently transferred to a PCI-capable hospital. Rescue PCI is associated with improved outcomes compared with conservative management in the event of failed reperfusion. Coronary angiography is generally recommended in all patients before discharge, even after successful thrombolysis. Patients with STEMI who present with heart failure or cardiogenic shock, or who develop these complications after thrombolytic therapy, are a particularly high-risk group (mortality rate >50%) and should be immediately transferred to a PCI-capable center.

Although thrombolytic therapy is potentially life-saving, it carries significant risks, primarily related to bleeding. Intracerebral hemorrhage is the most catastrophic complication of thrombolytic therapy and occurs in approximately 1% of patients. Relative and absolute contraindications to thrombolytic therapy are listed in **Table 8**.

Primary Percutaneous Coronary Intervention
PPCI refers to the process by which an emergency medical provider activates a team of providers to initiate emergent coronary angiography and PCI in patients with STEMI. Ideally, the time from first medical contact until PCI is less than 90 minutes. The amount of myocardial salvage is directly related to ischemic time; therefore, the quicker the artery can be opened, the better the final outcome. Because the rates of achieving vessel patency are higher and more reliable with

TABLE 8. Contraindications to Thrombolytic Therapy for ST-Elevation Myocardial Infarction

Absolute Contraindications

Any previous intracerebral hemorrhage

Known cerebrovascular lesion (e.g., arteriovenous malformation)

Ischemic stroke within 3 mo

Suspected aortic dissection

Active bleeding or bleeding diathesis (excluding menses)

Significant closed head or facial trauma within 3 mo

Relative Contraindications

History of chronic, severe, poorly controlled hypertension

Severe uncontrolled hypertension on presentation (SBP >180 mm Hg or DBP >110 mm Hg)[a]

History of ischemic stroke (>3 mo), dementia, or known intracranial abnormality

Traumatic or prolonged (>10 min) CPR or major surgery (<3 wk)

Recent (within 2-4 wk) internal bleeding

Noncompressible vascular puncture site

For streptokinase/anistreplase: previous exposure (>5 d) or previous allergic reaction to these agents

Pregnancy

Active peptic ulcer disease

Current use of anticoagulants: the higher the INR, the higher the bleeding risk

CPR = cardiopulmonary resuscitation; DBP = diastolic blood pressure; SBP = systolic blood pressure.

[a]Thrombolytic therapy can be considered if SBP can be reduced to <140 mm Hg and DBP to <90 mm Hg with initial medical therapy.

CONT.

PPCI than with thrombolysis, PPCI is the preferred method of treating STEMI when the patient presents to a hospital capable of performing PCI or can be transferred from an index hospital to a PCI-capable center quickly (time from first medical contact to PPCI of ≤120 minutes). Once the patient is in the catheterization suite, the initial focus is on quickly restoring flow to the acutely occluded artery. There is ongoing debate as to the timing and potential benefit of PCI of nonculprit vessels.

Patients undergoing PPCI should receive aspirin and heparin before thrombolytic therapy. During the procedure, patients generally receive intravenous heparin (with or without glycoprotein IIb/IIIa blockade) or bivalirudin. Most patients undergo stenting and receive loading doses of additional antiplatelet drugs (P2Y$_{12}$ inhibitors) (**Table 9**). Clopidogrel has historically been the most commonly prescribed P2Y$_{12}$ inhibitor. Compared with clopidogrel, prasugrel is more potent, has a quicker onset of action, and has a lower risk for thrombotic complications; however, prasugrel is also associated with an increased risk for bleeding. Prasugrel should not be used in patients with a history of stroke and those aged 75 years and older, and dosing must be adjusted for those weighing less than 60 kg (132 lb). Ticagrelor, a nonthienopyridine P2Y$_{12}$ inhibitor, also has greater potency and faster onset of platelet inhibition than clopidogrel. In the PLATO trial of patients with ACS, ticagrelor treatment resulted in significantly lower mortality rates compared with clopidogrel. Ticagrelor causes subjective dyspnea in some patients; this symptom is usually self-limited but occasionally causes drug discontinuation.

Medical Therapy

Medical therapies for the treatment of patients with ACS are summarized in **Table 10**.

All patients presenting with STEMI should receive aspirin and anticoagulation therapy. Regardless of the selected reperfusion strategy, patients should also be treated with a P2Y$_{12}$ inhibitor. Clopidogrel is indicated in patients receiving thrombolytic therapy, whereas clopidogrel, prasugrel, and ticagrelor are options for those undergoing PPCI (see Table 9).

β-Blockers decrease myocardial oxygen demand, reduce the incidence of ventricular arrhythmias, and improve long-term survival in patients with STEMI. Current guidelines suggest initiating these drugs within 24 hours of presentation. The COMMIT/CCS-2 trial demonstrated that intravenous metoprolol reduced the early risk for reinfarction and ventricular fibrillation in patients with acute MI but also resulted in a higher rate of cardiogenic shock. β-Blockers should not be given if there is evidence of hypotension, cardiogenic shock, pulmonary congestion, or atrioventricular block. In these cases, β-blockers may be withheld initially and introduced once the patient is stabilized.

ACE inhibitors are indicated in most patients with STEMI and particularly in patients with impaired left ventricular function, heart failure, or anterior wall infarction. ARBs may be used if the patient is intolerant of ACE inhibitors. These agents have shown significant early benefit and should be administered within the first 24 hours of presentation, assuming there are no contraindications.

Eplerenone, an aldosterone antagonist, has proved beneficial in patients with STEMI who have an ejection fraction less than or equal to 40% and either heart failure or diabetes; however, the treatment effects were demonstrated only when eplerenone was initiated within 1 week of presentation. Potassium levels must be carefully monitored, particularly in patients with pre-existing kidney dysfunction and those receiving ACE inhibitors or ARBs.

High-intensity statin therapy is indicated in patients with STEMI. Cholesterol levels may be transiently lower around the time of MI, and a low LDL cholesterol level should not dissuade clinicians from prescribing statins.

TABLE 9.	P2Y$_{12}$ Inhibitors Used in the Treatment of Patients with Coronary Artery Disease				
Drug	**Indications**	**Loading Dose**	**Maintenance Dose**	**Adverse Effects**	**Contraindications**
Clopidogrel	Stable CAD treated with PCI ACS	300-600 mg	75 mg/d	Increased bleeding risk	Known allergy to the drug
Ticagrelor	ACS	180 mg	90 mg twice daily[a]	Increased bleeding risk, dyspnea	Known allergy to the drug
Prasugrel	ACS treated with PCI[b]	60 mg	10 mg/d[c]	Increased bleeding risk	Known allergy to the drug, prior transient ischemic attack/stroke, age ≥75 y

ACS = acute coronary syndrome; CAD = coronary artery disease; PCI = percutaneous coronary intervention.

[a]Ticagrelor should be used with aspirin, 81 mg/d.

[b]Prasugrel should not be loaded "upstream" (before catheterization).

[c]Prasugrel, 5 mg/d, should be considered for those weighing less than 60 kg (132 lb) or at moderate to high risk for bleeding (e.g., patients with significant kidney function impairment).

TABLE 10. Medical Therapy for Acute Coronary Syndromes

Medication	Drugs in Class	Dosage	Indications	Comments
Antiplatelet Medications				
Aspirin	N/A	81-162 mg/d	All patients with ACS, unless intolerant or allergic	
Clopidogrel	N/A	75 mg/d	P2Y$_{12}$ inhibitor in combination with aspirin is indicated in all patients after ACS for at least 1 y	Clopidogrel is recommended as an alternative for patients with intolerance or allergy to aspirin
Prasugrel	N/A	5-10 mg/d	P2Y$_{12}$ inhibitor in combination with aspirin is indicated only in patients in whom PCI is performed for at least 1 y	Contraindicated with age >75 y or history of stroke/TIA Dosage adjustment to 5 mg/d should be considered for patients weighing <60 kg (132 lb)
Ticagrelor	N/A	90 mg twice daily	P2Y$_{12}$ inhibitor in combination with aspirin is indicated in all patients after ACS for at least 1 y	More rapid onset of action; does not require first-pass hepatic metabolism; no known genetic polymorphisms Decreased effectiveness with aspirin doses ≥100 mg
Cardioprotective Medications				
β-Blockers	Atenolol, metoprolol, carvedilol, nebivolol	Variable	All patients with prior MI or LV systolic dysfunction	Avoid in patients with cardiogenic shock, hypotension, or conduction disturbances
ACE inhibitors	Benazepril, captopril, enalapril, fosinopril, perindopril, trandolapril, lisinopril, ramipril, quinapril	Variable	All patients with LV systolic dysfunction, hypertension, diabetes mellitus, or kidney disease	Particularly beneficial in patients with anterior MI
Angiotensin receptor blockers	Losartan, valsartan, olmesartan, candesartan, irbesartan, telmisartan	Variable	All patients with LV systolic dysfunction, hypertension, diabetes, or kidney disease who are intolerant of ACE inhibitors	Should not be used in patients already taking an ACE inhibitor
Aldosterone inhibitor	Eplerenone	25-50 mg/d	STEMI patients with LVEF ≤40% and either clinical heart failure or diabetes	Caution is advised in patients with chronic kidney disease or hyperkalemia
High-intensity statin therapy	Atorvastatin	40-80 mg/d	For all patients with evidence of coronary artery disease and age ≤75 y	
	Rosuvastatin	20-40 mg/d		
Moderate-intensity statin therapy	Atorvastatin	10-20 mg/d	For all patients with evidence of coronary artery disease and age >75 y or otherwise intolerant of high-intensity statin therapy	
	Rosuvastatin	5-10 mg/d		
	Simvastatin	20-40 mg/d		
	Pravastatin	40-80 mg/d		
	Lovastatin	40 mg/d		
	Fluvastatin	40 mg twice daily		
Antianginal Medications				
Nitroglycerin	Nitrostat (SL)	0.4 mg every 5 min for a total of three doses	As part of multimodality treatment for ongoing chest pain	Avoid with SBP <90 mm Hg or ≥30 mm Hg below baseline, bradycardia, tachycardia, RV infarction, PDE-5 inhibitor use within the last 24-48 h, HCM, or severe AS
	Nitronal (IV)	Initial IV infusion rate of 5-10 µg/min	For persistent chest pain following three SL doses and as part of multimodality treatment for heart failure, hypertension	

(Continued on the next page)

TABLE 10.	Medical Therapy for Acute Coronary Syndromes *(Continued)*			
Medication	**Drugs in Class**	**Dosage**	**Indications**	**Comments**
Nondihydropyridine calcium channel blockers	Diltiazem, verapamil	Variable	Patients with NSTE-ACS who are intolerant of β-blockers or with angina refractory to nitrates and β-blockers	No benefit in STEMI patients May worsen clinical status with coincidental heart failure or LV dysfunction Avoid with evidence of heart failure, cardiogenic shock, or conduction abnormalities

ACS = acute coronary syndrome; AS = aortic stenosis; HCM = hypertrophic cardiomyopathy; IV = intravenous; LV = left ventricular; LVEF = left ventricular ejection fraction; MI = myocardial infarction; N/A = not applicable; NSTE-ACS = non-ST-elevation acute coronary syndrome; PCI = percutaneous coronary intervention; PDE = phosphodiesterase; RV = right ventricular; SBP = systolic blood pressure; SL = sublingual; STEMI = ST-elevation myocardial infarction; TIA = transient ischemic attack.

Intravenous nitroglycerin can be used to treat patients with STEMI and hypertension or heart failure; however, there is no role for the routine use of oral nitrates in the convalescent phase of STEMI. Calcium channel blockers and ranolazine also have no role in treating patients with STEMI.

Complications of STEMI

Arrhythmias commonly occur in the peri-infarct setting. Atrial fibrillation, which affects up to 10% to 20% of patients with STEMI, complicates management and may cause hemodynamic instability. Ventricular tachycardia and fibrillation may also occur during MI or after reperfusion. Repetitive and sustained bouts of postinfarct ventricular arrhythmias may warrant consultation with an electrophysiologist, as predischarge implantable cardioverter-defibrillator therapy has a role in treating late arrhythmias complicating STEMI. Routine suppression of ventricular ectopy with antiarrhythmic agents is generally not recommended and is associated with increased risk for ventricular arrhythmias. In particular, accelerated idioventricular rhythm, which commonly arises after reperfusion, is generally benign and transient, requiring no treatment. Atrioventricular blocks, including Wenckebach and complete heart block, may occur after inferior MIs. Temporary transvenous pacemakers are sometimes necessary, but permanent pacing is rarely required. Benign forms of vagally mediated heart block must be differentiated from Mobitz type 2 second-degree atrioventricular block, which is more frequently observed with anterior infarction and damage to the conduction system. Mobitz type 2 block may progress to complete heart block and necessitates permanent pacing.

Cardiogenic shock is a common complication of STEMI. It typically results from a large anterior MI due to severely reduced left ventricular systolic function and carries a mortality rate of 50% to 80%. Patients with cardiogenic shock, particularly those younger than 75 years, have a higher rate of survival if they receive emergent revascularization. In these cases, an intra-aortic balloon pump (IABP) or left ventricular assist device may be implanted temporarily, although limited data support their benefits in cardiogenic shock. Once the patient is stabilized, weening the patient from mechanical and inotropic support and gentle uptitration of afterload-reducing agents, such as captopril, can be attempted. β-Blockers should be avoided initially and can be introduced once the patient is stabilized. Diuretics should be used to treat pulmonary vascular congestion.

Approximately 10% to 20% of cases of anterior STEMI are complicated by left ventricular apical thrombus. Although not supported by rigorous studies, anticoagulation with warfarin is generally recommended for at least 3 months to reduce the risk for systemic embolization.

Rates of mechanical complications after STEMI, including left ventricular free wall rupture, right ventricular infarction, ventricular septal defect (VSD), and acute mitral regurgitation, are low; however, clinicians must be able to recognize these complications, given their highly morbid nature. Free wall rupture produces sudden-onset chest pain or syncope with rapid progression to pulseless electrical activity. It is more common in older adults, women, patients with anterior MI, those receiving anti-inflammatory agents, and patients with a significant delay in receiving reperfusion therapy (>12 hours). Surgery should be considered, but mortality rates, even among those who survive to the operating room, are very high.

Right ventricular infarction, typically indicated by ST-segment elevation in right-sided ECG leads (V_1 and V_4R), can complicate right coronary artery occlusion. It presents with hypotension, elevated jugular venous pressure, and an absence of findings on lung auscultation. Right ventricle pump dysfunction causes inadequate filling of the left ventricle, resulting in shock. Treatments include volume resuscitation and positive inotropes (dobutamine or dopamine) to bridge the right ventricle to recovery, which generally takes 2 to 3 days. Nitrates are contraindicated because they may worsen hypotension by reducing preload.

Acquired VSD from septal wall rupture may complicate inferior or anterior STEMI. With inferior STEMI, the VSD tends to be located in the inferior basal septum, whereas anterior STEMI generally leads to an apical VSD. VSDs typically occur within 3 to 5 days of STEMI presentation. Patients present with worsening heart failure and shock, and a harsh holosystolic murmur may be heard at the left lower sternal border. The diagnosis is confirmed with echocardiography. Although initial management may include afterload reduction with medical therapy and IABP support, the mortality rate in patients with medically treated postinfarct VSDs approaches 100%. Surgical closure should be considered; however, the mortality rate in surgical series is still high (approximately 50%). Patch closure can be very difficult owing to the necrotic tissue and inability to find viable myocardium to suture and patch. Percutaneous closure with a VSD occluder device is possible but often unsuccessful because of the nature of the defect, and residual shunting around the device is common.

Acute severe mitral regurgitation may occur as a result of papillary muscle rupture. Most often, the posteromedial papillary muscle ruptures with right coronary artery occlusion. This complication tends to occur several days after STEMI. Afterload reduction and IABP placement may be tried, but urgent surgical intervention is usually necessary. Acute severe mitral regurgitation may also result from left ventricular dysfunction and is often related to an inferior MI with restriction of the posterior mitral leaflet, termed functional ischemic mitral regurgitation. Ischemic mitral regurgitation is treated with revascularization and medical therapy.

KEY POINTS

- Primary percutaneous coronary intervention is preferred to thrombolytic therapy for the treatment of ST-elevation myocardial infarction.

- If primary percutaneous coronary intervention (PPCI) is not available within 120 minutes of first medical contact, patients with ST-elevation myocardial infarction should receive thrombolytic therapy and be urgently transferred to a PPCI-capable center.

- β-Blockers reduce the incidence of ventricular arrhythmias and improve long-term survival in patients with ST-elevation myocardial infarction; however, these agents are contraindicated when signs or symptoms of cardiogenic shock are present.

- All patients presenting with an ST-elevation myocardial infarction should be treated with aspirin, anticoagulation therapy, and a P2Y$_{12}$ inhibitor.

Non-ST-Elevation Acute Coronary Syndromes

NSTE-ACS is a common presentation of CAD. The chest pain associated with an NSTE-ACS is generally acute, is new in onset, and often occurs with rest or minimal exertion. The pathogenesis is plaque rupture within a coronary artery and transient or incomplete occlusion of the vessel. NSTEMI is differentiated from unstable angina by the presence of elevated serum cardiac biomarkers at the time of evaluation.

Risk Stratification

Many treatment options are available for patients with NSTE-ACS, and risk stratification tools can be used to aid in diagnostic and therapeutic decision making. The two most commonly used risk scores are the TIMI and GRACE risk models. The simpler of the two models, the TIMI risk score, predicts 14-day death, recurrent MI, and urgent revascularization rates (**Table 11**). The GRACE risk score (available at www.gracescore.org) is more complex, requiring a nomogram to calculate. It incorporates physical examination findings (heart rate, blood pressure, Killip class), clinical features (age, cardiac arrest at admission), electrocardiographic findings (ST-segment deviation), and biomarker variables (creatinine levels, elevated cardiac enzymes) to predict in-house and postdischarge death and MI risk. These scoring systems are useful in determining which patients may benefit most from more aggressive strategies, such as anticoagulation or an early invasive approach (**Figure 9**). An elevated troponin level is itself a powerful predictor of outcomes and identifies patients who will benefit from aggressive medical and invasive strategies (coronary angiography).

Medical Therapy

Medical therapies for patients with NSTE-ACS are similar to those for other ACS presentations; however, some unique features in this patient population are highly relevant to the

TABLE 11. TIMI Risk Score for Non-ST-Elevation Acute Coronary Syndromes

Prognostic Variables (1 Point Each)	
Age ≥65 y	
≥3 Traditional CAD risk factors[a]	
Documented CAD with ≥50% diameter stenosis	
ST-segment deviation	
≥2 Anginal episodes in the past 24 h	
Aspirin use in the past wk	
Elevated cardiac biomarkers (creatine kinase MB or troponin)	
TIMI Risk Score (Sum of Prognostic Variables)	
0-2	Low risk
3-4	Intermediate risk
5-7	High risk

CAD = coronary artery disease; TIMI = thrombolysis in myocardial infarction.

[a]Hypertension, hypercholesterolemia, diabetes mellitus, being a current smoker, family history of CAD.

Information from Antman EM, Cohen M, Bernink PJ, McCabe CH, Horacek T, Papuchis G, et al. The TIMI risk score for unstable angina/non-ST elevation MI: a method for prognostication and therapeutic decision making. JAMA. 2000;284:835-42. [PMID: 10938172]

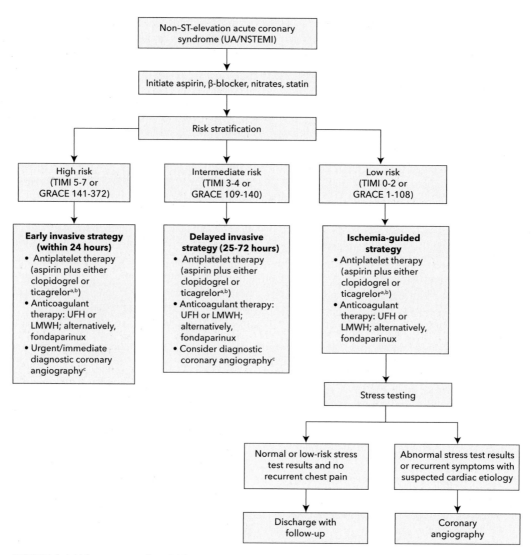

FIGURE 9. Initial management of non–ST-elevation acute coronary syndromes. LMWH = low-molecular-weight heparin; NSTEMI = non–ST-elevation myocardial infarction; UA = unstable angina; UFH = unfractionated heparin.

aClopidogrel or ticagrelor may be dosed at the time of hospital admission and diagnosis of acute coronary syndrome.

bIf coronary artery bypass grafting is required, clopidogrel or ticagrelor should be stopped, and surgery should be delayed for at least 5 days.

cIf the decision is made to withhold a P2Y₁₂ inhibitor until the time of angiography and a P2Y₁₂ inhibitor is desired, clopidogrel, ticagrelor, or prasugrel can be initiated.

Recommendations based on Amsterdam EA, Wenger NK, Brindis RG, Casey DE Jr, Ganiats TG, Holmes DR Jr, et al; ACC/AHA Task Force Members. 2014 AHA/ACC guideline for the management of patients with non-ST-elevation acute coronary syndromes: executive summary: a report of the American College of Cardiology/American Heart Association Task Force on Practice Guidelines. Circulation. 2014;130:2354-94. [PMID: 25249586] doi:10.1161/CIR.0000000000000133

treatment of this condition. Notably, thrombolytic therapy is not beneficial in patients with NSTE-ACS and is not recommended. Medical therapies for the treatment of NSTE-ACS are summarized in Table 10.

Antiplatelet Medications

Aspirin (162–325 mg) should be administered at presentation to all patients with definite or likely NSTE-ACS, followed by a daily dose of 81 to 162 mg. Early clopidogrel loading has been recommended in patients with NSTEMI; however, the optimal timing for loading of other oral antiplatelet agents is unclear. Prasugrel loading before coronary angiography is not beneficial. Clopidogrel

or ticagrelor therapy is recommended for 1 year after NSTE-ACS presentation, regardless of the treatment strategy. Prasugrel is indicated only in patients treated with PCI. Evidence supports continuing DAPT beyond 1 year in patients at high risk for recurrent vascular events (such as those with depressed left ventricular function, saphenous vein graft stenting, or diabetes) in whom the benefit exceeds the bleeding risk.

The use of intravenous glycoprotein IIb/IIIa inhibitors (eptifibatide, tirofiban) has decreased over the past decade. Although these drugs had been shown to improve outcomes in patients with NSTE-ACS (particularly higher-risk and troponin-positive patients), subsequent study demonstrated no benefit of upstream glycoprotein IIb/IIIa blockade and an increased risk for bleeding. These agents are generally reserved for use during PCI; however, given the advent of quicker-acting and more potent oral antiplatelet agents, administration of glycoprotein IIb/IIIa inhibitors in the setting of PCI has also significantly declined.

Anticoagulant Medications

Patients with definite NSTE-ACS should undergo anticoagulation. Intravenous unfractionated heparin and subcutaneous enoxaparin are most commonly used. Intravenous heparin is preferred in patients with kidney dysfunction because enoxaparin and similar agents are partially cleared by the kidneys. For patients proceeding to the catheterization laboratory, anticoagulant therapy should be provided until revascularization with PCI or CABG. In medically treated patients, anticoagulation is recommended for at least 48 hours and is generally continued until discharge.

Antianginal Medications

β-Blockers should be administered within 24 hours of NSTE-ACS because these agents reduce ventricular arrhythmias and long-term mortality. β-Blockers are not appropriate for patients with evidence of heart failure or shock at presentation. Likewise, these agents should not be given to patients with bradycardia, heart block, or a PR interval greater than 240 ms on ECG.

Calcium channel blockers are recommended for patients with NSTE-ACS intolerant of β-blocker therapy or in patients with angina symptoms despite therapy with nitrates and β-blockers. The nondihydropyridine calcium channel blockers reduce heart rate, blood pressure, and cardiac contractility, thereby reducing myocardial oxygen demand. However, because of these hemodynamic effects, use of these agents is also contraindicated in the setting of shock, pulmonary edema, or significant conduction disease. Importantly, short-acting dihydropyridine calcium channel blockers are contraindicated, owing to their ability to acutely lower the blood pressure and raise the heart rate.

Nitrates are primarily used to manage angina symptoms in patients with NSTE-ACS. Sublingual nitrates should be administered at presentation to relieve chest pain. For patients with persistent chest pain despite β-blockade, intravenous nitroglycerin can alleviate symptoms, particularly in those with hypertension. Patients receiving nitroglycerin infusions for a prolonged time will often require increased doses due to the development of nitrate tolerance. Nitrates should be avoided in patients who have had recent exposure (within 24-48 hours) to phosphodiesterase type 5 inhibitors such as sildenafil.

Patients with chest pain refractory to antianginal medications should be evaluated for noncardiac causes of chest pain and biomarker elevation, as well as for the possibility of severe underlying CAD or electrocardiographically silent coronary thrombosis.

Lipid-Lowering Medications

Statin therapy reduces mortality and adverse clinical event rates after ACS. High-intensity statin therapy is recommended because it improves outcomes compared with lower-intensity treatment. Initiating statins in the inpatient setting is associated with greater medication adherence. Furthermore, statin preloading before PCI has been associated with lower rates of periprocedural MI.

Invasive Versus Ischemia-Guided Treatment

Immediate invasive treatment (within 2 hours) is recommended for patients with NSTE-ACS who have hemodynamic instability, refractory chest pain, heart failure, or ventricular arrhythmias. In patients with an elevated clinical risk score, significant ST-segment deviation, or elevated cardiac biomarkers, cardiac catheterization is usually performed within 24 hours of presentation. The type of revascularization procedure (PCI or CABG) depends on the results of angiography.

An invasive strategy improves the composite clinical endpoint of death, recurrent MI, and repeat hospitalization compared with an ischemia-guided approach in high-risk and troponin-positive patients with NSTE-ACS. An invasive strategy is the favored approach, with the exception of patients with extensive noncardiac comorbid conditions (such as cancer), in whom the clinical benefits of revascularization may be lower, and patients with acute chest pain unlikely to be related to CAD.

With an ischemia-guided treatment strategy, patients undergo noninvasive stress testing before hospital discharge; cardiac catheterization is reserved for patients with active or intermittent ischemia, including those with angina despite medical therapy or evidence of ischemia on stress testing, and patients at very high clinical risk based on risk score. The ischemia-guided approach is appropriate for low-risk patients (TIMI score <2 or GRACE score <109).

KEY POINTS

- In patients with a non–ST-elevation acute coronary syndrome, initial risk stratification with the TIMI or GRACE risk scores aids in diagnostic and therapeutic decision making.
- Thrombolytic therapy is not indicated in patients with non–ST-elevation acute coronary syndromes. **HVC**
- The decision to pursue an invasive approach versus an ischemia-guided approach in patients with a non–ST-elevation acute coronary syndrome depends on the patient's risk for clinical events.
- Dual antiplatelet therapy is indicated for at least 1 year after a non–ST-elevation acute coronary syndrome (NSTE-ACS); clopidogrel and ticagrelor may be used in all patients with NSTE-ACS, whereas prasugrel may be used only in patients treated with percutaneous coronary intervention.

Acute Coronary Syndromes Not Associated with Obstructive Coronary Disease

Elevations in cardiac enzymes, particularly cardiac troponins, coupled with ECG changes provide excellent diagnostic discrimination for ACS. However, conditions not caused by acute coronary plaque rupture can present with similar findings, and treatment of these conditions with antithrombotic agents and revascularization is not beneficial or recommended.

Patients with accelerated hypertension, significant left ventricular hypertrophy, and cardiomyopathies may present with chest pain and elevated cardiac troponin levels caused by elevated left ventricular filling pressures or wall tension rather than plaque rupture. The ECG findings are often abnormal in these patients. Patients with supraventricular tachycardias, which may also dramatically increase the rate-pressure product, often present with chest pain, ST-segment depressions, and elevated cardiac enzyme levels, even if no CAD is present.

Coronary vasospasm is sudden constriction of a coronary artery. It may occur spontaneously or follow use of illicit substances (methamphetamines, cocaine) or prescription drugs (5-fluorouracil, bromocriptine). ECG abnormalities may be nonspecific or mimic STEMI patterns. Coronary vasospasm is a diagnosis of exclusion. Unless the patient has a history of vasospasm, patients often undergo coronary angiography, which may reveal normal findings or slowed coronary flow resulting from microvascular dysfunction. Provocative testing can be performed but is not usually indicated. Patients suspected of having vasospasm (or the related microvascular dysfunction) are usually treated empirically with nitrates and/or calcium channel blockers.

Takotsubo cardiomyopathy, alternatively termed stress cardiomyopathy or apical ballooning syndrome, is a relatively uncommon form of ACS (see Heart Failure). Patients present with acute chest pain, ECG changes (often ST-segment elevations), and elevated cardiac enzyme levels. Takotsubo cardiomyopathy most commonly occurs in women, and there is often, but not always, an antecedent psychological or physical stressor. Patients may initially be diagnosed with STEMI but found to have no significant coronary stenosis at the time of cardiac catheterization. Systolic apical ballooning and notable sparing of the base of the heart on echocardiography or ventriculography are characteristic of this syndrome.

Cardiac syndrome X is a poorly defined condition characterized by anginal chest pain in the presence of angiographically normal coronary arteries or insignificant CAD (<50% stenosis). Cardiac syndrome X is a frequent cause of chest pain syndromes in women, and patients often present without traditional risk factors for CAD. Several hypotheses have been proposed to explain the pathogenesis of this syndrome. One of the most accepted centers on microvascular dysfunction as the cause. Patients may be treated with β-blockers, calcium channel blockers, and nitrates.

Patients with chronic inflammatory muscle diseases or neuromuscular diseases may have elevated levels of cardiac troponin T due to expression of this enzyme in skeletal muscle. The cardiac troponin I level is normal in these cases, which can be helpful in differentiating ACS from these other entities.

Care After an Acute Coronary Syndrome

All patients with ACS should continue aspirin, preferably 81 mg/d, indefinitely. DAPT is recommended for at least 1 year (see Table 10). There is some evidence for extending DAPT beyond 1 year in stented and medically treated patients; however, the decision to prolong therapy should be individualized, with the risk for bleeding weighed against the risk for thrombosis. Statin therapy should continue indefinitely. β-Blockade and ACE inhibitor therapy should also be continued indefinitely in patients with left ventricular dysfunction; continuation of these medications is reasonable in patients with normal left ventricular function. Guidelines recommend avoiding NSAIDs if possible, owing to the increased cardiovascular risk associated with these drugs. Patients should be referred for cardiac rehabilitation, a medically observed exercise program, to improve functional capacity and risk factor profiles.

Management of Coronary Artery Disease in Special Populations

Women

Clinical Presentation

Women usually develop ischemic heart disease at an older age than men and more commonly present with stable CAD than an ACS. In women with typical angina symptoms, nonobstructive coronary stenoses are present on coronary angiography in more than 50% of cases, and microvascular dysfunction (endothelium-dependent or endothelium-independent) is thought to be a predominant cause of symptoms in these patients. In women with acute MI, the predominant symptom is chest pain or pressure; however, women can often have atypical symptoms, such as fatigue, dyspnea, nausea, or abdominal symptoms.

Several unique manifestations of cardiovascular disease, including spontaneous coronary artery dissection, takotsubo cardiomyopathy, and coronary vasospasm, occur primarily in women. Spontaneous coronary artery dissection is a common cause of chest pain among younger women who present with ACS. In many cases, spontaneous coronary artery dissection occurs in the peripartum period and is thought to be caused by hormonal changes, although the true cause is unknown. Given the preponderance of young women with this condition, minimizing radiation exposure and avoiding invasive angiography are recommended. This can typically be achieved with the use of supportive care with or without CT angiography. In severe cases, vessel occlusion causes STEMI and necessitates emergent revascularization.

Evaluation and Treatment

Noninvasive stress testing for the evaluation of CAD symptoms has a lower sensitivity and specificity in women than in men, and ST-segment deviation has a lower reported accuracy in women. Therefore, stress testing with imaging provides better accuracy in women (see Diagnostic Testing in Cardiology). Despite these differences, the same guideline recommendations apply to both women and men.

Reports from observational studies and substudies of randomized controlled trials suggest that women have worse outcomes after STEMI presentation. The cause of these worse outcomes is thought to be delays in recognition of CAD and longer overall ischemic time. Complication rates are also reported to be higher in women who undergo reperfusion therapy for STEMI. The COURAGE trial demonstrated that among patients with stable angina treated with revascularization, women had lower rates of overall mortality and nonfatal MI but a higher rate of complications compared with men. Overall, treatment guidelines do not differ for men and women.

Diabetes Mellitus
Risk and Evaluation
Diabetes has been proposed as a CAD equivalent because age-adjusted risk for CAD events is two- to threefold higher in patients with diabetes. Cardiovascular morbidity and mortality are also significantly higher in this population, especially in patients with type 2 diabetes. Much of the risk has been attributed to the higher incidence of known cardiovascular risk factors; however, evidence suggests that underlying vascular dysfunction may play an important role.

Patients with diabetes may present with atypical cardiac symptoms, such as dyspnea or nausea, requiring a high index of suspicion for CAD during their evaluation. The diagnostic accuracy of noninvasive stress testing in symptomatic patients with diabetes is similar to that in patients without diabetes. Although traditional risk factors for CAD should be aggressively managed in patients with diabetes, screening for CAD in asymptomatic persons is controversial, and routine stress testing is not recommended.

Medical Therapy and Secondary Prevention
Medical therapy for patients with diabetes and CAD includes aggressive risk factor reduction, glucose control, and antianginal therapy. The American College of Cardiology/American Heart Association recommend antihypertensive treatment with a target blood pressure below 130/80 mm Hg in patients with diabetes. In contrast, the American Diabetes Association recommends a systolic blood pressure goal of less than 140 mm Hg and a diastolic blood pressure goal of less than 90 mm Hg for most patients. Lower systolic and diastolic blood pressure targets may be appropriate for individuals at high risk for cardiovascular disease, if they can be achieved without undue treatment burden. ACE inhibitors and ARBs are preferred in the setting of hypertension because of their kidney-protective effects. High-intensity statin therapy is indicated in most patients with diabetes and CAD.

Aspirin is recommended for secondary prevention in all patients with diabetes and CAD. Primary prevention is recommended for patients with diabetes with a 10-year cardiovascular risk greater than 10% or one additional risk factor.

Tight glycemic control reduces microvascular complications; however, it does not reduce the risk for MI. In a recent study, liraglutide, a glucagon-like peptide-1 analogue, was associated with reduced risk for cardiovascular death in patients with type 2 diabetes and high cardiovascular risk. Initial studies suggested thiazolidinediones, specifically rosiglitazone, were associated with an elevated risk for cardiovascular events, although a subsequent clinical trial demonstrated no elevated risk for MI or death. Consequently, the FDA has removed the restriction on rosiglitazone use in patients with type 2 diabetes and CAD. Metformin does not have any cardiovascular effects, but caution should be exercised in patients undergoing coronary angiography, patients who have had an MI, and patients with heart failure because of concern for potentially fatal lactic acidosis.

Invasive Treatment
The choice of revascularization strategy (PCI or CABG) in patients with diabetes is based on many factors, including the severity and extent of CAD, comorbid conditions, and degree of atherosclerotic narrowing of small, distal vessels. Mortality rates are similar between the two procedures; however, CABG is generally preferred because it is associated with lower rates of repeat revascularization. In patients who undergo PCI, drug-eluting stent placement is recommended to reduce the occurrence of target vessel revascularization because of higher rates of restenosis in patients with diabetes.

> **KEY POINTS**
> - Stress testing is not routinely recommended in asymptomatic patients with diabetes mellitus to detect subclinical coronary artery disease.
> - Coronary artery bypass grafting is the preferred mode of revascularization in patients with diabetes mellitus.

HVC

Heart Failure
Pathophysiology of Heart Failure
Heart failure is a clinical syndrome characterized by signs and symptoms of fluid overload and decreased cardiac output. Heart failure can result from systolic or diastolic dysfunction. In cases of systolic dysfunction, multiple causes result in reduced stroke volume and ejection fraction, termed heart failure with reduced ejection fraction (HFrEF). Common causes of HFrEF include coronary artery disease (CAD), myocarditis, valvular heart disease, infiltrative processes, and hypertension. Diastolic dysfunction is usually characterized by a stiffened left ventricle with abnormal relaxation during diastole, resulting in an increase in left

ventricular preload. Ejection fraction classically remains normal in this setting, known as heart failure with preserved ejection fraction (HFpEF). Common causes of HFpEF include hypertension, aging, obesity, diabetes mellitus, and CAD. Often, patients with heart failure have concomitant systolic and diastolic dysfunction. The outcome of both processes is increased left ventricular filling pressures, which are transmitted to the lungs and subsequently to the right ventricle and the body. The increase in pressures causes the classic signs and symptoms of heart failure, including dyspnea, paroxysmal nocturnal dyspnea, orthopnea, peripheral edema, crackles on pulmonary auscultation, elevated jugular venous pressure, and an S_3.

In patients with heart failure, compensatory mechanisms activate to adapt to the reduction in cardiac output and elevated pressures. The heart dilates in response to an increase in preload to improve myocardial contraction (Frank-Starling mechanism). To combat the increase in wall stress that occurs with dilatation and high filling pressures, the myocytes hypertrophy, initially reducing wall stress but eventually leading to reduced left ventricular compliance. These changes improve or maintain stroke volume at first; however, in the long term, they contribute to worsening cardiac function.

Another compensatory mechanism is the upregulation of the renin-angiotensin-aldosterone system to produce angiotensin II and aldosterone. Angiotensin II causes vasoconstriction, which improves blood pressure and stimulates thirst. Aldosterone increases fluid retention by increasing sodium resorption. The adrenergic nervous system is stimulated, resulting in release of epinephrine, norepinephrine, and vasopressin. The hormones cause an increase in heart rate, contractility, and vascular resistance, and vasopressin causes additional water retention. These mechanisms improve blood pressure and forward flow initially; however, over time, they become deleterious. The increase in blood pressure causes an increase in afterload, leading to reduced stroke volume and increased ventricular preload. The increase in volume results in an increase in preload and left ventricular distention, followed by a rise in pulmonary pressures and enlarged heart size owing to both myocyte hypertrophy and elongation. Elevated levels of neurohormones also cause myocyte injury and adversely promote remodeling. The result is a cycle of slowly worsening left ventricular function with decreasing forward flow and increasing pulmonary and right-sided pressures.

KEY POINTS

- Common causes of heart failure with reduced ejection fraction include coronary artery disease, myocarditis, valvular heart disease, infiltrative processes, and hypertension.
- Heart failure with preserved ejection fraction is commonly caused by hypertension, aging, obesity, diabetes mellitus, or coronary artery disease.

Screening and Prevention

Patients at risk for heart failure (such as those with hypertension, diabetes, or vascular disease), but without heart failure symptoms or left ventricular dysfunction, should be screened with B-type natriuretic peptide (BNP) or N-terminal pro-B-type natriuretic peptide (NT-proBNP) measurement, followed by early intervention with appropriate therapy in those with elevated levels. BNP assays are typically used to establish or exclude heart failure as the cause of dyspnea. Small studies have shown that aggressive guideline-based medical therapy in patients with elevated BNP or NT-proBNP levels can help prevent future left ventricular dysfunction or new-onset heart failure. Additional research is needed to identify the effects of screening on mortality as well as the cost-effectiveness of such interventions.

Evidence has shown that heart failure incidence can also be reduced by significantly lowering blood pressure in at-risk patients. The American College of Cardiology (ACC), American Heart Association (AHA), and Heart Failure Society of America recommend targeting an optimal blood pressure of less than 130/80 mm Hg for heart failure prevention.

Diagnosis and Evaluation of Heart Failure

Clinical Evaluation

Clinical evaluation of patients suspected of having heart failure should include a comprehensive history and physical examination, focusing on assessment of fluid and perfusion status. Most patients with heart failure present with volume overload and normal cardiac output. The second most common presentation is low cardiac output with volume overload; rarely, patients have signs and symptoms of low cardiac output without volume overload. Volume overload is associated with crackles, jugular venous distention, peripheral edema, increased abdominal girth (ascites), dyspnea, orthopnea, and paroxysmal nocturnal dyspnea. Patients with heart failure typically develop exertional dyspnea first, followed by orthopnea and paroxysmal nocturnal dyspnea. Elevated jugular venous pressures and orthopnea are most predictive of an elevated pulmonary capillary wedge pressure, which suggests left-sided heart failure. Signs of low cardiac output include low pulse pressure, cool extremities, and reduced cognition. Although worsening kidney or liver function may be a sign of low cardiac output, end-organ dysfunction can also be caused by vascular congestion.

Diagnosis

Initial diagnostic testing should include electrocardiography to evaluate for ischemia and arrhythmia, chest radiography to exclude pulmonary causes of dyspnea, and a BNP or NT-proBNP assay to establish the presence and severity of heart failure. In patients with dyspnea, BNP can effectively differentiate cardiac from pulmonary causes. BNP levels are

---

elevated in patients with increased right or left ventricular filling pressures and systolic or diastolic heart failure (typically >400 pg/mL [400 ng/L]), whereas BNP levels are low to normal in patients with pulmonary disease (typically <100 pg/mL [100 ng/L]). Studies have shown that an elevated BNP level has a sensitivity for heart failure of 95% to 97% and a negative predictive value of 90% to 97%. Between 100 pg/mL and 400 pg/mL (100-400 ng/L), BNP concentrations are neither sensitive nor specific for excluding or confirming the diagnosis of heart failure. Other factors that increase BNP levels include kidney failure, older age, and female sex. BNP levels are reduced in patients with an elevated BMI.

Laboratory assessment should also include a complete blood count, serum electrolytes and kidney function tests, glucose and lipid levels, liver chemistry tests, and serum thyroid-stimulating hormone level. Thyroid-stimulating hormone measurement is indicated to evaluate for occult hypo- or hyperthyroidism as a reversible cause of heart failure. In hyperthyroidism in particular, the predominant manifestation of thyroid dysfunction may be cardiac symptoms, which will abate when the hyperthyroidism is treated.

Echocardiography is the primary diagnostic test in the evaluation of heart failure. An echocardiogram provides information on heart size, systolic and diastolic function, regional wall motion abnormalities, and valvular disease. Findings on echocardiography can provide information on underlying causes of heart failure as well. Regional wall motion abnormalities suggest CAD, and changes in the myocardium can suggest conditions such as cardiac amyloid. Echocardiography may also provide prognostic information, particularly in the setting of severely depressed ejection fraction.

Evaluation for Ischemia

CAD is the leading cause of heart failure in the United States (>50% of patients) and should be considered in all patients with newly diagnosed heart failure. The decision to evaluate for CAD depends on the patient's symptoms and risk factors (family history, male sex, diabetes, hypertension, tobacco use). Additionally, findings on electrocardiography and echocardiography may suggest an ischemic cause for left ventricular dysfunction. Patients with exertional chest pain, history of myocardial infarction, or other symptoms suggesting CAD should undergo further evaluation with stress testing or cardiac catheterization as clinically appropriate (see Diagnostic Testing in Cardiology). Identification of significant CAD is important, as left ventricular dysfunction caused by ischemia may improve or resolve with percutaneous or surgical revascularization.

Classification

The severity of heart failure is categorized according to the New York Heart Association (NYHA) functional classification (**Table 12**) and the ACC/AHA heart failure stages (**Table 13**). Patients can move back and forth between NYHA classes

TABLE 12. New York Heart Association Functional Classification

Class	Description
I	No limitations of physical activity
II	Slight limitation of physical activity
III	Marked limitation of physical activity
IIIA	Symptoms with less than ordinary activity
IIIB	Symptoms with minimal exertion
IV	Unable to carry on any physical activity without symptoms

TABLE 13. American College of Cardiology/American Heart Association Stages of Heart Failure

Stage	Description
Stage A	At risk for heart failure but without structural heart changes (e.g., patients with diabetes mellitus, coronary artery disease, hypertension, or vascular disease)
Stage B	Structural heart disease (e.g., reduced ejection fraction, left ventricular hypertrophy, chamber enlargement) but without heart failure symptoms
Stage C	Structural heart disease with current or prior heart failure symptoms
Stage D	Refractory heart failure requiring advanced intervention (e.g., biventricular pacemaker, left ventricular assist device, transplantation)

Information from Hunt SA, Abraham WT, Chin MH, Feldman AM, Francis GS, Ganiats TG, et al. 2009 Focused update incorporated into the ACC/AHA 2005 guidelines for the diagnosis and management of heart failure in adults: a report of the American College of Cardiology Foundation/American Heart Association Task Force on Practice Guidelines: developed in collaboration with the International Society for Heart and Lung Transplantation. Circulation. 2009;119:e391-479. [PMID: 19324966] doi:10.1161/CIRCULATIONAHA.109.192065

depending on fluid status and progression of heart failure; however, they may only progress in the ACC/AHA stages. Both the patient's functional class and stage affect the choice of therapy.

KEY POINTS

- B-type natriuretic peptide measurement is a sensitive and specific test for the diagnosis of heart failure in patients with dyspnea.
- In patients suspected of having heart failure, echocardiography should be performed to assess ejection fraction and identify possible causes of heart failure.

Medical Therapy for Systolic Heart Failure

The treatment of patients with HFrEF (systolic heart failure) includes treatment of acute exacerbations followed by long-term therapy to decrease morbidity and mortality and improve symptoms in patients with chronic heart failure.

ACE Inhibitors and Angiotensin Receptor Blockers

ACE inhibitors reduce morbidity and mortality in patients with HFrEF and are the cornerstone of long-term therapy for both symptomatic and asymptomatic patients. ACE inhibitors block the conversion of angiotensin I to angiotensin II, inhibiting the upregulation of the aldosterone pathway. The ATLAS trial examined the effects of low-dose versus high-dose ACE inhibitor therapy (lisinopril) in patients with systolic heart failure and found no difference in overall mortality; however, high-dose lisinopril was associated with a significant reduction in the composite endpoint of mortality and hospitalizations from heart failure and for any cause. On the basis of these results, the general consensus is to uptitrate ACE inhibitors to maximal doses or until the onset of symptomatic hypotension.

The primary adverse effects associated with the use of ACE inhibitors are kidney dysfunction, ACE inhibitor–induced cough, and angioedema. Although ACE inhibitors should be considered in every patient with HFrEF, elevations in creatinine levels may prevent use of maximal doses. Many physicians do not recommend increasing the dosage once the creatinine level rises to 2.5 mg/dL (221 µmol/L) or the estimated glomerular filtration rate falls below 30 mL/min/1.73 m². The estimated glomerular filtration rate should be monitored for decline during uptitration of ACE inhibitor or angiotensin receptor blocker (ARB) therapy and should be rechecked before discontinuation of these drugs, as other conditions or drugs may confound the assessment of kidney function. Hyperkalemia may also result from ACE inhibitor or ARB therapy in patients with pre-existing chronic kidney disease and may require dosage reduction or discontinuation. Development of ACE inhibitor–induced cough is the primary reason to switch a patient from an ACE inhibitor to an ARB. Although fewer data support the use of ARBs in asymptomatic patients with a reduced ejection fraction, there is general consensus that all patients who cannot tolerate ACE inhibitor therapy should receive an ARB. Patients who develop angioedema while taking an ACE inhibitor are often switched to an ARB; however, there are rare reports of ARB-induced angioedema, and patients should be informed of this risk.

Angiotensin Receptor–Neprilysin Inhibitor

The angiotensin receptor–neprilysin inhibitor (ARNI) valsartan-sacubitril belongs to a relatively new drug class that combines an ARB with a neprilysin inhibitor. Neprilysin is a neutral endopeptidase that degrades several vasoactive peptides, including natriuretic peptides and bradykinin. Inhibition of neprilysin increases levels of these substances, leading to enhanced diuresis, natriuresis, and myocardial relaxation. In the PARADIGM-HF trial, patients with symptomatic heart failure (elevated BNP or NT-proBNP level or a heart failure hospitalization within 12 months) and an ejection fraction below 40% were randomly assigned to receive valsartan-sacubitril or the ACE inhibitor enalapril. The patients who

received valsartan-sacubitril had a reduction in morbidity and mortality. However, 12% of patients withdrew from the trial during the run-in phase, primarily because of hypotension, kidney dysfunction, cough, and hyperkalemia. During the trial, 16.7% of patients had symptomatic hypotension, and in 4.8% of patients, creatinine level increased to higher than 2.5 mg/dL (221 µmol/L).

Guidelines currently recommend replacing an ACE inhibitor or ARB with valsartan-sacubitril in patients with chronic symptomatic HFrEF who tolerate ACE inhibitor or ARB therapy well. Caution should be used when initiating this drug in patients with hypotension or kidney impairment, and kidney function should be followed closely. Valsartan-sacubitril should not be administered concurrently with an ACE inhibitor or within 36 hours of the last dose of an ACE inhibitor owing to the risk for angioedema.

β-Blockers

β-Blockers should be initiated in all patients with HFrEF. β-Blockers improve remodeling, increase ejection fraction, and reduce hospitalization and mortality when added to ACE inhibitor and diuretic therapy. In contrast to ACE inhibitors, the benefits of β-blocker therapy do not appear to be a class effect, and one of the three agents shown to have a mortality benefit (bisoprolol, carvedilol, and metoprolol succinate) should be used.

β-Blockers are generally well tolerated, but they should be initiated only when the patient is euvolemic or nearly euvolemic. These agents have negative inotropic properties and may exacerbate heart failure in patients with volume overload. Consequently, β-blockers should be initiated at low doses and slowly uptitrated over weeks (not days) until the patient achieves a heart rate of around 60/min or has symptomatic hypotension (**Table 14**). In general, hospitalized patients should be started on β-blocker therapy before discharge. In patients with reactive airways disease or COPD, β-blocker therapy should not be initiated if the patient has bronchospasm or evidence of an exacerbation of pulmonary disease.

Initiating and Managing ACE Inhibitor and β-Blocker Therapy

ACE inhibitors and β-blockers are indicated in all patients with HFrEF. Either drug may be initiated first. Studies have shown that patients receive additive benefit from the second

TABLE 14.	Therapeutic Dosages of β-Blockers for Treatment of Heart Failure with Reduced Ejection Fraction	
Agent	**Target Dosage**
Carvedilol	25 mg twice daily (50 mg twice daily if weight >85 kg [187 lb])
Metoprolol succinate	200 mg daily
Bisoprolol	10 mg daily

agent regardless of which agent is started earlier. It is reasonable to select the first agent based on patient factors. For example, a β-blocker should be initiated first in patients with CAD or atrial fibrillation who require heart rate control. Conversely, an ACE inhibitor should be started first in patients with diabetes for the additional renal benefits. Regardless of the agent first initiated, the second drug should be started before the dosage of the first agent is maximized, especially if the patient has low blood pressure or is at risk for hypotension.

Recent guidelines recommend treating to a systolic blood pressure of less than 130/80 mm Hg in patients with HFrEF. Although randomized controlled trials have not specifically evaluated a goal blood pressure in patients with HFrEF, studies have shown that patients with lower blood pressure have fewer adverse cardiovascular events.

Diuretics

Loop diuretics are the mainstay of treatment for volume overload in patients with heart failure because of the increased potency of these agents compared with other diuretics. Of the four loop diuretics, furosemide is most commonly used; however, some studies have shown torsemide to be more effective, which may be attributable to its increased bioavailability and longer half-life. Occasionally, loop and thiazide diuretics are combined to potentiate diuresis. The lowest dosage that achieves euvolemia should be used. The primary side effects include hypokalemia and hypomagnesemia; therefore, electrolyte levels should be monitored.

Digoxin

Digoxin is used in patients with HFrEF and concomitant atrial fibrillation for rate control and in patients who continue to have symptoms of heart failure despite optimal therapy with ACE inhibitor and β-blocker therapies. Digoxin reduces the risk for hospitalization in patients with heart failure, and its discontinuation is associated with worsening heart failure symptoms. Unlike neurohumoral antagonists (including ACE inhibitors, β-blockers, and aldosterone antagonists), digoxin does not improve survival. The use of digoxin in patients with heart failure has decreased over the past 20 years, primarily because of its lack of mortality benefit and the dangerous side effects associated with digoxin toxicity. Digoxin should be managed carefully in patients with impaired kidney function, older adults, and women. It should be dosed to achieve a serum level of less than 1.0 ng/mL (1.28 nmol/L).

Aldosterone Antagonists

Aldosterone antagonists (spironolactone, eplerenone) reduce mortality and heart failure hospitalizations in patients with symptomatic heart failure (NYHA functional class II-IV symptoms) and patients with heart failure after an acute myocardial infarction. Despite their proven efficacy, they are underused, probably because of concerns of hyperkalemia and associated death raised by observational studies of spironolactone. Both drugs require that patients be monitored for hyperkalemia,

and these agents should be used carefully in patients with kidney dysfunction. In clinical trials, potassium supplementation was routinely discontinued at the beginning of therapy, and electrolyte measurement was repeated within 1 week of initiation.

Although spironolactone and eplerenone are both effective, their differences may guide drug selection. Spironolactone is a nonspecific antagonist that has antiandrogen and antiprogesterone side effects. It is extensively metabolized in the liver, and the half-life can increase in the setting of hepatic congestion. Eplerenone is a selective antagonist that is metabolized by cytochrome P-450 isoenzyme 3A4 (CYP3A4) and is subject to substantial drug interactions with both inhibitors and inducers of this isoenzyme.

Current guidelines recommend these agents as first-line therapy, along with ACE inhibitors and β-blockers, in patients with symptomatic heart failure. Generally, the doses of both the ACE inhibitor and β-blocker should be uptitrated to maximal levels before spironolactone or eplerenone is added. Aldosterone antagonists should not be considered diuretic therapy, and patients with volume overload will also need to be treated with a loop or thiazide diuretic.

Isosorbide Dinitrate-Hydralazine

Isosorbide dinitrate-hydralazine is superior to placebo in reducing hospitalization but inferior to ACE inhibitors for survival benefit in patients with symptomatic HFrEF. Therefore, this combination should be considered in patients intolerant of ACE inhibitors and ARBs, especially those with chronic kidney disease. In black patients with NYHA functional class III to IV symptoms, isosorbide dinitrate-hydralazine should be used in combination with optimal therapy, including ACE inhibitors, β-blockers, and aldosterone antagonists, to reduce mortality. Headache is a common adverse effect. Because many patients will not adhere to the dosage regimen of three doses daily, clinicians should strongly encourage patients to comply. Nonadherence issues may prompt clinicians to consider switching the patient to once-daily nitrate therapy, but once-daily therapy has not been studied in clinical trials to prove similar efficacy.

Calcium Channel Blockers

The nondihydropyridine calcium channel blockers verapamil and diltiazem both have detrimental effects in patients with systolic heart failure, probably related to negative inotropic effects, and these agents should not be used. Amlodipine and felodipine have shown neither benefit nor harm in patients with heart failure. Therefore, these two drugs are safe but should be used only in patients with hypertension despite therapy with other agents at maximal dosage.

Ivabradine

Ivabradine is a sinoatrial node modulator that selectively inhibits the I_f current in the sinoatrial node, causing a reduction in heart rate. It has no negative inotropic effects. In

CONT.

patients with chronic symptomatic heart failure and left ventricular ejection fraction less than or equal to 35% who are in sinus rhythm and taking maximally tolerated doses of a β-blocker, ivabradine reduces heart failure–associated hospitalizations and the combined endpoint of mortality and heart failure hospitalization. Ivabradine has been approved for use in the United States and should be considered for patients who have an elevated heart rate (≥70/min) in sinus rhythm despite maximally tolerated doses of β-blocker therapy. **H**

KEY POINTS

- Guidelines currently recommend replacing an ACE inhibitor or angiotensin receptor blocker (ARB) with valsartan-sacubitril in patients with chronic symptomatic heart failure with reduced ejection fraction who tolerate ACE inhibitor or ARB therapy well.

- β-Blockers are generally well tolerated in patients with heart failure, but these agents should be initiated only when the patient is euvolemic or nearly euvolemic.

- Ivabradine should be considered for patients with symptomatic heart failure and an ejection fraction less than or equal to 35% who have an elevated heart rate (≥70/min) in sinus rhythm despite maximally tolerated doses of β-blocker therapy.

- Aldosterone antagonists reduce mortality and heart failure hospitalizations in patients with symptomatic heart failure.

Management of Heart Failure with Preserved Ejection Fraction

The prototypical presentation of HFpEF is an elderly woman with long-standing hypertension associated with left ventricular hypertrophy; however, patients with CAD, diabetes, kidney disease, or other conditions may also present with signs and symptoms of heart failure and a normal ejection fraction. The primary therapies for HFpEF are diuretics to control symptoms of volume overload and antihypertensive agents to target a systolic blood pressure of less than 130 mm Hg in the setting of hypertension. In patients with worsened symptoms of heart failure and atrial fibrillation, restoration of sinus rhythm or rate control may reduce symptoms.

Despite many studies of therapeutic agents, no drug has been shown to reduce morbidity or mortality in patients with HFpEF, which may reflect the heterogeneity of etiology. The recent TOPCAT trial showed no difference in the primary combined endpoint of death, aborted cardiac arrest, or heart failure hospitalization in patients treated with spironolactone compared with those who received a placebo. In retrospective analysis, there was a mortality advantage with use of spironolactone in the United States, whereas in Europe, evidence showed spironolactone to be less effective. However, the clinical characteristics of the enrolled patients were statistically different in these two regions. Some clinicians have suggested

that spironolactone should be used routinely for this condition with no other proven treatments; however, spironolactone therapy for HFpEF is not supported by current evidence. **H**

KEY POINT

- The primary therapies for heart failure with preserved ejection fraction are diuretics to control symptoms of volume overload and antihypertensive agents to target a systolic blood pressure of less than 130 mm Hg.

Device Therapy

Implantable Cardioverter-Defibrillator Therapy for Prevention of Sudden Cardiac Death

Arrhythmias are a common cause of death in patients with heart failure, and implantable cardioverter-defibrillators (ICDs) improve survival when used for both primary and secondary prevention of arrhythmias. Current guidelines recommend ICD placement in patients receiving guideline-directed medical therapy who have an ejection fraction less than or equal to 35% and NYHA functional class II or III heart failure symptoms. Patients with class IV symptoms should only undergo ICD placement if they are candidates for heart transplant or left ventricular assist device (LVAD) placement. It is important to reassess both ejection fraction and symptoms after guideline-directed medical therapy (40 days after myocardial infarction, 3 months in all others). Many patients with new-onset heart failure experience substantial improvements in ejection fraction with medical therapy and may not require or benefit from ICD insertion.

Cardiac Resynchronization Therapy

Cardiac resynchronization therapy (CRT), or biventricular pacing, involves traditional pacing of the right ventricular apex and pacing of the left ventricular lateral wall via a lead inserted through the coronary sinus into a lateral cardiac vein. In patients with dyssynchrony (demonstrated in most trials by a widened QRS interval or left bundle branch block [LBBB]), CRT has improved ejection fraction, reduced heart failure symptoms, and reduced mortality. Retrospective analysis of many trials has shown that patients with LBBB are most likely to benefit from CRT. Based on these findings, CRT is indicated in patients with an ejection fraction less than or equal to 35%, NYHA functional class II to IV heart failure symptoms despite guideline-directed medical therapy, sinus rhythm, and LBBB with a QRS complex of 150 ms or greater. Patients with no LBBB but a QRS complex of 150 ms or greater may derive a lesser benefit from CRT. **H**

KEY POINTS

- Placement of an implantable cardioverter-defibrillator is recommended in patients with heart failure who have an ejection fraction less than or equal to 35% and New York Heart Association functional class II or III symptoms while taking guideline-directed medical therapy.

(Continued)

- Cardiac resynchronization therapy is indicated in patients with an ejection fraction less than or equal to 35%, New York Heart Association functional class II to IV heart failure symptoms despite guideline-directed medical therapy, sinus rhythm, and left bundle branch block with a QRS complex of 150 ms or greater.

Assessment of Chronic Heart Failure

Patients with chronic heart failure should be serially assessed for progression of disease in the outpatient setting. Each follow-up visit should include evaluation of current symptoms and functional capacity; assessment of volume status, electrolytes, and kidney function; and review of the patient's medication regimen for adequacy (both appropriate doses and the appropriate medications as heart failure progresses). Of equal or greater importance is repeated patient education, including reminding patients to take their medications as prescribed, measure their weight daily, avoid dietary sodium, watch their fluid intake, and exercise regularly. Patients who appropriately take their medications and avoid sodium and excess fluid intake can greatly improve their functional status.

Sleep disorders frequently occur in patients with heart failure and are often underdiagnosed. Recognizing these disorders and distinguishing between central and obstructive sleep apnea are important for improving quality of life in patients with heart failure and for potentially improving heart failure–related outcomes. Current guidelines support obtaining a formal sleep assessment in patients with symptomatic heart failure (NYHA functional class II-IV) and excessive daytime sleepiness or those who are suspected of having sleep-disordered breathing (see MKSAP 18 Pulmonary and Critical Care Medicine). Treatment with continuous positive airway pressure in patients with obstructive sleep apnea improves sleep quality and reduces the apnea–hypopnea index. In contrast, therapy for central sleep apnea with adaptive servoventilation has been shown to cause harm.

Serial B-Type Natriuretic Peptide Assessment

Measurement of BNP levels is helpful in determining whether dyspnea is related to heart failure or a different cause. For outpatients with chronic heart failure in whom volume status is uncertain on physical examination, BNP level can be useful in diagnosing fluid overload. BNP measurement in patients with stable heart failure also can provide information about prognosis and disease severity. However, serial measurements and treatment based on BNP levels have not been shown to reduce hospitalizations or mortality in patients with heart failure. Currently, BNP measurement should be used to aid in the diagnosis of heart failure and acute volume overload, but it should not be used serially in the inpatient or outpatient setting to guide care.

Echocardiography in Chronic Heart Failure

Echocardiography is the most common method for assessing left ventricular function. For patients with new-onset heart failure, guidelines suggest repeating assessment of left ventricular function after optimization of medical therapy. If the patient's ejection fraction is less than or equal to 35%, the patient may be a candidate for ICD or biventricular pacemaker placement. Current guidelines recommend routine echocardiography every 1 to 2 years in stable patients or when clinical status changes; however, routine echocardiography every 3 to 6 months is not indicated.

Assessing Prognosis

Many prognostic models have been developed to assist in predicting morbidity and mortality in patients with heart failure. These models are usually derived from retrospective analyses of clinical trials or large admission databases. To some extent, the models reflect the unique patient populations enrolled in clinical trials, which tend to have fewer comorbid conditions. Unfortunately, no one tool has been found to be more predictive than the others, and questions remain regarding the utility of these models for the individual patient. It has been suggested that these tools be used in addition to, not in place of, the clinician's judgment for heart failure management.

Clinical indicators associated with worse outcomes in the 1 to 2 years after diagnosis include heart failure hospitalization, poor exercise tolerance, ICD firings, serum sodium level less than 135 mEq/L (135 mmol/L), worsening kidney function, cardiac cachexia, required diuretic doses of more than 1 mg/kg, and symptomatic hypotension necessitating reduction in the dosage of heart failure medications. Heart failure hospitalizations are associated with a mortality rate of 10% to 20% over the next 6 months. In patients with poor prognosis, a frank discussion of advanced therapies, such as LVAD placement or heart transplantation, should occur. For patients who are ineligible for or uninterested in such therapies, end-of-life goals should be discussed, and palliative care or hospice should be considered.

- Serial B-type natriuretic peptide measurements should not be used to guide the care of patients with chronic heart failure. **HVC**

- Echocardiography should be performed every 1 to 2 years in stable patients with heart failure or when clinical status changes.

Inpatient Management of Heart Failure

Acute Decompensated Heart Failure

Initial management of patients hospitalized for acute decompensated heart failure should focus on identifying the cause of the heart failure exacerbation, determining the patient's

CONT.

current physiologic state, removing fluid to improve congestion, and optimizing medical therapy before discharge.

Determining the cause of acute heart failure can be challenging. Common causes include fluid overload in the setting of nonadherence to dietary fluid or salt intake recommendations and recurrent ischemia in patients suspected of having ischemic cardiomyopathy. Fluid overload can sometimes be related to an unintentional increase in foods with higher salt content or an inability to tolerate previous levels of fluid and salt intake due to progression of left ventricular dysfunction. Other causes of decompensation include hypertension, concurrent illness, and nonadherence to medication regimens, including but not limited to diuretics. An understanding of the cause of the decompensation may identify opportunities to prevent recurrence.

Patients hospitalized for heart failure should be evaluated for volume overload. Typical symptoms include orthopnea, paroxysmal nocturnal dyspnea, peripheral edema, weight gain, and progressive exertional dyspnea. On physical examination, jugular venous distention is usually present. Patients may have crackles (which are much more likely in acute than chronic heart failure), ascites, or peripheral edema. Perfusion should also be assessed, and patients may be classified as "warm" (adequate perfusion) or "cold" (inadequate perfusion). Signs and symptoms of poor perfusion include cool extremities, a narrow pulse pressure, poor mentation, and worsening kidney function. Intravenous inotropes or other advanced therapies should be considered in patients with signs of poor perfusion to help improve cardiac function.

Diuretic therapy is the principal treatment for patients with decompensated heart failure and fluid overload. A recent study evaluated different strategies for diuresis, including varied diuretic dosages and bolus versus continuous therapy. Administration of high-dose diuretics (2.5 times the outpatient oral daily dosage) was associated with increased diuresis but also transient worsening of kidney function. No differences were observed between bolus and continuous intravenous infusion groups, and length of stay did not differ regardless of the strategy used. Providing effective diuresis is essential and often requires intravenous administration. If the current dosage of loop diuretic is inadequate, increasing the dosage or adding a thiazide diuretic may be considered. Notably, administering low-dose dopamine to improve diuresis and preserve kidney function offers no benefit.

In patients with acute kidney dysfunction at the time of admission, it is still important to treat with diuretic therapy. The most likely cause of the dysfunction is poor kidney perfusion due to vascular congestion, and kidney function will often improve with diuresis. In contrast, withholding ACE inhibitors and aldosterone antagonists may be reasonable until kidney function improves. If a patient receiving diuretic therapy develops worsening kidney function when approaching euvolemia, withholding diuretics for 1 day to allow extravascular fluid to redistribute into the vascular space should be considered. Once euvolemia has been achieved, creatinine often also increases, which may indicate decongestion.

Standard heart failure therapy, including ACE inhibitor or ARB therapy, β-blockers, and aldosterone antagonists, should either be maintained throughout hospitalization or be restarted before discharge. If β-blockers are discontinued upon admission because of signs of low cardiac output, therapy should not be reinitiated until the patient nears euvolemia. If the patient is admitted with volume overload without signs of low cardiac output, β-blocker therapy can usually be maintained at the same or a lower dosage during hospitalization.

BNP level should be measured upon admission and before discharge for prognostic purposes because high levels are linked with increased mortality and rehospitalization. Likewise, patients with BNP levels that fail to decrease during an admission have a higher mortality rate. Serum troponin measurement upon admission can also be used for prognostication; patients with elevated troponin levels have worse clinical outcomes and a higher risk for death. Currently, there are no absolute cutoff values for these biomarkers, and measurement data should be used in combination with clinical judgment in advising the patient with heart failure.

Cardiogenic Shock

Cardiogenic shock is characterized by signs and symptoms of low cardiac output and end-organ compromise, with acute worsening of kidney and liver function. Patients with cardiogenic shock often require intravenous inotropic agents to improve hemodynamic status, including increasing cardiac output and urine output (**Table 15**). Routine use of invasive pulmonary artery catheterization to monitor hemodynamics does not improve survival or reduce future hospitalization in patients with decompensated heart failure. Therefore, pulmonary artery, or "right heart," catheterization should be used only when hemodynamic and volume status is not evident from physical examination findings or other noninvasive tests, or when hemodynamic data may lead to advanced mechanical circulatory support or consideration of heart transplantation.

The use of percutaneous mechanical support during acute exacerbation has greatly increased in the past few years. Intra-aortic balloon pumps, percutaneous ventricular assist devices, and extracorporeal membrane oxygenators can be quickly placed to support the critically ill patient. Treatment by a team composed of a heart failure physician, critical care physician, and cardiac surgeon is suggested to rapidly deploy therapy and care for the patient in the following days. Decisions regarding longer-term options for advanced heart failure (heart transplantation or permanent or "destination" LVAD) are an important aspect in the use of mechanical support in the acute setting. In patients who do not show clinical improvement, there should be daily discussions about treatment options and goals of care, including

TABLE 15. Intravenous Vasoactive Medications Used for Treatment of Cardiogenic Shock

Medication	Mechanism	Inotropy	Vasodilation
Milrinone	Phosphodiesterase inhibition	++	+
Dobutamine	β_1, β_2 Receptor agonism	++	(+) (at low dose)
			− (vasoconstriction, at high dose)
Nesiritide	Natriuretic peptide receptor agonism	0	++
Sodium nitroprusside	Nitric oxide production	0	++
Nitroglycerin	Nitric oxide production	0	++ (mainly venous)
Vasopressin	Arginine vasopressin receptor (V receptor) agonism	−	− (vasoconstriction)
Dopamine	Dopaminergic receptor (D receptor) agonism	+	− (vasoconstriction, at high dose)
	β_1 Receptor agonism at intermediate dose		
	α_1 Receptor agonism at high dose		
Norepinephrine	α_1, α_2 Receptor agonism greater than β_1 receptor agonism	+	− (vasoconstriction)

Strength of effect: ++ indicates very strong; + indicates strong; (+) indicates weak; 0 indicates neutral; − indicates opposite effect.

transplantation, permanent device placement, or palliative care or hospice.

Strategies to Prevent Readmission

The first step in preventing heart failure readmission is to treat any reversible causes of the exacerbation. Medication reconciliation before discharge should ensure that the patient is taking the appropriate medications, particularly those that reduce mortality and morbidity in heart failure. Patients should not be discharged until they have achieved euvolemia with diuresis. Patients should be educated on heart failure physiology, the importance of medication and dietary adherence, signs and symptoms of worsening heart failure, and when to contact a physician. Finally, an early follow-up appointment (within 7 days) should be scheduled to review the medication list, assess the patient's volume status and adherence to diet and medications, and reinforce patient education points.

KEY POINTS

- Management of patients with acute decompensated heart failure focuses on identifying the cause of the heart failure exacerbation, determining the patient's current physiologic state, treating fluid overload, and optimizing medical therapy before discharge.

- In patients hospitalized with acute heart failure, scheduling an early follow-up appointment (within 7 days) to review the medication list, assess the patient's volume status and adherence to diet and medications, and reinforce patient education points reduces the risk for heart failure readmission.

- Routine invasive pulmonary artery catheterization for hemodynamic monitoring is not recommended in patients with decompensated heart failure.

Advanced Refractory Heart Failure

Once heart failure has progressed to ACC/AHA stage D, characterized by persistent severe symptoms despite maximum therapy, advanced treatments should be considered. Cardiac transplantation remains the gold standard therapy for patients with end-stage heart failure. Unfortunately, because of a lack of appropriate donors, fewer than 3000 heart transplantations are performed in the United States each year. Indications for transplantation generally include age younger than 65 to 70 years, no medical contraindications (such as diabetes with end-organ complications, malignancies within 5 years, kidney dysfunction, or other chronic illnesses that will decrease survival), and good social support and adherence. The use of an LVAD as "destination therapy" should be considered for patients who are not transplant candidates. Many patients awaiting transplant also require an LVAD for support until an organ becomes available. Hospice may be considered as an option in shared decision-making discussions.

Mechanical Circulatory Support

In the past 10 years, clinical outcomes of patients with advanced heart failure have markedly improved with the use of LVADs. With newer continuous-flow devices, patients have 1-year survival approximating that of cardiac transplant recipients and substantial improvements in functional capacity and quality of life. Because these devices provide continuous flow, most patients no longer have a palpable pulse, and blood pressure must be measured by Doppler. Typical therapy includes anticoagulation to prevent pump thrombus formation, continued heart failure therapy with ACE inhibitors (or ARBs) and β-blockers, and management of fluid overload with diuretics.

LVADs are associated with important complications related to both the driveline, which passes through the skin and connects the internal pump to a power source, and the pump itself. Major complications include hemorrhagic and thrombotic strokes; skin infections; pump thrombosis; and gastrointestinal bleeding, which is usually associated with small bowel arteriovenous malformations. Despite these complications, LVADs have been associated with survival of more than 10 years in some patients.

Management of Posttransplant Patients

Most patients who undergo heart transplantation quickly recover physical activity and have normal quality of life, with a mean survival of more than 11 years. The most frequent complication within the first year after transplant is infection. Cytomegalovirus (CMV) infection is common, and patients at moderate risk (CMV-positive donor/CMV-positive recipient) and high risk (CMV-positive donor/CMV-negative recipient) often receive antiviral prophylaxis for 6 months. Incidence of rejection is highest in the first 6 months after transplantation. Because most patients with rejection are asymptomatic, regularly scheduled endomyocardial biopsies are often performed to detect rejection for the first few years after transplant. Severe rejection is characterized by signs of acute heart failure and atrial arrhythmias (typically atrial flutter) or conduction abnormalities. Early complications related to immunosuppressive therapy include hypertension (more than 90% of patients) and diabetes (15%-20% of patients). Long-term complications after transplantation include CAD and an increased incidence of malignancies, including skin cancer (common) and B-cell lymphoma related to immunosuppressive therapy (less common).

When new drugs are added to a transplant patient's medication regimen, careful attention is essential to avoid drug-drug interactions. Cyclosporine and tacrolimus, two agents commonly used for immunosuppression, are metabolized by the CYP3A4 system. Many drugs increase or decrease the metabolism of cyclosporine and tacrolimus, and conversely, these agents may alter the metabolism of other drugs. An extensive list of drugs that can interact through the CYP3A4 isoenzyme can be found at medicine.iupui.edu/clinpharm/ddis.

KEY POINTS

- Patients with severe heart failure symptoms despite maximal medical therapy are candidates for advanced treatment, including placement of a left ventricular assist device and heart transplantation.
- Cardiac transplantation is the gold standard therapy for patients with end-stage heart failure.
- Endomyocardial biopsy should be routinely performed after heart transplantation to diagnose rejection.

Specific Cardiomyopathies

For a discussion of hypertrophic cardiomyopathy and restrictive cardiomyopathy, refer to Myocardial Disease. Peripartum cardiomyopathy is discussed in Pregnancy and Cardiovascular Disease.

Takotsubo Cardiomyopathy

Takotsubo cardiomyopathy, also known as stress cardiomyopathy or apical ballooning syndrome, is a clinical syndrome associated with reduced ejection fraction, elevated cardiac enzyme levels, and signs of ischemia on electrocardiography. It typically occurs in older women and is usually precipitated by a stressful physical or emotional event, such as the death of a loved one, sudden surprise, or other acute stressors. The exact mechanism of takotsubo cardiomyopathy is unknown, but the condition is postulated to result from a reversible toxic effect of very high catecholamine levels on the myocardium. On cardiac imaging, wall motion abnormalities that do not follow a coronary artery territory (typically, apical dyskinesis or ballooning) are often found with preservation of basal wall motion. Because these acute events often resemble an acute coronary syndrome, emergent coronary angiography is often performed and demonstrates nonobstructive CAD. Treatment is largely supportive and is similar to that for other heart failure syndromes (diuretics, ACE inhibitors, β-blockers). Most patients will recover cardiac function over the course of a few weeks to months. As with other forms of new-onset heart failure, repeat echocardiography should be performed in 3 to 6 months to evaluate recovery. If a patient has recovery of function, it is unclear for how long medical therapy should be continued, but most clinicians continue therapy for at least 1 year.

Acute Myocarditis

Myocarditis is a clinical syndrome of acute-onset heart failure. Causes include viral, bacterial, or other infections; toxins; and immunologic syndromes. The classic form is viral in origin and is usually preceded by a typical upper respiratory tract infection caused by adenovirus, echovirus, or coxsackievirus. Although the pathogenesis is not completely understood, it is thought that acute viral infection causes early destruction of the myocytes, followed by an immune response that causes further destruction.

Clinically, patients may be asymptomatic or have a viral prodrome with fever, myalgia, and muscle soreness. Patients may also present with acute heart failure symptoms. Echocardiography is useful to assess for other causes of heart failure. Definitive diagnosis may require cardiac magnetic resonance imaging or endomyocardial biopsy. Anti-inflammatory agents are not of benefit in the treatment of acute myocarditis. Standard therapy for heart failure is recommended. Prognosis depends on the clinical presentation.

Giant Cell Myocarditis

Giant cell myocarditis is an acute and frequently fatal form of myocarditis that typically occurs in younger persons. It is often rapidly progressive and can cause both left and right ventricular dysfunction. Giant cell myocarditis is also associated with an increased incidence of high-grade atrioventricular block and ventricular arrhythmias. Unlike in acute myocarditis, aggressive immunosuppressive therapy has some benefit and should be initiated in these patients. For this reason, patients with acute heart failure unresponsive to usual care or with accompanying arrhythmias should undergo endomyocardial biopsy for diagnosis. Initial biopsy findings may be negative because of the patchy nature of the inflammation. Patients with giant cell myocarditis often require percutaneous or surgical ventricular support until they recover or need heart transplantation or LVAD placement. If giant cell myocarditis is suspected, prompt transfer to a hospital equipped with mechanical support should be considered because patients can progress from feeling well to moribund within hours.

Tachycardia-Mediated Cardiomyopathy

Tachycardia-mediated cardiomyopathy has been associated with both supraventricular and ventricular arrhythmias. Reversible causes of tachycardia, such as hyperthyroidism, should be ruled out. Importantly, heart rate control improves left ventricular function in these patients. The primary treatments are medications, such as β-blockers, and catheter-directed ablation. In patients with atrial fibrillation associated with rapid ventricular response, there is no evidence that converting to sinus rhythm is more efficacious than controlling the heart rate. In patients with ventricular arrhythmias or frequent premature ventricular contractions, cardiomyopathy is generally thought to develop when the burden of premature ventricular contractions is more than 10,000/day; ablation, especially if the premature ventricular contractions are unifocal, should be considered.

Arrhythmias

Introduction

Arrhythmias are traditionally categorized as supraventricular or ventricular based upon simple electrocardiographic (ECG) findings. Supraventricular arrhythmias originate from the atrium or atrioventricular (AV) node and are characterized by normal-appearing QRS complexes unless complicated by an aberrant ventricular condition. Ventricular arrhythmias originate below the AV node and are characterized by abnormal-appearing and prolonged QRS complexes. Disruptions in rhythm and rate occur in seven basic patterns: early beats, bigeminal beats, grouped beats, pauses, bradycardia, tachycardia, and chaotic rhythms. This section provides an approach to bradycardia and tachycardia and discusses the diagnosis and management of specific rhythm disorders.

Approach to Bradycardia

Clinical Presentation and Evaluation

Bradycardia (heart rate <60/min) may be asymptomatic or associated with symptoms of lightheadedness, syncope, exertional intolerance, dyspnea, and fatigue. It can result from disease in the sinus node, AV node, or His-Purkinje system, or from dysfunction of the autonomic system.

Diagnostic evaluation consists of a thorough history, physical examination, focused laboratory testing (electrolyte levels, thyroid function testing), and resting 12-lead ECG. It is important to identify severe or unstable conduction abnormalities that require urgent intervention. The evaluation should also include investigation for extrinsic and reversible causes of bradycardia, including ischemia, myocarditis, endocarditis, hypothyroidism, electrolyte disturbances, and medication use (especially β-blockers and digoxin). Clues from the history and physical examination may suggest Lyme disease, elevated intracranial pressure, or typhoid as other potential causes of bradycardia. Additional testing may include exercise treadmill testing to assess chronotropic competence and ambulatory ECG monitoring (see Diagnostic Testing in Cardiology).

Sinus Bradycardia

Sinus bradycardia is defined as the presence of sinus rhythm with a heart rate below 60/min. Sinus bradycardia may be appropriate in trained athletes and during sleep. Inappropriate or pathologic sinus bradycardia is most commonly caused by sinus node dysfunction due to age-related myocardial fibrosis. Less commonly, sinus node dysfunction may result from right coronary ischemia; intracranial hypertension; postoperative scarring or fibrosis from cardiothoracic surgery; or infiltrative or inflammatory disorders, such as sarcoidosis. The most common extrinsic cause is medication use.

Atrioventricular Block

AV block may be classified as first degree, second degree, or third degree. First-degree AV block is defined by a delay in AV conduction (PR interval >200 ms). In large cohort studies, first-degree AV block has been associated with an increased risk for atrial fibrillation and all-cause mortality.

In second-degree AV block, only some P waves conduct to the ventricles. Mobitz type 1 second-degree (Wenckebach) AV block is characterized electrocardiographically by a PR interval that progressively prolongs until a beat is dropped (**Figure 10**). Mobitz type 2 second-degree AV block is typified by ECG findings of grouped beating and progressive shortening of the RR intervals (**Figure 11**). The PR interval does not lengthen in Mobitz type 2 before nonconducted atrial beats. When 2:1 block is present, the Mobitz type cannot be determined. Mobitz type 2 AV block usually occurs below the AV node and has a higher risk for progression to complete heart block.

In third-degree AV block, also termed complete heart block, no P waves conduct to the ventricles. AV dissociation is observed on the ECG (**Figure 12**).

Treatment

In patients with symptomatic bradycardia and hemodynamic distress, atropine should be administered. If atropine is

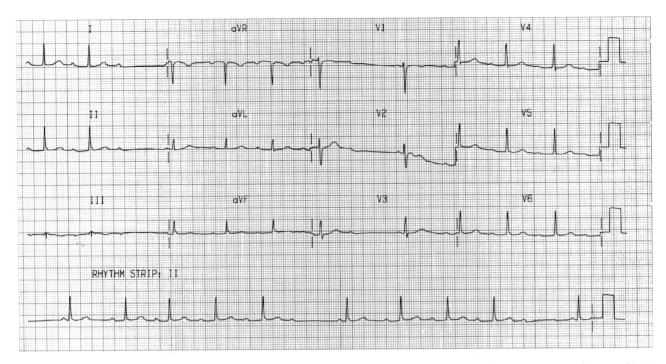

FIGURE 10. Electrocardiogram showing Mobitz type 1 second-degree atrioventricular block (Wenckebach block), which manifests as a progressive prolongation of the PR interval until there is a dropped ventricular beat.

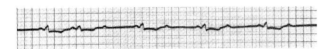

FIGURE 11. Electrocardiogram showing Mobitz type 2 second-degree atrioventricular block. P waves are blocked intermittently, and the PR interval is fixed. Note the wide QRS complexes, which are also more consistent with block below the compact atrioventricular node.

ineffective, dopamine or epinephrine infusions can be given until transcutaneous pacing or a temporary pacing wire (preferred) can be placed. Temporary pacing is indicated in cases of hemodynamically unstable bradycardia or asystole. In some unique circumstances, prophylactic temporary pacing may be considered, including in patients undergoing transcatheter aortic valve replacement with high-risk features for heart block (such as right bundle branch block).

In hemodynamically stable patients, reversible and extrinsic causes of bradycardia should always be addressed before more invasive measures, such as permanent pacing, are considered. Common indications for permanent pacing include the following:

- Symptomatic bradycardia without reversible cause
- Asymptomatic bradycardia with significant pauses (>3 seconds in sinus rhythm) or heart rate less than 40/min
- Atrial fibrillation with pauses of 5 seconds or longer
- Alternating bundle branch block
- Asymptomatic complete heart block or Mobitz type 2 second-degree AV block

The various types of implanted cardiac electronic devices, their functions, and their general indications are reviewed in **Table 16**. Patients with left bundle branch block or right bundle branch block with or without a prolonged PR interval do not require permanent pacing because intraventricular conduction delays have a low risk for progressing to complete heart block (1%-3% per year). **H**

KEY POINT

- Permanent pacing is indicated for symptomatic bradycardia with no underlying reversible cause and in asymptomatic patients who have atrioventricular and infranodal conduction disturbances that have a high risk for progressing to complete heart block or asystole.

Approach to the Patient with Tachycardia

Clinical Presentation and Evaluation

Patients with tachycardia (heart rate >100/min) may be asymptomatic or experience tachypalpitations, a sensation of skipped beats, lightheadedness or dizziness, chest discomfort, dyspnea, exertional intolerance, fatigue, progressive heart failure, near-syncope, or syncope. In asymptomatic patients, tachycardia may be discovered incidentally during routine ECG, monitoring in the setting of hospitalization, or other medical care.

ECG documentation of tachycardia and correlation with symptoms is the key component of the diagnostic evaluation.

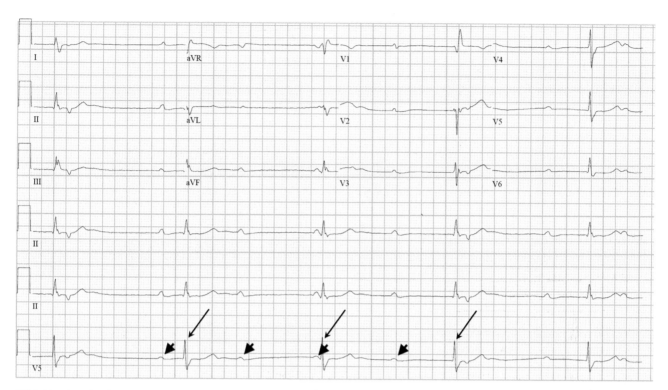

FIGURE 12. In this electrocardiogram, the P waves (*short arrows*) and the QRS complexes (*long arrows*) are not associated with each other, indicating the presence of complete heart block.

TABLE 16.	Cardiac Implantable Electronic Devices for Treatment of Cardiac Rhythm Disorders					
			Functions		
Device	**Components**	**Indications**	**Pacemaker Function**	**Antitachycardia Pacing**	**Defibrillation**
Transvenous pacemaker	Pulse generator and intravascular leads (single- or dual-chamber)	Sinus node dysfunction, atrioventricular block, nonreversible symptomatic bradycardia	Yes	No	No
Leadless pacemaker	Pulse generator with tines implanted directly into the cardiac chamber; no leads	Atrial fibrillation with bradycardia, paroxysmal sinus node dysfunction (e.g., brief sinus pauses)	Yes (ventricular sensing and pacing only)	No	No
Implantable cardioverter-defibrillator	Defibrillator and intravascular leads (single- or dual-chamber)	Monitoring and treatment of ventricular arrhythmias	Yes	Yes	Yes
Subcutaneous implantable cardioverter-defibrillator	Defibrillator and a single lead that are entirely under the skin (extravascular); no transvenous leads	Monitoring and treatment of ventricular arrhythmias	No	No	Yes
Cardiac resynchronization therapy-pacing (CRT-P)	Pulse generator and intravascular leads, including a pacing lead in the coronary sinus to pace the left ventricle	Restoring electrical synchrony in patients with symptomatic heart failure (left ventricular ejection fraction ≤35% and left bundle branch block)	Yes	No	No
Cardiac resynchronization therapy-defibrillator (CRT-D)	Defibrillator and intravascular leads, including a pacing lead in the coronary sinus to pace the left ventricle	Restoring electrical synchrony between the ventricles in patients with heart failure; monitoring and treating ventricular arrhythmias	Yes	Yes	Yes

After a thorough history and physical examination, a 12-lead ECG should be obtained in all patients with stable tachycardia. A 12-lead ECG recorded during symptoms, although often not possible to obtain, is far superior to most forms of ambulatory monitoring in terms of diagnostic value (see Diagnostic Testing in Cardiology for strategies for selecting an appropriate monitoring device). Thyroid function testing and echocardiography may be considered in selected patients with tachycardia.

Sinus Tachycardia

Sinus tachycardia (sinus rhythm with a heart rate >100/min) is the most common tachycardia and is typically the result of physiologic demand or distress, including exercise, pain, fever, anemia, or anxiety. Diagnostic evaluation and treatment are guided by the underlying cause.

Inappropriate sinus tachycardia (IST) is a disorder characterized by an elevated resting heart rate, with exaggerated increases in heart rate with light activity. The sinus rate typically decreases during sleep, which can be documented with ambulatory ECG monitoring. IST frequently presents in women in their second to fourth decades and appears to be more common in health care professionals. Symptoms vary and can include palpitations, lightheadedness, syncope (or near-syncope), dyspnea, and fatigue. The diagnosis of IST is based on the exclusion of other causes of tachycardia, such as hyperthyroidism, anemia, pheochromocytoma, and structural heart disease. First-line therapy is removal of aggravating factors and exercise therapy. In patients with bothersome and persistent symptoms, pharmacologic therapy with β-blockers, calcium channel blockers, or ivabradine (in refractory cases) can be considered.

Postural orthostatic tachycardia syndrome (POTS) is another condition that often presents with tachycardia. POTS is a form of dysautonomia characterized by orthostatic intolerance and excessive tachycardia, particularly with standing. Diagnostic criteria for POTS include an increase in heart rate of 30/min or more, or an increase to greater than 120/min, within 10 minutes of standing. The diagnosis is often confirmed with tilt-table testing. Behavioral modification, compression stockings, exercise training, and increased fluid intake are important components of therapy. Medical therapy for POTS is highly variable and may include, but is not limited to, β-blockers, fludrocortisone, selective serotonin reuptake inhibitors, midodrine, and pyridostigmine.

Supraventricular Tachycardias

Paroxysmal supraventricular tachycardias (SVTs), including atrioventricular nodal reentrant tachycardia (AVNRT), accessory pathway–mediated tachycardias, and atrial tachycardia, are frequently the cause of palpitations in younger persons. The accessory pathway may result from anterograde conduction, manifesting as a delta wave on ECG or retrograde conduction (so-called concealed accessory pathway). Management of these arrhythmias is discussed later in this chapter.

Other Tachycardias

Older patients with palpitations are more likely to have atrial fibrillation, atrial flutter, or ventricular tachycardia (VT), often due to underlying cardiovascular disease. VT is often associated with hemodynamic compromise; however, some VT can be well tolerated, particularly in patients with normal ventricular function. Evidence of hemodynamic compromise, including syncope, may also be present in patients with atrial tachyarrhythmias. For further discussion of the clinical presentation and management of these conditions, refer to the Atrial Fibrillation, Atrial Flutter, and Ventricular Arrhythmias sections later in the chapter.

KEY POINT

- Sinus tachycardia is the most common tachycardia and is typically the result of physiologic demand or distress, including exercise, pain, fever, anemia, or anxiety.

Antiarrhythmic Drugs

Antiarrhythmic agents are used to treat and suppress arrhythmias. These medications have traditionally been organized according to primary mechanism of action by using the Vaughan-Williams classification system (Table 17); however, most antiarrhythmic drugs exert their effects through several mechanisms.

Class I and class III antiarrhythmic drugs are the most effective antiarrhythmic drugs. Class IA agents are indicated for specific conditions (see Table 17). These medications have been associated with ventricular proarrhythmia, sudden death, and increased mortality in patients with coronary artery disease or structural heart disease. Class II agents (β-blockers) and class IV agents (nondihydropyridine calcium channel blockers) are commonly used to inhibit arrhythmia induction and AV conduction in patients with supraventricular or atrial arrhythmias. Class III agents sotalol and dofetilide are used to treat atrial and ventricular arrhythmias. Class III antiarrhythmic therapy should be initiated in an in-patient setting, with regular assessment of the corrected QT (QTc) interval. Ibutilide is an intravenous class III potassium channel blocker that is used for pharmacologic cardioversion of atrial fibrillation.

Amiodarone is among the most effective and commonly used antiarrhythmic drugs. This multichannel blocker is frequently used to treat patients with recurrent VT or atrial fibrillation. Amiodarone has no significant risk for proarrhythmia but is associated with thyroid, liver, lung, and eye toxicities, as well as neurologic side effects. Monitoring thyroid and liver function every 6 months is recommended in patients receiving amiodarone. Patients should also undergo annual pulmonary function testing and ophthalmologic examination. Amiodarone interacts with many drugs, including warfarin, statins, and digoxin. Dronedarone, another multichannel blocker, can be used in patients with intermittent atrial fibrillation and no overt heart failure.

TABLE 17.	Antiarrhythmic Medications					
Classification	**Mechanism of Action**	**Individual Agents/ Examples**	**Effects**	**Use**	**Side Effects**	**Contraindications**
Class IA	Sodium channel blockade with some potassium channel blockade	Quinidine, procainamide, disopyramide	Decreases speed of depolarization and prolongs repolarization	Preexcited atrial fibrillation (procainamide), Brugada syndrome (quinidine), SVT, atrial fibrillation, ventricular arrhythmias	Anticholinergic effects, including increased heart rate, dry mouth, urinary retention, blurry vision, and constipation Lupus-like syndrome (procainamide)	Ischemic or structural heart disease, second- or third-degree AV block without a pacemaker, prolonged QT interval, advanced kidney impairment
Class IB	Sodium channel blockade	Lidocaine, mexiletine, phenytoin	Decreases speed of depolarization	Ventricular arrhythmias	Headache, dizziness, or other neurologic symptoms Seizures (lidocaine toxicity)	Advanced liver disease
Class IC	Sodium channel blockade	Flecainide, propafenone	Decreases speed of depolarization and shortens repolarization	Atrial fibrillation, SVT, ventricular arrhythmias	Headache, dizziness, or other neurologic symptoms	Ischemic or structural heart disease, sinus node dysfunction, second- or third-degree AV block or bundle branch disease without a pacemaker
Class II	β-Adrenergic blockade	Metoprolol, propranolol, carvedilol, atenolol, bisoprolol	Decreases sympathetic tone; suppresses automaticity, sinoatrial conduction, and AV conduction	Rate control of atrial arrhythmias, SVT, ventricular arrhythmias	Fatigue, drowsiness, dizziness, hair loss, cold hands and feet, depression, erectile dysfunction, bronchospasm	Severe asthma, cardiogenic shock, second- or third-degree AV block, preexcitation
Class III	Potassium channel blockade	Sotalol, dofetilide, ibutilide	Prolongs action potential duration	Atrial fibrillation, atrial flutter, ventricular arrhythmias, pharmacologic cardioversion of atrial fibrillation (ibutilide)	Headache, dizziness, bradycardia, fatigue, dyspnea (sotalol) Headache, dizziness, diarrhea; rarely, torsades de pointes (dofetilide)	CrCl <40 mL/min/1.73 m², QTc interval >440 ms, sinus bradycardia <50/min, second- or third-degree AV block without a pacemaker
Class IV	Calcium channel blockade (nondihy-dropyridines)	Verapamil, diltiazem	Suppresses sinoatrial and AV conduction	SVT, rate control of atrial arrhythmias, triggered arrhythmias (outflow tract VTs)	Dizziness, constipation, dependent edema, nausea	Significant sinus node dysfunction, second- or third-degree AV block without a pacemaker, preexcitation
Multichannel blockers	Several mechanisms, including potassium, sodium, and calcium channel blockade	Amiodarone, dronedarone	Multiple mechanisms, although they act principally by extending repolarization	Atrial arrhythmias, ventricular arrhythmias	Fatigue, dizziness, nausea, vomiting, constipation or diarrhea, tremor *Hypo + HypER Thyroid*	Advanced liver, lung, or thyroid disease (amiodarone) Advanced liver disease, permanent atrial fibrillation, recent decompensated or advanced heart failure (NYHA functional class III-IV) (dronedarone)

(Continued on the next page)

TABLE 17. Antiarrhythmic Medications *(Continued)*

Classification	Mechanism of Action	Individual Agents/ Examples	Effects	Use	Side Effects	Contraindications
Late sodium channel blockers	Late sodium channel blockade	Ranolazine	Shortens action potential duration and prevents calcium overload	Atrial fibrillation, ventricular arrhythmias	Dizziness, nausea, headache, constipation, hypoglycemia	Advanced liver disease, use of strong CYP3A4 inhibitors or inducers
Adenosine receptor agonists	A_1-receptor agonism	Adenosine	Slows or blocks sinoatrial and AV node conduction	Termination of SVT	Flushing, dyspnea, chest pain, hypotension, dizziness, nausea	Severe asthma, cardiac transplantation
Cardiac glycoside	Increases vagal activity	Digoxin	Slows AV node conduction	Rate control of atrial fibrillation	Nausea, vomiting, dizziness, blurry vision and yellow halos, thrombocytopenia	Advanced kidney impairment (requires dose adjustment)

AV = atrioventricular; CrCl = creatinine clearance; CYP3A4 = cytochrome P450 3A4; NYHA = New York Heart Association; QTc = corrected QT; SVT = supraventricular tachycardia; VT = ventricular tachycardia.

Ranolazine, digoxin, and adenosine are excluded from the Vaughan-Williams classification. Ranolazine is used to treat angina and decreases the risk for atrial fibrillation and ventricular arrhythmias. Digoxin is a positive inotropic agent that also increases vagal activity, leading to a lower resting heart rate. It can be used for rate control in patients with atrial fibrillation. Adenosine is used in the acute treatment of arrhythmias to interrupt AV conduction and terminate SVT.

Administering adenosine can also help in determining the type of arrhythmia.

Atrial Fibrillation

Atrial fibrillation is defined by the presence of disorganized atrial activity with an irregularly irregular ventricular response on ECG (**Figure 13**). It is the most common

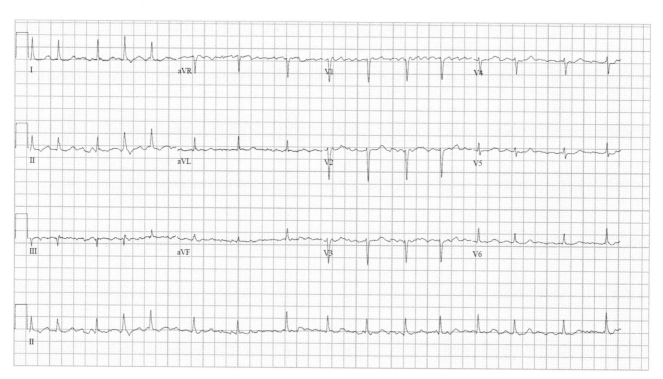

FIGURE 13. Electrocardiogram demonstrating atrial fibrillation. No clear P waves are seen, and the ventricular response is irregular.

↑ RISK FOR:
- STROKE
- HF
- DEMENTIA

WORKUP: TTE
TSH, T4
SLEEP SCREEN

Arrhythmias

sustained arrhythmia, affecting more than 33 million persons worldwide. Lifetime risk for atrial fibrillation is 25% in patients older than 40 years. Incidence is strongly associated with and increases with age. Accordingly, atrial fibrillation is particularly common in the elderly, occurring in 10% of persons older than 80 years. Atrial fibrillation is associated with an increased risk for adverse cardiac events, including a five-fold increased risk for stroke, as well as increased risk for heart failure and dementia. Among patients aged 55 years and older who have a cryptogenic ischemic neurologic event, such as a stroke or transient ischemic attack, occult intermittent atrial fibrillation is thought to be present in up to 25% of cases, and 30-day ambulatory ECG monitoring is indicated for detection.

Atrial fibrillation is usually the result of long-standing risk factors, such as diabetes mellitus, obesity, hypertension, coronary artery disease, heart failure, and obstructive sleep apnea. It may also be caused by reversible or acute physiologic insults, including cardiac surgery, pulmonary embolism, or hyperthyroidism. When there are no identified risk factors, a predisposing genetic background is often present. *CAUSES*

Clinical Presentation

Patients with atrial fibrillation may be asymptomatic or experience palpitations, lightheadedness or dizziness, dyspnea, exercise intolerance, chest pain, near-syncope, or, rarely, syncope. In some cases, atrial fibrillation can lead to hemodynamic compromise, especially in patients with advanced diastolic dysfunction or restrictive cardiomyopathy. Patients with atrial fibrillation uncommonly present with tachycardia-induced cardiomyopathy, characterized by asymptomatic left ventricular dysfunction or overt heart failure. [H]

Atrial fibrillation is categorized according to its duration. Paroxysmal atrial fibrillation stops spontaneously within 7 days of onset, whereas persistent atrial fibrillation lasts for 7 days or more. Long-standing persistent atrial fibrillation is continuous, with a duration of more than 1 year.

Acute Management

Immediate cardioversion is indicated in patients with hypotension, acute myocardial ischemia, or decompensated heart failure. R wave synchronization during cardioversion is necessary to avoid an "R-on-T" event and provocation of ventricular fibrillation (VF). [H]

In stable patients, the primary goals of therapy are to prevent stroke, control heart rate, and minimize or eliminate symptoms. Upon diagnosis, reversible causes must be ruled out. All patients should undergo thyroid function testing to evaluate for hyperthyroidism. Patients with risk factors for or symptoms suggestive of sleep apnea should undergo testing (see MKSAP 18 Pulmonary and Critical Care Medicine). Echocardiography is indicated to evaluate for potential valvular or other structural heart disease. Echocardiography can also be used to assess left atrial size, which helps determine

the severity of the underlying atrial myocardial dysfunction. Transesophageal echocardiography is often used before elective (nonemergent) cardioversion to exclude the presence of *TEE* left atrial thrombus or left atrial appendage thrombus if the patient has not received adequate anticoagulation therapy (3 weeks' duration) before the procedure.

Anticoagulation [H]

In patients who are not undergoing cardioversion, intravenous anticoagulation is usually unnecessary; however, oral anticoagulation should be initiated if the patient has sufficient risk factors for stroke. The most common method of assessing stroke risk in nonvalvular atrial fibrillation is by calculating the CHA_2DS_2-VASc score (**Table 18**). Patients with valvular atrial fibrillation (mechanical prosthesis or rheumatic mitral stenosis) require oral anticoagulation regardless of the presence or absence of other risk factors. *w/ WARFARIN*

If cardioversion is planned, the duration of atrial fibrillation guides therapy. Patients with atrial fibrillation with a known duration of less than 48 hours have a low risk for thrombus formation and subsequent stroke, and preprocedural anticoagulation is not needed. In patients in whom the duration of atrial fibrillation is unclear or in whom atrial fibrillation has lasted longer than 48 hours, anticoagulation therapy for 3 weeks is required before cardioversion. In the absence of preprocedural anticoagulation, transesophageal echocardiography can be performed to exclude the presence of

UNCLEAR OR >48hr = 3 WKS AC

TABLE 18. CHA_2DS_2-VASc Score, Adjusted Stroke Rates, and Antithrombotic Therapy Recommendations		
CHA_2DS_2-VASc Score[a]	Incidence of Ischemic Stroke/100 Patient-Years[b]	Antithrombotic Therapy[c]
0	0.2	None
1	0.6	None or aspirin or OAC
2	2.2	OAC
3	3.2	OAC
4	4.8	OAC
5	7.2	OAC
6+	10.3	OAC

OAC = oral anticoagulation.

[a]CHA_2DS_2-VASc scoring (maximum 9 points): One point each is given for heart failure, hypertension, diabetes mellitus, vascular disease (prior myocardial infarction, peripheral artery disease, aortic plaque), female sex, and age 65 to 74 years. Two points each are given for previous stroke/transient ischemic attack/thromboembolic disease and age ≥75 years.

[b]Data from Friberg L, Rosenqvist M, Lip GY. Evaluation of risk stratification schemes for ischaemic stroke and bleeding in 182 678 patients with atrial fibrillation: the Swedish Atrial Fibrillation cohort study. Eur Heart J. 2012;33:1500-10. [PMID: 22246443] doi:10.1093/eurheartj/ehr488

[c]Recommendations from January CT, Wann LS, Alpert JS, Calkins H, Cigarroa JE, Cleveland JC Jr, et al; ACC/AHA Task Force Members. 2014 AHA/ACC/HRS guideline for the management of patients with atrial fibrillation: a report of the American College of Cardiology/American Heart Association Task Force on Practice Guidelines and the Heart Rhythm Society. Circulation. 2014;130:e199-267. [PMID: 24682347] doi:10.1161/CIR.0000000000000041

CONT. left atrial appendage thrombus and facilitate urgent cardioversion. Regardless of the duration or nature of atrial fibrillation, all patients who undergo cardioversion must receive anticoagulation therapy for at least 4 weeks following the procedure owing to an increased risk for thromboembolic events after sinus rhythm is restored. **H**

Cardioversion and Rate Control

Pharmacologic or electrical cardioversion should be pursued in patients with significant symptoms despite rate control. In patients without structural heart disease, class IC agents or ibutilide can be considered for pharmacologic cardioversion. Patients treated with ibutilide should be monitored on telemetry for a minimum of 6 hours or until the QTc returns to baseline, owing to a small risk for torsade de pointes.

Heart rate control is necessary in patients with rapid ventricular rates to improve cardiac function and alleviate symptoms. Acutely, the goal heart rate should be between 60/min and 110/min. Commonly used medications include AV nodal blockers, such as metoprolol or diltiazem. Intravenous or oral administration may be appropriate depending on a patient's symptoms. In patients with left ventricular dysfunction, calcium channel blockers should be avoided. Digoxin can be used as adjunctive therapy to improve rate control, especially in patients with heart failure.

[handwritten margin note: AVOID CCB IN LV DYSFUNCTION]

Long-Term Management
Anticoagulation

Arterial thromboembolic events are the most serious complication of atrial fibrillation. In nonvalvular atrial fibrillation patients, the absolute risk for stroke is approximately 4% per year; however, the presence of comorbidities (such as heart failure, hypertension, diabetes, or vascular disease) can increase the risk 15- to 20-fold. Hypertension is associated with an increased risk for both atrial fibrillation and stroke; therefore, blood pressure control is critical in the management of atrial fibrillation.

H Stroke prevention with antithrombotic therapies is dependent on the patient's risk for stroke and risk for bleeding. Although several risk stratification scores are available, current guidelines recommend the use of the CHA_2DS_2-VASc score in patients with nonvalvular atrial fibrillation. Adjusted stroke rates and recommendations for antithrombotic therapy based on the CHA_2DS_2-VASc score are shown in Table 18. Patients with nonvalvular atrial fibrillation who have a CHA_2DS_2-VASc score of 2 or higher should be treated with anticoagulation to prevent stroke. Patients with valvular atrial fibrillation (rheumatic heart disease, mitral stenosis, and valve replacement) should receive warfarin. Non–vitamin K antagonist oral anticoagulants (NOACs) are not approved for use in valvular atrial fibrillation. However, patients with atrial fibrillation and other valvular lesions (aortic valve disease, mitral regurgitation, and tricuspid regurgitation) are eligible for NOAC therapy.

Bleeding scores, such as the ATRIA, HAS-BLED, and ORBIT scores, may be used to identify patients with significant bleeding risk based on patient characteristics, including anemia, hypertension, labile INR, older age, kidney insufficiency, and treatment with antiplatelet medications. Reversible risk factors for bleeding should be addressed in patients receiving anticoagulants. Concomitant antiplatelet therapy should be avoided unless the patient has recent active coronary artery disease (acute coronary syndrome or revascularization within the past year). *[handwritten: ANTIPLT TX]*

Several oral anticoagulants are available for stroke prevention in patients with atrial fibrillation. Vitamin K antagonism with dose-adjusted warfarin is an effective, low-cost therapy; however, warfarin has limitations, including the need for frequent monitoring and adjustment and numerous food and drug interactions. The safety and efficacy of warfarin therapy depend on the time the patient is in the therapeutic range (INR 2-3).

Four NOACs are approved for the prevention of stroke in atrial fibrillation (**Table 19**). Dabigatran, an oral direct thrombin inhibitor, is superior to warfarin for the prevention of ischemic stroke and results in less intracranial bleeding. Patients taking dabigatran have a higher risk for gastrointestinal bleeding relative to warfarin and may experience dyspepsia. Rivaroxaban, a direct factor Xa inhibitor, is noninferior to warfarin in the prevention of stroke or systemic embolism and is associated with less intracranial and fatal bleeding. As with dabigatran, patients taking rivaroxaban have a higher risk for gastrointestinal bleeding compared with those taking warfarin. Apixaban, another oral factor Xa inhibitor, is superior to warfarin for the prevention of stroke and confers less risk for major bleeding, including intracranial bleeding. Edoxaban is noninferior to warfarin for stroke prevention and is associated with less major bleeding. All of the NOACs have shorter half-lives than warfarin; however, there are no quick, readily available serum assays to accurately determine anticoagulant activity. Reversal agents and antidotes continue to be developed for these agents. Andexanet alfa is being evaluated for reversal of factor Xa inhibition, for use in patients treated with rivaroxaban, apixaban, or edoxaban. Idarucizumab is a dabigatran-reversal agent available for emergency invasive or surgical procedures or in cases of uncontrolled or life-threatening bleeding.

Approximately 10% to 25% of patients with atrial fibrillation have contraindications to oral anticoagulation or discontinue therapy for various reasons, including bleeding events. In patients who are at moderate to high risk for stroke (CHA_2DS_2-VASc score ≥3), left atrial appendage occlusion to prevent stroke and systemic thromboembolism can be considered. Occlusion of the left atrial appendage can be achieved percutaneously with a self-expanding device that is implanted in the left atrial appendage or with surgical closure. Left atrial

TABLE 19. Anticoagulants Approved for Stroke Prevention in Atrial Fibrillation

Medication	Frequency	Type of AF	Cautions and Dosing
Warfarin (vitamin K antagonist)	Dosing adjusted to INR	Valvular[a] or nonvalvular	Avoid in pregnancy Caution with idiopathic thrombocytopenic purpura, heparin-induced thrombocytopenia, liver disease, protein C or S deficiency Many drug interactions
Dabigatran (direct thrombin inhibitor)	Twice daily	Nonvalvular	Caution with P-glycoprotein inhibitors ↑RISK OF GI BLEED Reduce dose with CrCl 15-30 mL/min/1.73 m²
Rivaroxaban (factor Xa inhibitor)	Once daily	Nonvalvular	Avoid with CrCl <30 mL/min/1.73 m², moderate liver ↑ GI BLEED impairment, strong P-glycoprotein inhibitors, and strong cytochrome P-450 inducers and inhibitors ↓ ICH + FATAL BLEED Reduce dose with CrCl 30-50 mL/min/1.73 m²
Apixaban (factor Xa inhibitor)	Twice daily	Nonvalvular	Avoid with strong P-glycoprotein inhibitors or strong ↓STROKE cytochrome P-450 inducers and inhibitors ↓ MAJOR BLEED Reduce dose with two of the following criteria: creatinine ≥1.5 mg/dL 133 (μmol/L), age ≥80 years, or weight ≤60 kg (132 lb)
Edoxaban (factor Xa inhibitor)	Once daily	Nonvalvular	Avoid with strong cytochrome P-450 inducers and inhibitors Reduce dose with CrCl 30-50 mL/min/1.73 m², weight ≤60 kg (132 lb), or concomitant use of verapamil or quinidine (potent P-glycoprotein inhibitors) ↓ MAJOR BLEED

AF = atrial fibrillation; CrCl = creatinine clearance.

[a]Valvular atrial fibrillation refers to atrial fibrillation in the presence of a mechanical heart valve, rheumatic mitral valve disease, and/or mitral stenosis.

appendage occlusion has a lower risk for intracranial bleeding compared with dose-adjusted warfarin. **H**

Rate Versus Rhythm Control

Studies have not demonstrated that sinus rhythm restoration is superior to rate control alone. Consequently, the decision to initiate a rate or rhythm control strategy is predominantly based on symptoms, patient age, and patient preference. Rate control can be used to manage asymptomatic patients, with a resting heart rate goal of less than 80/min. A goal of less than 110/min may be considered in select patients without left ventricular dysfunction. β-Blockers, calcium channel blockers, and digoxin can be used to control the ventricular rate in patients with atrial fibrillation. Combination therapy may be needed to adequately control heart rate. Aside from resting heart rate assessment, evaluation of the heart rate with activity, such as with a 6-minute walk test, stress test, or 24-hour ambulatory ECG monitoring, should be performed.

A rhythm control strategy can improve quality of life in patients who continue to have symptoms despite adequate rate control. Because the long-term effects of rate control are unknown, rhythm control is often pursued in younger patients (aged <50 years) with minimal symptoms. Rhythm control may require cardioversion in addition to antiarrhythmic therapy. Antiarrhythmic drug selection is guided by the patient's comorbid conditions and safety considerations. Patients with infrequent atrial fibrillation who have no structural heart disease or conduction disease often benefit from a "pill-in-the-pocket" approach. With this strategy, patients take a class IC drug (flecainide or propafenone) at the onset of an episode of atrial fibrillation. These patients should be receiving β-blocker or calcium channel blocker therapy or should take one of these medications before taking the "pill in the pocket." Pill-in-the-pocket therapy should be initiated in a monitored setting to ensure patient safety.

Nonpharmacologic Strategies

Catheter ablation with pulmonary vein isolation is an effective rhythm control therapy in patients with recurrent symptomatic atrial fibrillation despite antiarrhythmic drug therapy. Catheter ablation is most effective in patients without significant left atrial enlargement and multiple comorbid conditions. Seventy percent to 90% of patients with paroxysmal atrial fibrillation are symptom-free 1 year after the procedure; however, success rates vary. Complications include thromboembolism (0.5%-1% risk), tamponade, and vascular complications (such as insertion hematoma, pseudoaneurysm, arteriovenous fistula, and retroperitoneal bleeding). Longer-term complications, such as pulmonary vein stenosis, are uncommon.

AV node ablation is an option in patients with atrial fibrillation who have continued symptomatic tachycardia despite rate and rhythm control therapy. Therapeutic ablation of the

ABLATION COMPLICATIONS

AV node requires implantation of a permanent pacemaker. These patients remain in atrial fibrillation and still require anticoagulation.

KEY POINTS

- Immediate cardioversion to sinus rhythm is indicated in patients with atrial fibrillation who have hypotension, acute myocardial ischemia, or decompensated heart failure, regardless of atrial fibrillation duration.

- Current guidelines recommend calculation of the CHA_2DS_2-VASc score for stroke risk stratification in patients with nonvalvular atrial fibrillation; patients with a CHA_2DS_2-VASc score of 2 or higher should be treated with oral anticoagulation to prevent stroke.

- A rhythm control strategy can improve quality of life in patients with atrial fibrillation who continue to have symptoms despite adequate heart rate control.

Atrial Flutter — RHYTHM CONTROL w/ ABLATION

Atrial flutter is an organized macro-reentrant tachycardia with discrete regular atrial activity on ECG, usually with a rate of 250/min to 300/min. Typical atrial flutter is characterized electrocardiographically by a sawtooth pattern with inverted flutter waves in leads II, III, and aVF and positive flutter waves in lead V_1 (**Figure 14**). Typical atrial flutter is the result of counterclockwise reentry around the tricuspid annulus. In atypical flutter, the circuit can travel in a clockwise direction or can

occur in other locations in the right and left atria. Atypical flutter may occur after ablation or after congenital or valvular cardiac surgery.

Management of atrial flutter is similar to atrial fibrillation management; however, a rhythm control strategy is favored in atrial flutter because rate control may be difficult and often requires high doses of more than one AV nodal blocker. Catheter ablation is the definitive treatment for typical atrial flutter, owing to a very high success rate (>95%) and low complication rate. Oral anticoagulation in patients with atrial flutter is approached in the same manner as in patients with atrial fibrillation. Patients with atrial flutter and sufficient stroke risk (CHA_2DS_2-VASc score ≥2) require oral anticoagulation to prevent stroke and systemic embolism. **H**

KEY POINT

- Catheter ablation is the definitive treatment of typical atrial flutter, owing to a very high success rate (>95%) and low complication rate.

Supraventricular Tachycardias
Clinical Presentation

SVTs are rapid heart rhythms that arise from the atrium or require conduction through the AV node. Atrial fibrillation and atrial flutter are technically SVTs, although the term generally pertains to paroxysmal SVTs. SVTs can affect all age groups but frequently occur in younger patients. Prevalence is higher in women than in men. SVTs usually occur in the

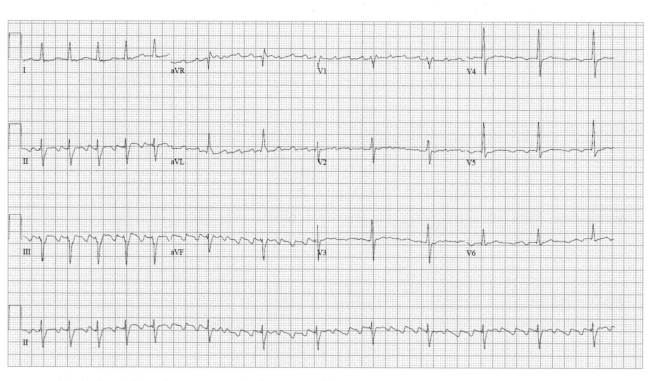

FIGURE 14. In this electrocardiogram demonstrating typical atrial flutter, negatively directed sawtooth waves are seen in the inferior leads, and positive waves are seen in lead V_1. In the bottom rhythm strip, 2:1 and 4:1 conduction patterns are seen.

absence of structural heart disease, although echocardiography should be performed to exclude underlying cardiac dysfunction or structural defects. Patients often have repeated episodes of tachycardia and may report palpitations, a sensation of pounding in the neck, fatigue, lightheadedness, chest discomfort, dyspnea, presyncope, and, less commonly, syncope.

The ECG typically demonstrates a narrow-complex tachycardia; however, wide QRS complexes (>120 ms) may be present in cases of bundle branch block, aberrancy, pacing, or anterograde accessory pathway conduction (antidromic tachycardia). SVTs may be classified electrocardiographically according to the relationship of the P wave and the QRS complex. Short-RP tachycardias (RP interval < PR interval) feature a P wave that closely follows the QRS complex, whereas long-RP tachycardias feature a P wave that is more than half the distance between the RR interval (RP interval > PR interval). Short-RP tachycardias include typical AVNRT, AVRT, and junctional tachycardia. Long-RP tachycardias include atypical AVNRT, sinus tachycardia, and atrial tachycardia.

Vagal maneuvers, including the Valsalva maneuver (bearing down), carotid sinus massage, or facial immersion in cold water, are first-line therapy to restore sinus rhythm in patients with SVT. Adenosine can be used to terminate SVT and simultaneously help diagnose its cause. Tachycardias that terminate with adenosine are typically AV node dependent (AVNRT and AVRT), whereas continued atrial activity (P waves) during AV block is consistent with atrial flutter or atrial tachycardia.

ADENOSINE FOR Tx + DX

Atrioventricular Nodal Reentrant Tachycardia

AVNRT accounts for two thirds of all cases of SVT, not including cases of atrial fibrillation and flutter. AVNRT is the result of a reentrant circuit within the AV node that uses both the fast and slow pathways. Typical AVNRT involves conduction down the slow pathway and back up to the atrium over the fast pathway (slow-fast). This conduction pattern results in a short RP interval with a retrograde P wave inscribed very close to the QRS complex (**Figure 15**). Atypical AVNRT occurs when the impulse travels down the fast pathway and returns to the atrium via the slow pathway (fast-slow), resulting in a long RP interval.

AVNRT may be terminated with vagal maneuvers or adenosine. AV nodal blocking therapy with β-blockers or calcium channel blockers is used to prevent recurrent AVNRT. In patients with recurrent AVNRT and patients who do not tolerate or prefer to avoid long-term medical therapy, catheter ablation should be considered. Catheter ablation of AVNRT has a high success rate, although it is associated with a 1% risk for injury to the AV node necessitating pacemaker implantation.

Atrioventricular Reciprocating Tachycardia

AVRT is an accessory pathway (bypass tract)–mediated tachycardia that is often observed as preexcitation on ECG (**Figure 16**). Early ventricular activation over the accessory pathway causes shortening of the PR interval, and the initial part of the QRS complex is slurred because of premature ventricular depolarization in the myocardial tissue adjacent to the accessory pathway. In AVRT, the tachycardia can conduct anterograde over the AV node (orthodromic AVRT) or anterograde over the accessory pathway (antidromic AVRT). Orthodromic AVRT is the most

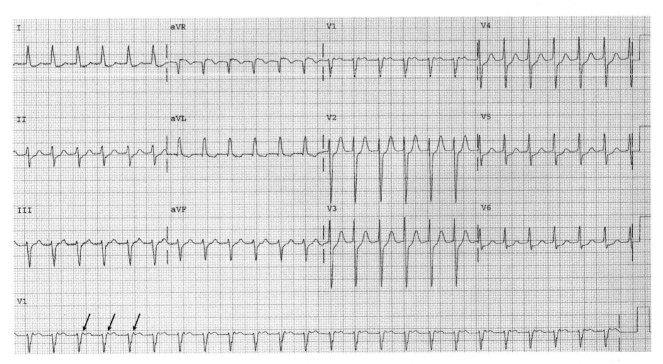

FIGURE 15. Electrocardiogram showing atrioventricular nodal reentrant tachycardia characterized by a short RP interval with a retrograde P wave inscribed very close to the QRS complex, which is best seen in V₁ (appearing as a pseudo r′ wave [*arrows*]).

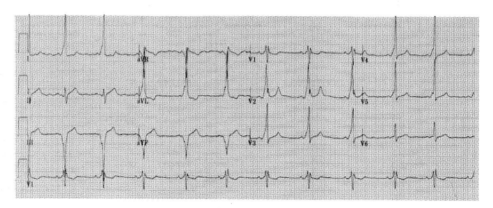

FIGURE 16. Electrocardiogram demonstrating sinus rhythm with preexcitation as indicated by the presence of a delta wave. The slurring of the QRS upstroke represents premature depolarization of the ventricular tissue adjacent to the accessory pathway.

CONT.

common type of AVRT, accounting for more than 90% to 95% of cases. This type of AVRT has a narrow QRS complex, owing to conduction over the AV node and the His-Purkinje system. Antidromic AVRT is characterized by a wide, slurred QRS complex resulting from conduction over the bypass tract and activation of the ventricle without use of the specialized conduction system. Adenosine can be given to terminate orthodromic AVRT; however, adenosine and other AV nodal blockers are contraindicated in cases of antidromic AVRT.

Wolff-Parkinson-White (WPW) syndrome is defined by symptomatic AVRT with evidence of preexcitation on resting ECG (delta wave). It is often seen in patients with Ebstein anomaly. Atrial fibrillation occurs in up to one third of patients with WPW syndrome. Rapid conduction over an accessory pathway in atrial fibrillation can result in VF and sudden cardiac death (SCD), although this occurs in less than 1% of cases of WPW syndrome.

In patients with preexcitation on ECG, stress testing can effectively risk-stratify patients; patients in whom preexcitation is lost during exercise are generally at low risk for ventricular arrhythmia and SCD. Electrophysiology testing is also helpful in determining the risk for SCD and in localizing the pathway to facilitate catheter ablation. Catheter ablation is first-line therapy for patients with WPW syndrome and has a high success rate; however, ablation success is dictated by the location of the bypass tract. Antiarrhythmic therapy is considered second-line therapy. In patients with accessory pathways close to the AV node, antiarrhythmic drug therapy is particularly useful because catheter ablation carries an unacceptable risk for iatrogenic heart block.

In asymptomatic patients with preexcitation on ECG, management is controversial. Invasive testing is generally not required, unless the patient has a high-risk occupation, such as a commercial airline pilot. ◨

Premature Atrial Contractions and Atrial Tachycardia

Premature atrial contractions (PACs) are early isolated beats that arise from the atria. They are exceedingly common, and their frequency increases with age. During ambulatory ECG monitoring, only 1% of persons have no PACs. High PAC burden is associated with increased risk for atrial fibrillation. Symptomatic PACs are typically treated with β-blockers or calcium channel blockers.

Atrial tachycardia can arise in the presence or absence of structural heart disease. β-Blocker or calcium channel blocker therapy is first-line treatment for symptomatic atrial tachycardia. Second-line treatment consists of catheter ablation or antiarrhythmic drug therapy. Ablation success rates are generally lower in patients with atrial tachycardia than in patients with other SVTs.

Multifocal atrial tachycardia is typified by three or more P-wave morphologies and a heart rate greater than 100/min (**Figure 17**). It is usually seen in patients with end-stage COPD.

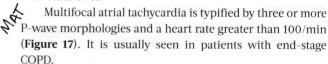

KEY POINTS

- Vagal maneuvers, including the Valsalva maneuver, carotid sinus massage, or facial immersion in cold water, may restore sinus rhythm in patients with supraventricular tachycardia.

- Patients with recurrent atrioventricular nodal reentrant tachycardia are treated with atrioventricular nodal blocking agents (β-blockers or calcium channel blockers) or catheter ablation.

- First-line therapy for patients with Wolff-Parkinson-White syndrome is catheter ablation; antiarrhythmic therapy is reserved for second-line therapy.

Wide-Complex Tachycardia

A wide-complex tachycardia is any tachycardia with a QRS complex of 120 ms or greater. Differential diagnoses include SVT with aberrancy, preexcited tachycardia (antidromic tachycardia), ventricular paced rhythm, and VT.

In adult patients with structural heart disease, 95% of wide-complex tachycardias are VT. Several important clinical

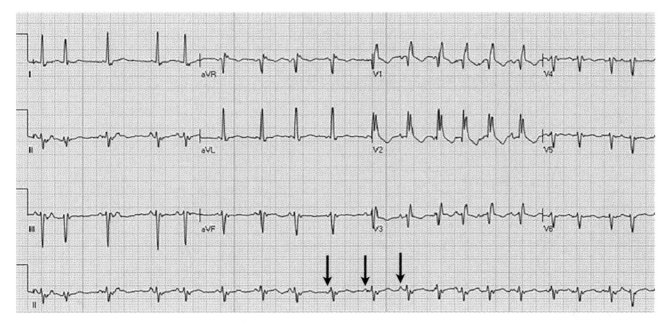

FIGURE 17. Electrocardiogram showing multifocal atrial tachycardia typified by three or more P-wave morphologies (*arrows*).

and ECG features can distinguish VT from other conditions. Wide-complex tachycardias that are positive in lead aVR, have a QRS morphology that is concordant (all predominantly positive or negative) in the precordial leads, have QRS morphology other than typical right or left bundle branch block, and exhibit extreme axis deviation ("northwest" axis) are usually VT. AV dissociation, fusion beats, and capture beats are all highly suggestive of VT (**Figure 18**). When the origin of a wide-complex tachycardia cannot be determined, VT should be assumed until expert consultation can be obtained. **H**

Ventricular Arrhythmias
Premature Ventricular Contractions

Premature ventricular contractions (PVCs) occur in up to 75% of healthy persons. Symptoms include palpitations or the

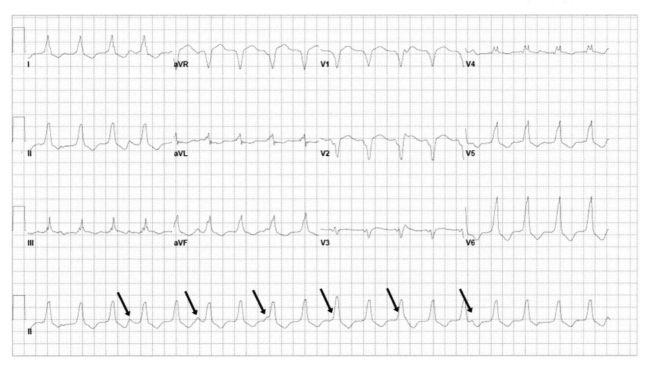

FIGURE 18. Electrocardiogram demonstrating a regular monomorphic wide-complex tachycardia in a left bundle branch block pattern. The presence of atrioventricular dissociation confirms the diagnosis of ventricular tachycardia. The arrows identify nonconducting P waves.

perception of skipped beats. Forceful beats are caused by increased cardiac filling during the pause following the PVC. PVCs are more common in patients with hypertension, left ventricular hypertrophy, previous myocardial infarction, and other forms of structural heart disease, such as nonischemic cardiomyopathy.

In the absence of high-risk features (syncope, a family history of premature SCD, structural heart disease), reassurance is appropriate management. PVCs require treatment when symptoms are bothersome or frequent (>10% of all beats or 10,000 PVCs per day). Tachycardia-induced cardiomyopathy may result from frequent PVCs (see Heart Failure).

First-line treatment for PVC suppression is β-blocker or calcium channel blocker therapy. β-Blockers are preferred in patients with ventricular dysfunction. If PVCs persist despite β-blockade or calcium channel blockade, antiarrhythmic drug therapy may be used. The selection of an antiarrhythmic medication for PVC suppression depends on many factors, including kidney function and comorbid conditions. In young healthy patients without structural heart disease, class IC drugs are usually effective. Amiodarone is most commonly used in patients with structural heat disease, particularly heart failure. Catheter ablation should be considered in patients with continued frequent PVCs despite medical therapy, those who cannot tolerate medical therapy, and patients who develop PVC-related left ventricular dysfunction.

Ventricular Tachycardia with Structural Heart Disease

In ischemic and nonischemic cardiomyopathy, the presence of myocardial scar tissue facilitates a reentry circuit and the development of VT. VT is usually regular and monomorphic in patients with ventricular scarring. Sustained VT (≥30 seconds) can lead to hypotension, syncope, VF, and cardiac arrest; however, short episodes of VT (nonsustained) or slow sustained VT may be well tolerated or cause no symptoms.

Evaluation with resting ECG, exercise treadmill testing (to provoke arrhythmias), and cardiac imaging (to identify structural heart disease) is indicated in all patients with VT. Patients with ischemic cardiomyopathy who present with VT should be considered for angiography and revascularization if appropriate. Cardiac magnetic resonance imaging clarifies the extent and pattern of myocardial scarring, which can be helpful in refining the cause of the cardiomyopathy and can assist in determining prognosis. For example, patients with a higher burden of myocardial scarring have higher risk for recurrent arrhythmia.

β-Blockers and ACE inhibitors reduce the risk for SCD in patients with prior myocardial infarction and cardiomyopathy. In those with recurrent VT despite β-blocker therapy, antiarrhythmic drug therapy with amiodarone may be considered. Catheter ablation should be considered in patients with recurrent VT despite medical therapy. ICD placement is indicated for secondary prevention of SCD in patients with structural heart disease or cardiomyopathy who have sustained VT/VF,

provided that reversible causes have been excluded (such as acute coronary ischemia or cocaine ingestion).

Idiopathic Ventricular Tachycardia

Idiopathic VT (so-called normal heart VT) occurs in the absence of structural heart disease, typically arising from the outflow tracts, fascicles, and papillary muscles. Patients with idiopathic VT usually present with palpitations in the third to fifth decades of life. Episodes of syncope are uncommon. Arrhythmic events are often triggered by stress, emotion, or exercise. These tachycardias are responsive to adenosine.

Calcium channel blockers, especially verapamil, and β-blockers are first-line treatment for idiopathic VT. Catheter ablation can be considered if symptoms continue despite these therapies. ICDs are contraindicated in patients with hemodynamically stable idiopathic VT, owing to the benign prognosis and efficacy of other therapies.

KEY POINT

- The primary treatment for patients with premature ventricular contractions (PVCs) without high-risk features (syncope, a family history of premature sudden cardiac death, structural heart disease) is reassurance; treatment is reserved for those with bothersome symptoms or frequent PVCs.

HVC

Inherited Arrhythmia Syndromes

Patients younger than age 40 years with unexplained SCD, unexplained near drowning, or recurrent exertional syncope, who do not have ischemic or other structural heart disease, should be evaluated for inherited arrhythmia syndromes. Additionally, unexplained premature death (age <35 years) or sudden death in a first-degree family member (age <40 years) should raise suspicion for an inherited arrhythmia syndrome and prompt referral to a cardiovascular specialist, with genetic counseling and genetic testing as indicated by clinical findings. The diagnosis of inherited arrhythmia syndromes can be complicated because of variable penetrance and expressivity of these disorders. Characteristic findings and treatments for these syndromes are reviewed in **Table 20**.

Long QT syndrome is among the most common inherited arrhythmias, affecting between 1 in 1000 and 1 in 5000 persons. Prolongation of the QTc interval has many causes, most of which are acquired, such as medication use, structural heart disease, and electrolyte abnormalities. Drugs that have been implicated in QT prolongation include antiarrhythmic agents, antibiotics (including some macrolides and fluoroquinolones), antipsychotic drugs, and antidepressants. A list of drugs categorized by their potential to cause QT prolongation is available at crediblemeds.org. The presence of a prolonged QTc interval (>440 ms in men and >460 ms in women) alone is insufficient to diagnose long QT syndrome. Diagnosis requires the presence of a QTc interval greater than 500 ms on repeated 12-lead ECGs accompanied by unexplained syncope or ventricular

TABLE 20. Inherited Arrhythmia Syndromes

Disorder	Presenting Symptoms and Characteristic Findings	Treatment[a]
Long QT syndrome	Syncope, QTc interval usually >460 ms, torsades de pointes	β-Blockers, ICD, exercise restriction
Short QT syndrome	Syncope, QT interval <340 ms, atrial fibrillation, VT, VF	ICD in all patients
Brugada syndrome	Syncope, VF, coved ST-segment elevation in early precordial leads (V_1 through V_3)	ICD + QUINIDINE IF PERSISTANT
Catecholaminergic polymorphic VT	Syncope, polymorphic or bidirectional VT during exercise or emotional distress	β-Blockers, verapamil, flecainide, ICD, exercise abstinence
Early repolarization syndrome	Syncope, inferior and lateral early repolarization on ECG, VF	ICD
ARVC/D	Syncope, palpitations, T-wave inversions in leads V_1 through at least V_3, monomorphic VT, abnormal signal-averaged ECG, frequent PVCs, and abnormal right ventricular size and function on echocardiography or CMR imaging	ICD, β-blockers, antiarrhythmic medications, exercise abstinence

ARVC/D = arrhythmogenic right ventricular cardiomyopathy/dysplasia; CMR = cardiac magnetic resonance; ECG = electrocardiography; ICD = implantable cardioverter-defibrillator; PVC = premature ventricular contraction; QTc = corrected QT; VF = ventricular fibrillation; VT = ventricular tachycardia.

[a]Treatment recommendations for ICDs in inherited arrhythmia syndromes are guided by risk stratification with criteria that are often disease specific. Additionally, antiarrhythmic drugs are often required in several syndromes for recurrent ventricular arrhythmias.

arrhythmia. Patients with a QTc interval greater than 500 ms are at greatest risk for SCD. β-Blockers are first-line therapy; however, patients with cardiac arrest or those who have recurrent events (syncope or VT) refractory to β-blocker therapy are candidates for ICD placement. These patients should not participate in competitive athletics.

Short QT syndrome is a rare and genetically heterogeneous disorder characterized by a short QT interval (QT <340 ms or QTc <350 ms). It is inherited in an autosomal dominant pattern. Patients can present with atrial and ventricular arrhythmias (including atrial fibrillation, polymorphic VT, and VF) and syncope. Patients with short QT syndrome are considered to be at very high risk for SCD; therefore, ICD placement is recommended in all patients.

Brugada syndrome is distinguished by right precordial ECG abnormalities, including ST-segment coving (concave or linear downsloping ST segment) in leads V_1 to V_3 with or without right bundle branch block, VF, and cardiac arrest (**Figure 19**). Brugada syndrome has an increased prevalence in men and persons of Asian descent. Arrhythmic events in patients with Brugada syndrome are more common at night during sleep. Abnormalities on ECG can be intermittent and may be elicited by fever or pharmacologic challenge with sodium channel blockade (such as with procainamide infusion). Patients with syncope or ventricular arrhythmia should undergo ICD implantation. Quinidine may be beneficial in patients with recurrent ventricular arrhythmias and/or ICD shocks.

Catecholaminergic polymorphic VT is a rare disorder characterized by intracellular calcium overload, polymorphic ventricular arrhythmias, and cardiac arrest. The arrhythmias are usually triggered by high-adrenergic states, including

strong emotion and exercise. These arrhythmias can also be provoked with epinephrine infusion. β-Blocker therapy and ICD placement are treatments. Patients with catecholaminergic polymorphic VT should avoid exercise.

Early repolarization syndrome should be strongly suspected in patients with unexplained VF arrest, particularly when provoked during exercise. Early repolarization (J-point elevation) is a common and usually benign ECG finding; however, the presence of inferior and lateral early repolarization of more than 1 mm in a patient with VF and/or cardiac arrest should be considered early repolarization syndrome. ICD implantation is indicated in patients with VF or cardiac arrest.

Hypertrophic cardiomyopathy or arrhythmogenic right ventricular cardiomyopathy/dysplasia (ARVC/D) can often present as SCD in young persons. Hypertrophic cardiomyopathy and arrhythmic risk stratification are discussed in Myocardial Disease. Most patients with ARVC/D present between puberty and young adulthood; however, it can also occur in older age. Patients with ARVC/D usually present with frequent ventricular ectopy and/or monomorphic VT, although severe cases can present with heart failure. The diagnosis is established by ECG abnormalities, family history, the presence of arrhythmias, and structural abnormalities of the right ventricle. Cardiac magnetic resonance imaging can demonstrate enlargement (segments of poorly contracting heart muscle), focal aneurysms, and wall motion abnormalities in the right ventricle (hypokinesis). ARVC/D is usually progressive, and patients with ARVC/D should abstain from vigorous exercise. Patients with ARVC/D and cardiac arrest or risk factors (nonsustained VT, inducible VT) should be offered ICD implantation. β-Blockers are first-line therapy for ventricular arrhythmia, although antiarrhythmic

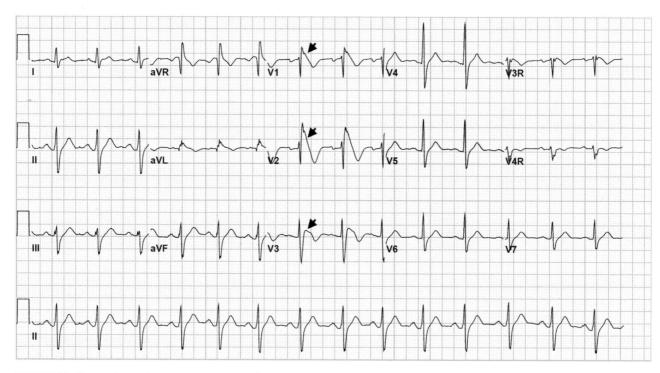

FIGURE 19. Electrocardiogram demonstrating a type 1 Brugada pattern, ≥2 mm J-point elevation, ST-segment coving (concave or linear downsloping ST segment) (*arrowheads*), and T-wave inversions in leads V_1 to V_3.

therapy with sotalol or amiodarone or catheter ablation is often required for recurrent VT.

> **KEY POINT**
>
> • Unexplained premature death (at age <35 years) or sudden death in a first-degree family member should raise suspicion for an inherited arrhythmia syndrome and prompt referral to a cardiovascular specialist.

Sudden Cardiac Arrest

Epidemiology and Risk Factors

SCD is defined as an instantaneous fatal event or collapse within 1 hour of symptom onset in an apparently healthy person. In patients in whom death was unwitnessed, SCD is considered to have occurred if the patient was known to be alive and well within the past 24 hours. VT and VF are the most common causes of SCD.

In the United States, more than 350,000 episodes of SCD occur each year. The annual risk for SCD is 1:1000 in the general population. The highest incidence occurs in patients with pre-existing structural heart disease, although left ventricular function is normal in most patients experiencing SCD. Risk factors include heart failure, diminished left ventricular function, previous myocardial infarction, unexplained syncope, left ventricular hypertrophy, nonsustained ventricular arrhythmia, chronic kidney disease, and sleep apnea. It is important to distinguish between myocardial infarction and SCD when a family history of cardiac disease is obtained.

Acute Management

Cardiac arrest necessitates immediate cardiopulmonary resuscitation (CPR) and advanced cardiac life support. Basic life support guidelines emphasize the importance of immediate, rapid, and sustained chest compressions in caring for individuals with cardiac arrest. Following activation of the emergency medical system and request for an automated external defibrillator, the patient's pulse should be checked immediately. Chest compressions should be initiated if no definite pulse is detected within 10 seconds. High-quality CPR (30 compressions and 2 breaths per cycle if no advanced airway is present) includes adequate depression of the lower sternum at a rate of at least 100 compressions per minute with adequate time for chest recoil. Interruptions in chest compressions should be minimized. Once an airway has been secured, breaths should be delivered at a rate of 1 breath per 6 seconds (10/min) to avoid breath stacking and increased thoracic pressure, which impedes cardiac output. Defibrillation should occur as soon as possible in patients with a shockable rhythm because time to defibrillation is an important determinant of the likelihood of survival to hospital discharge.

According to the 2015 American Heart Association advanced cardiovascular life support guidelines, the presence or absence of a shockable rhythm guides management after CPR has been initiated. In patients with asystole or pulseless electrical activity, CPR is continued with reassessment of rhythm status for a shockable rhythm every 2 minutes. Epinephrine should be administered intravenously to increase coronary perfusion. Vasopressin is no longer recommended because it provides no advantages over epinephrine. Likewise, atropine should not be used for the treatment of asystole or pulseless electrical activity arrest. Any reversible causes (such as tamponade) should be identified and treated.

Patients with VT/VF should be shocked, followed by immediate resumption of CPR and reassessment of the rhythm in 2 minutes. Epinephrine should be administered after the second shock and every 3 to 5 minutes thereafter. Amiodarone should be given as a bolus if VT/VF continues despite three shocks and epinephrine administration. A second dose of amiodarone can be given if VT/VF persists.

Device Therapy for Prevention of Sudden Death

ICDs have demonstrated efficacy in the primary and secondary prevention of SCD. Patients with sustained ventricular arrhythmias (>30 seconds) or cardiac arrest without a reversible cause have a class I recommendation for secondary prevention ICD placement. Patients with heart failure who meet specific criteria should undergo ICD placement for primary prevention (see Heart Failure). Patients with heart failure and interventricular conduction defects (predominantly left bundle branch block) often benefit from cardiac resynchronization therapy or cardiac resynchronization therapy in combination with a defibrillator.

Patients with ICDs need to avoid strenuous upper extremity exercises, including weight lifting, because of concern for lead stress and subsequent fracture. Inappropriate detection of VT/VF and shocks can result from electromagnetic interference; therefore, patients need to avoid devices that pose risks, such as arc welding equipment and high-voltage machinery. Patients with ICDs who are undergoing invasive procedures or surgery should be evaluated by their electrophysiologist for device reprogramming recommendations.

In the past, ICDs were implanted almost exclusively by using a transvenous approach. New techniques allow for implantation of defibrillators in the lateral chest at the midaxillary line adjacent to the heart with tunneling of the lead under the skin next to the sternum. Subcutaneous defibrillators have several advantages, including reduced risk for device infection.

KEY POINT

- Implantable cardioverter-defibrillators are effective for primary and secondary prevention of sudden cardiac death.

Device Infection

Device infections have many different forms, ranging from pocket infections to endocarditis. Most infections are due to *Staphylococcus epidermidis* and *Staphylococcus aureus*. Symptoms of cardiac device infection include fever, chills, malaise, lassitude, and failure to thrive, particularly in the elderly.

Physical examination of the pocket may reveal erythema, swelling, drainage, or wound dehiscence. In patients suspected of having device infection, several blood cultures, an erythrocyte sedimentation rate, and a C-reactive protein level

should be obtained. A transesophageal echocardiogram should be obtained to evaluate for intracardiac or lead vegetations. Aspirating the device pocket is never indicated because this can damage the leads or introduce infection in a sterile or uninfected pocket. PET-CT can also identify infection of the device pocket or leads if other testing is inconclusive.

Treatment of cardiac device infection includes complete extraction of all hardware, debridement of the pocket, sustained antibiotic therapy, and reimplantation at a new location after infection has been eradicated.

Valvular Heart Disease
General Principles

Valvular heart disease (VHD) is characterized by underlying functional or anatomic abnormalities in the cardiac valves that result in regurgitation or stenosis. VHD is common, occurring in approximately 20 million persons in the United States. Although there are congenital forms, VHD is largely age dependent, and 3% to 6% of those aged 65 years and older are affected.

A thorough history and physical examination are essential in evaluating for VHD. Many heart valve lesions are slowly progressive, and patients may unconsciously limit their activity in response to a worsening of underlying VHD. The most common symptom is exertional dyspnea. Other symptoms include angina, syncope, palpitations, lower extremity edema, and ascites, depending on the lesion and severity. Typical physical examination findings for valvular and other cardiac lesions are described in **Table 21**. Twelve-lead electrocardiography, chest radiography, and transthoracic echocardiography (TTE) with two-dimensional imaging may be performed to evaluate for VHD.

For clinical monitoring and timing of intervention, VHD is classified into four stages (A to D), which consider the presence of symptoms, severity of the lesion, ventricular response to the volume or pressure overload caused by the lesion, effect on the pulmonary or systemic circulation, and heart rhythm changes (**Table 22**). Surveillance intervals for echocardiographic evaluation based on disease severity are listed in **Table 23** on page 58.

Surgery can be a life-saving intervention in select patients, and surgical risk calculation is a key component of the patient evaluation. Surgical risk is determined through an assessment of the patient's age, morbidities, frailty, and impediments specific to the procedure being considered (for example, prior chest radiation therapy for a sternotomy approach). Risk calculators derived from national databases can assist in estimating risk for morbidity and mortality for various surgical valve procedures. One such calculator, the Society of Thoracic Surgery Adult Cardiac Surgery Risk Calculator, is available at riskcalc.sts.org. Although risk calculators contain many data input fields, it is important to note that frailty and some other important patient and procedural characteristics are not part of these online assessment tools.

TABLE 21. Valvular and Other Cardiac Lesions and Their Associated Examination Findings

Cardiac Condition	Characteristic Murmur	Location	Radiation	Associated Findings	Severity and Pitfalls
Aortic stenosis	Midsystolic; crescendo-decrescendo	RUSB	Right clavicle, carotid, apex	Enlarged, nondisplaced apical impulse; S_4; bicuspid valve without calcification will have systolic ejection click followed by murmur	Severe aortic stenosis findings may include decreased A_2; high-pitched, late-peaking murmur; diminished and delayed carotid upstroke Radiation of murmur down the descending thoracic aorta may mimic mitral regurgitation
Aortic regurgitation	Diastolic; decrescendo	LLSB (valvular) or RLSB (dilated aorta) (heard best sitting and leaning forward)	None	Enlarged, displaced apical impulse; S_3 or S_4; increased pulse pressure; bounding carotid and peripheral pulses	Acute severe regurgitation murmur may be masked by tachycardia and short duration of murmur Severity in chronic regurgitation is difficult to assess by auscultation
Mitral stenosis	Diastolic; low-pitched, decrescendo	Apex (heard best in left lateral decubitus position)	None	Loud S_1; tapping apex beat; opening snap after S_2 if leaflets mobile; irregular pulse if atrial fibrillation present	Interval between S_2 and opening snap is short in severe mitral stenosis Intensity of murmur correlates with transvalvular gradient P_2 may be loud if pulmonary hypertension present
Mitral regurgitation	Systolic; holo-, mid-, or late systolic	Apex	Axilla or back; occasionally anteriorly to precordium	Systolic click in mitral valve prolapse; S_3; apical impulse hyperdynamic and may be displaced if dilated left ventricle; in mitral valve prolapse, Valsalva maneuver moves onset of clicks and murmur closer to S_1; handgrip maneuver increases murmur intensity	Acute severe regurgitation may have soft or no holosystolic murmur, mitral inflow rumble, or S_3
Tricuspid regurgitation	Holosystolic	LLSB	LUSB	Merged and prominent c and v waves in jugular venous pulse; murmur increases during inspiration	Right ventricular impulse below sternum Pulsatile, enlarged liver with possible ascites Murmur may be high-pitched if associated with severe pulmonary hypertension
Tricuspid stenosis	Diastolic; low-pitched, decrescendo; increased intensity during inspiration	LLSB	None	Elevated central venous pressure with prominent a wave, signs of venous congestion (hepatomegaly, ascites, edema)	Low-pitched frequency may be difficult to auscultate, especially at higher heart rate
Pulmonary valve stenosis	Systolic; crescendo-decrescendo	LUSB	Left clavicle	Pulmonic ejection click after S_1 (diminishes with inspiration)	Increased intensity of murmur with late peaking
Pulmonary valve regurgitation	Diastolic; decrescendo	LLSB	None	Loud P_2 if pulmonary hypertension present	Murmur may be minimal or absent if severe due to minimal difference in pulmonary artery and right ventricular diastolic pressures

(Continued on the next page)

TABLE 21. Valvular and Other Cardiac Lesions and Their Associated Examination Findings *(Continued)*

Cardiac Condition	Characteristic Murmur	Location	Radiation	Associated Findings	Severity and Pitfalls
Innocent flow murmur	Midsystolic; grade 1/6 or 2/6 in intensity	RUSB	None	Normal intensity of A_2; normal splitting of S_2; no radiation	May be present in conditions with increased flow (e.g., pregnancy, fever, anemia, hyperthyroidism)
Hypertrophic obstructive cardiomyopathy	Systolic; crescendo-decrescendo	LLSB	None	Enlarged, hyperdynamic apical impulse; bifid carotid impulse with delay; increased intensity during Valsalva maneuver or with squatting to standing	Murmur may not be present in nonobstructive hypertrophic cardiomyopathy
Atrial septal defect	Systolic; crescendo-decrescendo	RUSB	None	Fixed split S_2; right ventricular heave; rarely, tricuspid inflow murmur	May be associated with pulmonary hypertension with increased intensity of P_2, pulmonary valve regurgitation
Ventricular septal defect	Holosystolic	LLSB	None	Palpable thrill; murmur increases with handgrip maneuver, decreases with amyl nitrite	Murmur intensity and duration decrease as pulmonary hypertension develops (Eisenmenger syndrome) Cyanosis if Eisenmenger syndrome develops

A_2 = aortic component of S_2; LLSB = left lower sternal border; LUSB = left upper sternal border; P_2 = pulmonic component of S_2; RLSB = right lower sternal border; RUSB = right upper sternal border.

TABLE 22. Stages of Progression of Valvular Heart Disease

Stage	Definition	Description
A	At risk	Patients with risk factors for development of VHD
B	Progressive	Patients with progressive VHD (mild to moderate severity and asymptomatic)
C	Asymptomatic severe	Asymptomatic patients who have the criteria for severe VHD: C1: Asymptomatic patients with severe VHD in whom the left or right ventricle remains compensated C2: Asymptomatic patients with severe VHD, with decompensation of the left or right ventricle
D	Symptomatic severe	Patients who have developed symptoms as a result of VHD

VHD = valvular heart disease.

Reproduced with permission from Nishimura RA, Otto CM, Bonow RO, Carabello BA, Erwin JP 3rd, Guyton RA, et al; American College of Cardiology/American Heart Association Task Force on Practice Guidelines. 2014 AHA/ACC guideline for the management of patients with valvular heart disease: executive summary: a report of the American College of Cardiology/American Heart Association Task Force on Practice Guidelines. J Am Coll Cardiol. 2014;63:2438-88. [PMID: 24603192] doi:10.1016/j.jacc.2014.02.537. Copyright 2014, Elsevier.

Therefore, a comprehensive, holistic approach is required for determining patient surgical risk and candidacy. Frailty, which is variably defined as a geriatric syndrome characterized by declines in several physiologic systems and processes, portends an increased risk for mortality in patients undergoing surgery and can be measured preoperatively (see MKSAP 18 General Internal Medicine).

For all patients in whom surgical or interventional therapy is being considered, a multidisciplinary approach with a heart team consisting of cardiologists, surgeons, and interventional cardiologists is recommended. Evaluations in centers with specialized expertise in VHD (for example, a Heart Valve Center of Excellence) is also advised for patients in whom intervention is being considered when (1) there are no symptoms; (2) multiple or complex morbidities are present; or (3) surgical valve repair is favored over valve replacement.

Medical therapy, although often effective for symptom palliation, has not been shown to prevent progression of VHD or improve long-term survival in patients with VHD.

KEY POINTS

- Many heart valve lesions progress slowly, leading patients to unconsciously limit their activity in response; therefore, a careful history and detailed physical examination are essential.

- For all patients with valvular heart disease in whom surgical or interventional therapy is being considered, a multidisciplinary approach with a heart team consisting of cardiologists, surgeons, and interventional cardiologists is recommended.

- Medical therapy, although often effective for symptom palliation, has not been shown to prevent progression of valvular heart disease or improve long-term survival in patients with valvular heart disease.

TABLE 23. Serial Evaluation of Asymptomatic Patients with Left-Sided Valvular Conditions

Factors Considered	Lesion Severity	Frequency of Evaluation
Aortic Stenosis		
Stenosis severity; rate of progression; LV systolic function; ascending aorta dilation if associated with bicuspid aortic valve	At risk (V_{max} <2 m/s)	
	Mild (V_{max} 2.0-2.9 m/s or mean gradient <20 mm Hg)	Clinical evaluation yearly; echo every 3-5 y
	Moderate (V_{max} 3.0-3.9 m/s or mean gradient 20-39 mm Hg)	Clinical evaluation yearly; echo every 1-2 y
	Severe (V_{max} ≥4 m/s or mean gradient ≥40 mm Hg, AVA ≤1.0 cm^2)	Clinical evaluation yearly; echo every 6-12 mo
	Very severe (V_{max} ≥5 m/s or mean gradient ≥60 mm Hg)	Clinical evaluation yearly; echo every 6-12 mo
Aortic Regurgitation		
Regurgitation severity; rate of progression; LV ejection fraction; LV chamber size; ascending aorta dilation if bicuspid aortic valve	Mild (VC <0.3 cm, ERO <0.10 cm^2, RV <30 mL/beat, RF <30%); normal EF	Clinical evaluation yearly; echo every 3-5 y
	Moderate (VC 0.3-0.6 cm, ERO 0.10-0.29 cm^2, RV 30-59 mL/beat, RF 30%-49%)	Clinical evaluation yearly; echo every 1-2 y
	Severe (VC >0.6 cm, ERO >0.3 cm^2, RV ≥60 mL/beat, RF ≥50%)	
	EF ≥50%; LVESD ≤50 mm	Clinical evaluation every 6-12 mo; echo every 6-12 mo, more frequently for dilating LV
	EF <50%; LVESD >50 mm	Clinical evaluation every 6-12 mo; echo every 6-12 mo, more frequently for dilating LV
Mitral Stenosis		
Stenosis severity	Mild and moderate (MVA >1.5 cm^2, diastolic pressure half-time <150 ms)	Clinical evaluation yearly; echo every 3-5 y
	Severe (MVA ≤1.5 cm^2, diastolic pressure half-time ≥150 ms or ≥220 ms with very severe stenosis, PASP >30 mm Hg)	Clinical evaluation yearly; echo every 1-2 y for MVA 1.0-1.5 cm^2, every year for MVA <1.0 cm^2
Mitral Regurgitation		
Regurgitation severity; rate of progression; EF; LV chamber size	At risk (VC <0.3 cm)	Clinical evaluation yearly; echo only if symptomatic
	Mild and moderate (VC <0.7 cm, ERO <0.40 cm^2, RV <60 mL/beat, RF <50%)	Clinical evaluation yearly; echo every 3-5 y for mild severity, every 1-2 y for moderate severity
	Severe (VC ≥0.7 cm, ERO ≥0.4 cm^2, RV ≥60 mL/beat, RF ≥50%)	Clinical evaluation every 6-12 mo; echo every 6-12 mo, more frequently for dilating LV

AVA = aortic valve area; echo = echocardiography; EF = ejection fraction; ERO = effective regurgitant orifice; LV = left ventricular; LVESD = left ventricular end-systolic dimension; MVA = mitral valve area; PASP = pulmonary artery systolic pressure; RF = regurgitant fraction; RV = regurgitant volume; VC = vena contracta width; V_{max} = maximum aortic jet velocity.

Recommendations based on Nishimura RA, Otto CM, Bonow RO, Carabello BA, Erwin JP 3rd, Guyton RA, et al; American College of Cardiology/American Heart Association Task Force on Practice Guidelines. 2014 AHA/ACC guideline for the management of patients with valvular heart disease: executive summary: a report of the American College of Cardiology/American Heart Association Task Force on Practice Guidelines. J Am Coll Cardiol. 2014;63:2438-88. [PMID: 24603192] doi:10.1016/j.jacc.2014.02.537

Aortic Stenosis

Clinical Presentation and Evaluation

Aortic stenosis may be congenital, such as in persons with a bicuspid aortic valve, or acquired. The most common cause is degeneration of the valve that occurs with aging; severe lesions occur in approximately 3% of persons aged 65 years and older (**Figure 20**). Other causes include rheumatic disease and chest radiation. Although rheumatic disease of the mitral valve frequently occurs in isolation, rheumatic aortic valve disease almost never occurs without mitral valve involvement. Chest radiation (for example, mantle therapy for non-Hodgkin lymphoma) commonly causes a mixture of both valvular stenosis and regurgitation.

Aortic stenosis results in chronic pressure overload of the left ventricle (LV), leading to concentric LV hypertrophy and myocardial interstitial fibrosis. Diastolic dysfunction follows, with eventual systolic heart failure and pulmonary congestion. Exertional dyspnea, syncope, and angina are the most common presenting symptoms; however, symptoms may not

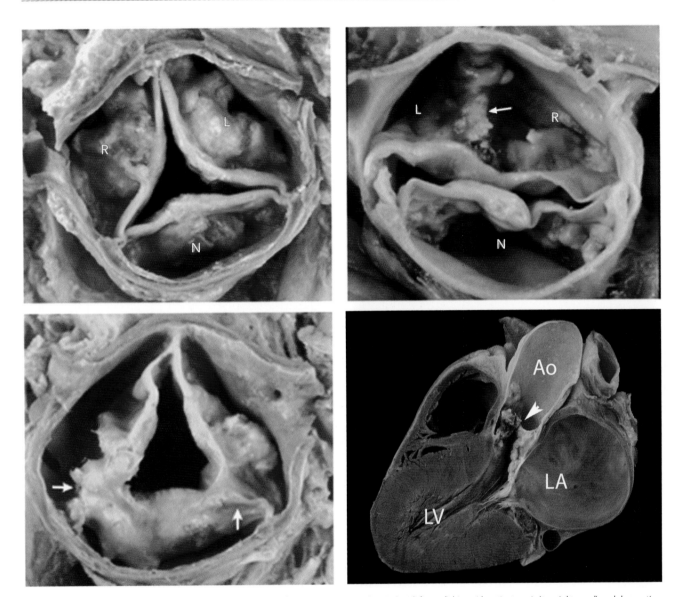

FIGURE 20. Aortic stenosis. Gross specimens showing pathology of degenerative aortic stenosis (*top left panel*), bicuspid aortic stenosis (*top right panel*), and rheumatic aortic disease (*bottom left panel*). The raphe between the left (L) and right (R) aortic cups is fused in this case of bicuspid aortic stenosis (*arrow in top right panel*). Fusion of the commissures is a distinctive feature of rheumatic disease (*arrows in bottom left panel*). Gross specimen showing severe left ventricular (LV) hypertrophy as a result of pressure overload from severe aortic stenosis (*arrowhead in bottom right panel*). Ao = ascending aorta; LA = left atrium; N = noncoronary cusp.

Images courtesy of Dr. William Edwards, Mayo Clinic.

appear until stenosis is severe. The disease typically progresses with a decrease in the aortic valve area of approximately 0.12 cm² per year, but the rate depends on patient age, underlying severity of the stenosis, and comorbid conditions, such as kidney failure and hypertension. Among asymptomatic patients with severe aortic stenosis, 75% will die or develop symptoms within 5 years. Once symptoms occur in patients with severe aortic stenosis, life expectancy is generally only 1 to 2 years. Thus, serial evaluation every 6 to 12 months is recommended for patients with severe disease (see Table 23).

In patients with severe aortic stenosis, the characteristic physical findings include a late-peaking systolic murmur, a diminished or absent aortic component of the S₂, and a delay

in the carotid upstroke (pulsus tardus) that may be accompanied by a decreased pulse amplitude due to low cardiac output (pulsus parvus). Physical findings that suggest severe aortic stenosis should be promptly evaluated (see Table 21).

The primary imaging modality for the evaluation of aortic stenosis is TTE (**Figure 21**). Echocardiography can determine the cause and severity of aortic stenosis (such as the gradient and valve area) as well as LV function and wall thickness. In some patients, echocardiography may underestimate the severity of aortic stenosis. Further evaluation with cardiac catheterization, during which the cardiac output and the gradient across the aortic valve can be measured, is required when there are discrepancies between the findings on physical

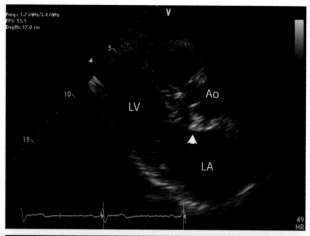

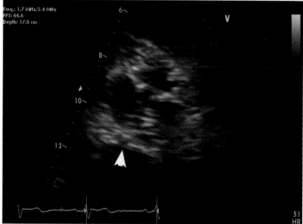

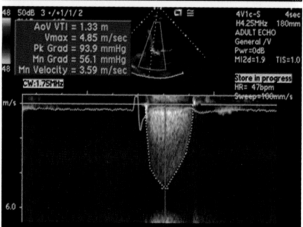

FIGURE 21. Echocardiographic findings in aortic stenosis. Calcific aortic stenosis (*arrowhead*) is present in parasternal long-axis (*top panel*) and short-axis (*middle panel*) views. Left ventricular (LV) hypertrophy is also present. Doppler echocardiogram shows a mean aortic gradient of 56 mm Hg, consistent with severe aortic stenosis (*bottom panel*). Ao = ascending aorta; LA = left atrium.

area and either low velocity or low gradient: patients with severe LV dysfunction and low cardiac output and patients with preserved LV function and paradoxical low-flow, low-gradient aortic stenosis. In the former group, dobutamine echocardiography or an invasive hemodynamic study is needed to distinguish true aortic stenosis from pseudostenosis. With pseudostenosis, dobutamine increases cardiac output and the opening forces on the aortic valve, causing the valve area to increase out of the severe range. With true aortic stenosis, the calculated valve area remains in the severe range with dobutamine administration, and the aortic valve gradient and velocity increase with increased stroke volume. In patients with paradoxical low-flow, low-gradient aortic stenosis, low stroke volume (<35 mL/m^2) results from a combination of small LV size and high aortic impedance to flow (hypertension). Determination of lesion severity in paradoxical aortic stenosis requires consideration of the hemodynamics, valve morphology (such as degree of degeneration), presence of LV hypertrophy, and clinical presentation of the patient. In patients with either low-flow, low-gradient severe aortic stenosis or paradoxical low-flow, low-gradient severe aortic stenosis, observational studies have shown improved survival with aortic valve replacement compared with medical therapy.

Management

Aortic valve replacement is a life-prolonging procedure in patients with severe aortic stenosis. The indications for aortic valve replacement in severe aortic stenosis are (1) the presence of symptoms (such as dyspnea, angina, presyncope, or syncope), (2) LV systolic dysfunction (ejection fraction <50%) in an asymptomatic patient, or (3) a concomitant cardiac surgical procedure for another indication (such as simultaneous coronary artery bypass grafting or ascending aorta surgery). Aortic valve replacement may be considered in asymptomatic patients with abnormal results on supervised exercise testing, such as those with poor exercise tolerance, abnormal electrocardiographic changes, or hypotension during testing.

Aortic valve replacement can be performed with open cardiac surgery (surgical aortic valve replacement [SAVR]) or via transcatheter approach (transcatheter aortic valve replacement [TAVR]) (**Figure 22**). SAVR and TAVR have similar procedural and long-term survival rates, with expected operative mortality rates of 1% to 3%. The choice between surgical and transcatheter interventions is based on the presence of symptoms and the patient's surgical risk, as determined through comprehensive assessment by a multidisciplinary heart team. TAVR is currently indicated for symptomatic patients with trileaflet aortic stenosis who are at intermediate or high surgical risk and who do not have concomitant severe aortic regurgitation. Randomized trials comparing TAVR with SAVR in low-risk patients are ongoing.

Although the pathophysiology of aortic stenosis is known to be inflammatory, randomized trials of medical therapy, specifically statins, have not found this therapy to be effective in slowing disease progression. For patients with coexistent

examination and the echocardiographic results in symptomatic patients being considered for surgery.

Severe aortic stenosis is typically defined by a small valve area (≤1.0 cm^2) and either high peak velocity (>4 m/s) or high mean gradient (>40 mm Hg). There are two patient subsets in which severe aortic stenosis may be present with a small valve

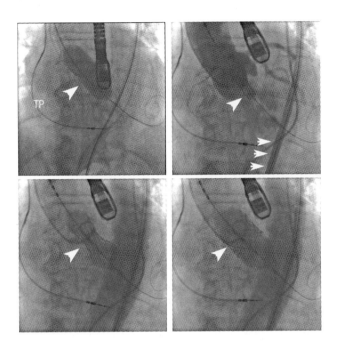

FIGURE 22. Transcatheter aortic valve replacement. *Top left panel:* Balloon aortic valvuloplasty (*arrowhead*) is first performed. *Top right panel:* Using a transfemoral approach (*arrows*), a transcatheter aortic valve (*arrowhead*) is positioned at the aortic annulus using aortography. *Bottom left panel:* The prosthesis (*arrowhead*) is then slowly inflated using rapid pacing from a temporary pacemaker (TP), which creates ventricular standstill. *Bottom right panel:* The prosthesis is fully deployed.

hypertension or heart failure, guideline-directed medical therapy is recommended. Vasodilators should be used with caution in patients with aortic stenosis and heart failure symptoms. In select cases, balloon valvuloplasty may be used to bridge patients to therapy with TAVR or SAVR.

KEY POINTS

- The most common cause of severe aortic stenosis is degeneration of the aortic valve.
- The characteristic physical findings of severe aortic stenosis include a late-peaking systolic murmur, a diminished or absent aortic component of the S_2, and a weak and delayed carotid upstroke.
- Echocardiography is accurate for defining the severity of aortic stenosis in most patients; when there is a discrepancy between the clinical and echocardiographic findings, cardiac catheterization should be considered in patients who are surgical candidates.
- Aortic valve replacement is a life-prolonging intervention in patients with severe aortic stenosis; the patient's surgical risk and the presence of symptoms determine whether aortic valve replacement is performed using open surgery or a transcatheter approach.
- Transcatheter aortic valve replacement is indicated for symptomatic patients with trileaflet aortic stenosis who are at intermediate or high surgical risk and who do not have concomitant severe aortic regurgitation.

Aortic Regurgitation

Clinical Presentation and Evaluation

Aortic regurgitation may be caused by aortic root pathology or intrinsic valve disease and can manifest acutely or chronically. Causes of chronic aortic regurgitation include ascending aortic dilatation and valve abnormalities due to bicuspid disease, calcific degeneration, rheumatic involvement, or chest radiation. Causes of acute aortic regurgitation are endocarditis, blunt chest trauma, iatrogenic causes (such as complications of balloon aortic valvuloplasty), and aortic dissection.

In chronic aortic regurgitation, volume overload causes progressive LV dilatation and eccentric hypertrophy. Chronic aortic regurgitation may be tolerated for many years but can eventually lead to symptoms, including shortness of breath, fatigue, or angina. Physical findings result from the large stroke volume and LV dilatation and include bounding peripheral pulses, displacement of the LV apex, and a diastolic decrescendo murmur heard either along the right sternal border (suggesting root pathology) or left sternal border (suggesting valve pathology) (see Table 21). The large forward stroke volume can also result in an early-peaking systolic ejection murmur. In patients with acute regurgitation, the abrupt onset of volume overload may not be well tolerated, and these patients can present with acute heart failure or even cardiogenic shock. Additionally, patients with acute regurgitation may not have bounding pulses because stroke volume has not markedly increased, and murmurs may be softer or shorter in duration, owing to the rapid equalization of pressures between the aorta and LV.

TTE is recommended for the evaluation of aortic regurgitation and LV function. When endocarditis is suspected and transthoracic imaging is suboptimal, transesophageal echocardiography (TEE) is advised. As an alternative, cardiac magnetic resonance (CMR) imaging and invasive angiography also can be used to determine the severity of regurgitation. Criteria for severe aortic regurgitation include a jet width that occupies 65% of the LV outflow tract or more, vena contracta greater than 0.6 cm, holodiastolic flow in the descending aorta, regurgitation volume of 60 mL or more, and effective regurgitant orifice area of 0.3 cm² or greater. The LV is also typically dilated in chronic aortic regurgitation. For patients suspected of having an aortic root abnormality, an evaluation with CMR imaging, CT, or TEE is recommended.

Management

Acute aortic regurgitation due to aortic dissection is a surgical emergency. For other acute causes, the indications for surgery depend on severity, presence of symptoms, and the hemodynamic stability of the patient. In cases of chronic aortic regurgitation, surgery with traditional open aortic valve replacement is advised for patients with symptoms (typically, dyspnea or angina), those with LV dysfunction (ejection fraction <50%), or patients undergoing other cardiac surgery. Surgical treatment of aortic regurgitation is reasonable in cases of significant LV

CONT.

dilatation (end-systolic diameter >50 mm or indexed end-systolic dimension >25 mm/m^2). Aortic valve repair without valve replacement may be performed in centers of expertise. Follow-up of asymptomatic patients is based on severity of regurgitation and other factors (see Table 23).

Medical therapy, preferably with dihydropyridine calcium channel blockers (nifedipine, isradipine, felodipine, nicardipine, nisoldipine, lacidipine, and amlodipine), ACE inhibitors, or angiotensin receptor blockers, is recommended in patients with chronic aortic regurgitation in the setting of hypertension. In the absence of hypertension, medical therapy is appropriate for symptomatic patients who are not surgical candidates.

KEY POINTS

- Characteristic physical findings of chronic aortic regurgitation include bounding peripheral pulses, displacement of the left ventricular apex, and a diastolic decrescendo murmur heard along the right sternal border or left sternal border.

- Emergent surgery is indicated for patients with acute aortic regurgitation due to aortic dissection.

- In cases of chronic aortic regurgitation, surgery with traditional open aortic valve replacement is advised for patients with symptoms, those with left ventricular dysfunction, or patients undergoing other cardiac surgery.

- Medical therapy with dihydropyridine calcium channel blockers, ACE inhibitors, or angiotensin receptor blockers is recommended for patients with aortic regurgitation and hypertension; in the absence of hypertension, medical therapy is appropriate in symptomatic patients who are not surgical candidates.

Bicuspid Aortic Valve Disease

Bicuspid aortic valve disease affects approximately 1% to 2% of the general population. Bicuspid morphology leads to abnormal shear forces and predisposes to early degeneration of the valve, resulting in stenosis in most patients (up to 75%) (see Figure 20) and pure regurgitation in a small minority of patients (2%-10%). Patients with a bicuspid aortic valve typically present with an incidental systolic ejection murmur in adolescence or young adulthood and gradually progress to severe disease in the fifth or sixth decade of life. More than one third of those older than 70 years with severe aortic stenosis have an underlying bicuspid valve.

A bicuspid aortic valve is often accompanied by abnormalities in the aortic arch, independent of the severity of aortic stenosis or regurgitation, and may be associated with aneurysms, dissection, or coarctation. Therefore, in patients with a bicuspid aortic valve, the aortic arch should be examined for aortopathy with CMR imaging, echocardiography, or cardiac CT; serial imaging is indicated if abnormalities are detected. The imaging modality and frequency depend on several factors, including the location and severity of the abnormalities, age of the patient, family history, and candidacy for surgery (see Diseases of the Aorta). Importantly, bicuspid aortic valve disease is heritable, and first-degree relatives should be screened for its presence with echocardiography.

Management of bicuspid aortic valve disease depends on the predominant lesion type (aortic stenosis or regurgitation) and its severity. In patients with a bicuspid valve who are undergoing surgery for severe aortic stenosis or regurgitation, surgical repair of the ascending aorta is advised when the aortic diameter is greater than 4.5 cm. In the absence of surgical indications for a stenotic or regurgitant aortic valve, surgical repair of the ascending aorta or aortic sinuses is advised when the aortic diameter is greater than 5.5 cm or when the diameter is greater than 5.0 cm with additional risk factors for dissection (family history, rate of progression ≥0.5 cm/year).

No medical therapies slow aortic dilatation in patients with aortopathy and a bicuspid aortic valve. Blood pressure should be controlled in patients with concomitant hypertension.

KEY POINTS

- Bicuspid morphology predisposes to early degeneration of the aortic valve, resulting in stenosis in most patients and pure regurgitation in few patients.

- Patients with a bicuspid aortic valve typically present with an incidental systolic ejection murmur in adolescence or young adulthood and gradually progress to severe disease in the fifth or sixth decade of life.

- Management of bicuspid aortic valve disease follows the recommendations for the predominant valve lesion type (aortic stenosis or regurgitation) and severity of the valvular disease.

Mitral Stenosis
Clinical Presentation and Evaluation

The leading cause of mitral stenosis is rheumatic heart disease, which has a higher predilection for women than men (female-to-male ratio of 4:1). Although relatively uncommon in the United States, rheumatic heart disease is frequent in populations with limited access to treatment for streptococcal pharyngitis. Rheumatic heart disease results in fusion of the mitral commissures and, in more advanced forms, calcification of the valve and abnormalities in the subvalvular apparatus (**Figure 23**). Other causes of mitral stenosis are parachute mitral valve, chest radiation, and severe mitral annular calcification. Mitral annular calcification is more common in the elderly and is associated with inflammatory disorders, peripheral artery disease, and chronic kidney disease.

The natural history of mitral stenosis is characterized by a slow progression over decades, with gradual enlargement of the left atrium (LA) and preservation of LV function. Symptoms

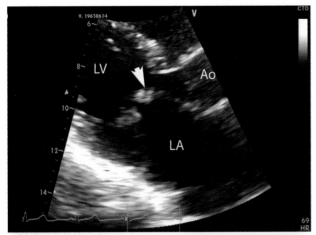

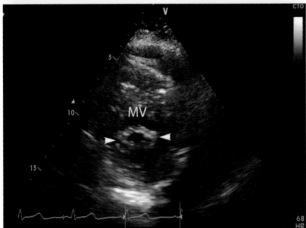

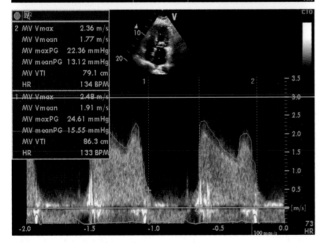

FIGURE 23. Rheumatic mitral stenosis. *Top panel:* Diastolic doming (*arrowhead*) is present with a "hockey stick" deformity from mitral stenosis. *Middle panel:* Commissural fusion (*arrowheads*) of the mitral valve (MV) is present. *Bottom panel:* Doppler echocardiogram showing a mitral gradient of 13 mm Hg, consistent with severe stenosis. Ao = ascending aorta; LA = left atrium; LV = left ventricle.

of mitral stenosis may arise from low cardiac output (fatigue), pulmonary congestion (dyspnea), and pulmonary hypertension with right-sided heart failure (lower extremity edema). Symptoms typically occur with exertion because exercise shortens diastolic filling time and increases the transvalvular

flow and diastolic mitral gradient, leading to worsening of LA hypertension. Symptoms may first occur during pregnancy owing to increased blood volume and cardiac output. Patients can also present with systemic embolization, atrial fibrillation, or, in severe cases, hemoptysis. Heart failure is the cause of death in approximately 60% of patients with mitral stenosis, and thromboembolism is the cause in most others.

On physical examination, the findings of mitral stenosis when the valve is pliable include a tapping LV impulse in the precordium, a loud S_1, an increased pulmonic component of S_2, a diastolic opening snap, and a diastolic rumble or low-pitched murmur at the apex (see Table 21). Signs of pulmonary or systemic congestion may be present depending on the severity of the lesion and the patient's volume status.

TTE is highly accurate for assessing mitral stenosis severity, pulmonary pressures, and right ventricular function (see Table 23). Additional imaging or cardiac catheterization is rarely required. Severe mitral stenosis is defined by a mitral valve area of 1.5 cm² or less, which usually corresponds to a mean mitral gradient of more than 5 to 10 mm Hg at a normal heart rate. In patients with a discrepancy between the clinical findings and the echocardiographic findings, stress echocardiography with pharmacologic or physical stressors should be pursued to assess the response of the mitral gradient and pulmonary pressures.

Management

The procedure of choice for patients with significant rheumatic mitral stenosis and a pliable mitral valve is percutaneous balloon mitral commissurotomy (PBMC). PBMC is indicated for symptomatic patients with severe mitral stenosis and favorable valve morphology. PBMC may be considered in asymptomatic patients with critical mitral stenosis when the valve area is less than 1.0 cm². In patients with LA thrombus, moderate mitral regurgitation, or a severely calcified valve, PBMC should not be performed. In appropriately selected patients, success rates with PBMC are 95%, and complications occur in less than 5% of patients. Surgery for mitral stenosis should be performed in patients with severe symptoms (New York Heart Association functional class III or IV) and a nonpliable valve or concomitantly in patients undergoing other cardiac surgical procedures.

Nearly 50% of patients with mitral stenosis have atrial fibrillation, and without anticoagulation therapy, these patients have a risk for thromboembolism of 20% to 25%. Patients with mitral stenosis and atrial fibrillation should receive warfarin, with a goal INR of 2.0 to 3.0. Other indications for anticoagulation are a history of LA thrombus or systemic embolization. Notably, clinical trials of non–vitamin K antagonist oral anticoagulants in atrial fibrillation excluded patients with mitral stenosis; therefore, the efficacy and safety of these agents in this population have not been demonstrated.

Because the mitral gradient is heavily dependent on transvalvular flow, medical therapy with negative chronotropic agents, diuretics, and long-acting nitrates can be effective for symptom palliation in patients who are not candidates for interventional or surgical therapy.

Mitral Regurgitation

Clinical Presentation and Evaluation

Mitral regurgitation may arise from any portion of the complex valve apparatus (such as the leaflets, annulus, chordae, papillary muscles, or LV free walls) and may present acutely or chronically. Causes of acute mitral regurgitation are infective endocarditis, papillary muscle ischemia or rupture, trauma (for example, injury from PBMC), or degenerative disease with chordal rupture and flail leaflet. Chronic mitral regurgitation is classified as primary or secondary. Chronic primary mitral regurgitation relates to processes involving any portion of the mitral annulus. Common causes of primary mitral regurgitation are mitral valve prolapse (also known as myxomatous or degenerative mitral valve disease), radiation therapy, rheumatic disease, and cleft mitral valve. Chronic secondary mitral regurgitation involves causes other than the annulus, such as ventricular dysfunction. H

Mitral regurgitation results in volume overload with LV dilatation and LA hypertension, which may progress and cause pulmonary hypertension and right ventricular failure. In acute mitral regurgitation, heart failure symptoms often occur abruptly because there has not been time for adaptive chamber dilatation, and patients may present with cardiogenic shock. The systolic murmur in acute mitral regurgitation may be brief because of the rapid equalization of LA and LV pressures. Echocardiography with color flow imaging can underestimate the severity of the regurgitation. Thus, when acute mitral regurgitation is suspected, comprehensive assessment to identify the potential causes should be pursued, and additional imaging with TEE should be considered. Aggressive evaluation and accurate diagnosis are crucial for patients with acute mitral regurgitation.

Chronic primary mitral regurgitation is predominantly caused by mitral valve prolapse, which affects approximately 2% of the general population or roughly 500,000 persons in the United States. Echocardiography in patients with chronic primary mitral regurgitation may show a range of abnormalities, including prolapse, gross degeneration of one or both leaflets (Barlow syndrome), or chordal rupture with flail leaflet

(**Figure 24**). Barlow syndrome is more common in young adult patients. In patients who are relatively older, fibroelastic deficiency predominates and frequently results in chordal rupture. The mitral valve apparatus is normal in patients with chronic secondary mitral regurgitation (**Figure 25**). In these patients, ventricular dysfunction causes mitral regurgitation through papillary muscle displacement and tethering of the mitral leaflets, which impairs coaptation.

The physical examination in patients with chronic mitral regurgitation is notable for a blowing holosystolic murmur at the apex. In patients with mitral valve prolapse, one or more systolic clicks may precede the murmur, and variation in severity, preload, and afterload can lead to differences in murmur onset (holosystolic, midsystolic, or late systolic). In patients with LV dilatation, the apical impulse may be displaced laterally, and an S_3 may be audible, especially in patients with secondary mitral regurgitation due to LV dysfunction.

TTE readily assesses the severity of primary mitral regurgitation, with a high degree of accuracy and precision. Severe primary mitral regurgitation is defined by using several parameters; the most common is an effective regurgitant orifice area of 0.4 cm² or larger, regurgitant volume of 60 mL or more, or vena contracta of 0.7 cm or larger. In some instances, TEE may be required to further elucidate the mechanism of the mitral regurgitation, particularly when surgical or interventional therapy is planned. TEE may be especially useful in evaluating for acute mitral regurgitation, in which rapid systolic equalization of LV and LA pressures can pose challenges for both the bedside examination and TTE imaging. H

Appropriate follow-up of asymptomatic patients with mitral regurgitation is outlined in Table 23.

Management

Medical therapy and surgical intervention can be life-saving in patients with acute severe mitral regurgitation. Vasodilator therapy with a titratable drug, such as nitroprusside, decreases aortic impedance and mitral regurgitation, thereby improving forward cardiac output. An intra-aortic balloon pump can be used to decrease afterload and augment systemic and coronary perfusion pressures. Prompt surgical correction should be considered for all patients with acute severe mitral regurgitation. H

Patients with chronic severe primary mitral regurgitation generally do poorly without surgery, particularly when there are significant symptoms, flail leaflet, or LV dilatation. In one study of 458 patients with asymptomatic severe primary mitral regurgitation, the 5-year survival rate was only 58%. Surgical treatment with repair of the mitral valve is indicated for chronic severe primary mitral regurgitation in (1) symptomatic patients with left ventricular ejection fraction (LVEF) greater than 30%, (2) asymptomatic patients with LV dysfunction (LVEF of 30%-60% and/or LV end-systolic diameter ≥40 mm), or (3) patients undergoing another cardiac surgical procedure. Surgical repair is reasonable in asymptomatic patients with preserved LV function when the expected repair success rate is

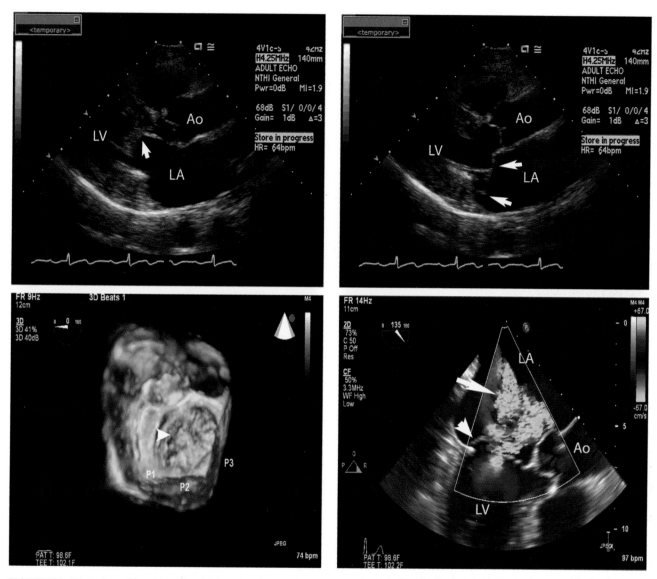

FIGURE 24. Mitral valve prolapse. Echocardiogram showing normal opening of the mitral valve (*arrow, top left panel*), which then prolapses into the left atrium during systole (*arrows, top right panel*). In a different patient with myxomatous degeneration, a flail portion of the posterior mitral valve is present (*bottom panels*); torn chordae are seen (*arrowheads*), leading to severe regurgitation seen on color flow imaging (*arrow, bottom right panel*). Ao = ascending aorta; LA = left atrium; LV = left ventricle.

greater than 95% and the operative risk is less than 1% or when serial imaging studies have demonstrated a progressive increase in LV size or decrease in LVEF. Mitral valve repair should also be considered in asymptomatic patients with chronic severe primary mitral regurgitation who have new-onset atrial fibrillation or pulmonary hypertension (pulmonary artery systolic pressure >50 mm Hg). Surgical repair is preferred over replacement in all patients, and patients should be referred to a surgical center with expertise in valve repair. Medical therapy with vasodilators in patients with primary mitral regurgitation is not beneficial in the absence of symptoms or LV dysfunction.

For patients who are not surgical candidates, mitral valve repair with a catheter-based clip device was approved by the FDA in 2013. The percutaneously delivered clip improves coaptation of the mitral valve leaflets, leading to increased valve closure and a reduction in regurgitation. In selected patients with primary mitral regurgitation, success rates with implantation of the device are approximately 90%, with a procedural mortality of approximately 2%.

In patients with chronic secondary mitral regurgitation, the primary goal of therapy is to address the underlying ventricular dysfunction with guideline-directed medical therapy and, if indicated, cardiac resynchronization therapy (see Heart Failure). Guideline-directed medical therapy for ventricular dysfunction includes ACE inhibitors, angiotensin receptor blockers, an angiotensin receptor–neprilysin inhibitor, β-blockers, diuretics, and/or aldosterone antagonists. Benefits of valve repair or replacement in patients with secondary mitral regurgitation are less certain, although studies have

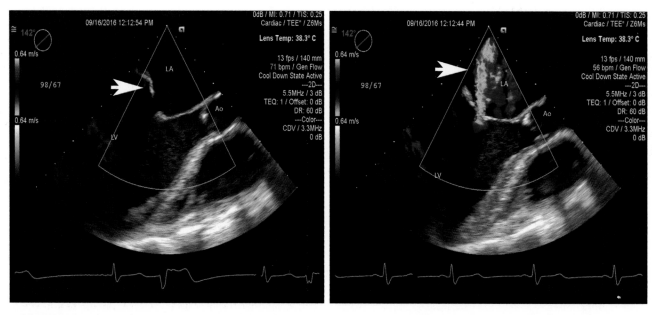

FIGURE 25. Secondary mitral regurgitation in a patient with prior inferior myocardial infarction. Tethering of the posterior leaflet (*arrow*) is present due to the prior infarction and left ventricular remodeling (*left panel*). Mitral regurgitation (*arrow*) is evident on color flow imaging (*right panel*). Ao = ascending aorta; LA = left atrium; LV = left ventricle.

demonstrated favorable LV remodeling after surgery. Surgery for secondary mitral regurgitation is generally advised for those undergoing concomitant cardiac surgical procedures (for example, coronary artery bypass grafting), but mitral regurgitation may recur after repair because of primary LV dysfunction. Trials of transcatheter mitral valve replacement for patients with secondary mitral regurgitation and high surgical risk are ongoing.

KEY POINTS

- Patients with acute mitral regurgitation may present with acute heart failure; these patients may be difficult to diagnose clinically or with echocardiography.

- The most common cause of chronic primary mitral regurgitation is mitral valve prolapse.

- Surgery for chronic severe primary mitral regurgitation is indicated in the presence of symptoms, left ventricular dilatation, or need for concomitant cardiac surgery.

- Surgical repair is preferred over replacement in patients with chronic primary mitral regurgitation, and patients should be referred to a surgical center with expertise to improve the chances of repair.

- Transcatheter mitral valve repair with implantation of a clip device is indicated for patients with chronic primary mitral regurgitation who are at high surgical risk.

- Patients with chronic secondary mitral regurgitation should be treated with guideline-directed medical therapy for ventricular dysfunction, although surgical intervention may be considered for those undergoing concomitant cardiac surgery.

Tricuspid Valve Disease

Tricuspid regurgitation, the most common form of tricuspid valve disease, is frequently functional and clinically asymptomatic. Causes of tricuspid regurgitation include cor pulmonale (or pulmonary hypertension) with right ventricular failure, pacemaker or defibrillator lead placement, trauma, congenital abnormalities, and infective endocarditis. When symptomatic, patients can present with fatigue from low cardiac output and symptoms and signs of right-sided failure, such as elevated jugular venous pulse (a large c-v wave), a palpable right ventricular lift, hepatic congestion with pulsatile liver, and peripheral edema. The murmur of tricuspid regurgitation is typically a holosystolic murmur heard along the left sternal border that increases during inspiration due to increased venous return.

Tricuspid regurgitation should be evaluated by TTE, which also allows assessment of right ventricular function and estimation of pulmonary pressures. In patients with tricuspid regurgitation due to pacemaker or defibrillator lead placement, TEE may be required to more clearly evaluate the regurgitant murmur.

Medical therapy with loop diuretics and aldosterone antagonists is effective in improving symptoms of right-sided congestion; however, caution should be exercised to minimize the potential for creating a low-flow state with impaired cardiac output. Surgery is recommended for patients with severe tricuspid regurgitation who are undergoing left-sided valve surgery. Additionally, surgery may be considered in patients with symptomatic tricuspid regurgitation who are unresponsive to medical therapy or have right-sided heart failure.

Tricuspid stenosis is nearly always caused by rheumatic disease. Other causes include radiation therapy, carcinoid syndrome, and medication use (for example, the ergot agents pergolide or cabergoline). Symptoms of tricuspid stenosis (fatigue, cold skin) are typically overshadowed by those caused by the left-sided abnormalities of coexistent rheumatic mitral disease. Findings on physical examination include those of right-sided congestion (elevated jugular venous pulse, hepatic congestion, peripheral edema) and a diastolic rumble. Surgery for tricuspid stenosis is typically performed in concert with therapy for rheumatic mitral disease.

KEY POINTS

- Loop diuretics and aldosterone antagonists can improve symptoms of right-sided congestion in patients with significant tricuspid regurgitation.

- Tricuspid valve surgery is recommended for patients with severe tricuspid regurgitation undergoing left-sided valve surgery and may be considered in select cases of severe tricuspid regurgitation that are refractory to medical therapy.

Prosthetic Valves

The choice of prosthesis for a patient undergoing surgical valve replacement is complex. Factors to consider are the patient's age, the expected durability of the prosthesis, the surgical risk for reoperation in the event of degeneration, and the ability and willingness of the patient to take warfarin for anticoagulation. The American College of Cardiology/American Heart Association VHD guideline recommends a mechanical valve prosthesis in patients younger than 50 years, bioprosthesis in patients older than 70 years, and either a bioprosthesis or mechanical valve prosthesis in those age 50 to 70 years. However, the final decision on valve type should be reached through a shared decision-making process between the care provider and patient. The patient should thoroughly understand the risks and benefits as well as have decision-making capacity. Additional considerations include the expected durability of bioprostheses (15 years) and that structural deterioration of the valve is more common in younger patients. In those younger than 60 years, approximately 40% of valves have evidence of clinically severe deterioration by 15 years.

Immediately after implantation, all patients should undergo echocardiography to document the baseline hemodynamic performance of the valve, and repeat evaluations should be performed for signs or symptoms of prosthetic dysfunction. Annual evaluation is recommended for all patients with a bioprosthesis beginning at 10 years after surgery. Data on long-term durability of TAVR prostheses are currently limited to a follow-up of 5 years; however, thus far, valve durability is not different from surgical prostheses.

Lifelong warfarin anticoagulation is indicated in all patients with a mechanical valve prosthesis. In recent VHD guidelines, the goal INR for warfarin anticoagulation in patients with a mechanical prosthesis has shifted from a range to a single value. This change was made to minimize the time the patient spends at the low and high ends of a target range because drifting above and below the range can be deleterious. The use of a single-value INR target can pose logistic challenges for testing and warfarin adjustments, and in those instances, recommendations to improve processes and enhance patient understanding and motivation should be considered.

In patients with a mechanical aortic valve prosthesis (bileaflet or current-generation single-tilting disc) with no additional risk factors for thromboembolism (history of embolization, hypercoagulable disorder, LV dysfunction, atrial fibrillation), the goal INR for warfarin anticoagulation is 2.5. In patients with a mechanical aortic valve prosthesis with risk factors for thromboembolism, an older-generation aortic valve prosthesis (ball-in-cage), or any mitral prosthesis, the target INR is 3.0. Because of the risk for valve thrombosis, direct thrombin inhibitors and factor Xa inhibitors should not be used for anticoagulation therapy in patients with a mechanical valve prosthesis. Oral anticoagulation with warfarin should be considered for at least 3 months and as long as 6 months after implantation of a mitral or aortic bioprosthesis. An INR of 2.5 should be targeted in these patients.

Aspirin (75-100 mg/d) is highly recommended in addition to warfarin therapy for patients with a mechanical prosthesis based on the results of randomized trials, which showed reduction in the risk for embolic events, including stroke (1.3% per year versus 4.2% per year; $P < 0.027$) and death (2.8% per year versus 7.4% per year; $P < 0.01$). For all patients with a bioprosthesis, low-dose aspirin is generally recommended. H

KEY POINTS

- A shared decision-making process should guide the choice of prosthetic valve type.

- Echocardiographic evaluation of prosthetic valve function is recommended at baseline and in patients with symptoms or signs suggesting prosthetic dysfunction.

- Annual echocardiographic evaluation is recommended for all patients with a bioprosthesis beginning at 10 years after surgery.

- Lifelong warfarin anticoagulation is indicated in all patients with a mechanical valve prosthesis.

- Antiplatelet therapy with low-dose aspirin is strongly recommended for patients with a mechanical prosthesis and is reasonable for patients with a bioprosthesis.

Infective Endocarditis

Diagnosis and Management

Infective endocarditis is a life-threatening disorder that involves native valvular structures or implanted cardiovascular devices. Such devices include cardiac valve prostheses, permanent pacemakers, implanted cardioverter-defibrillators, and occluders for repair of congenital lesions (such as atrial septal defect and ventricular septal defect occluders). Risk factors for infective endocarditis include advanced ~~age, diabetes~~ mellitus, ~~immunosuppression, injection drug use, congenital heart~~ disease, ~~cardiac transplantation with valvulopathy,~~ and an ~~implanted cardiovascular device.~~ Early diagnosis, targeted antimicrobial therapy, and consideration of early surgical intervention are paramount to the evaluation and treatment of infective endocarditis.

Infective endocarditis is diagnosed with the modified Duke criteria. Definite infective endocarditis requires either pathological confirmation (microorganisms demonstrated by culture or histologic examination of a vegetation, a vegetation that has embolized, or an intracardiac abscess specimen; or a vegetation or intracardiac abscess confirmed by histological examination showing active endocarditis) or clinical criteria consisting of ~~two major~~ criteria, ~~one major criterion plus three min~~or criteria, or ~~five minor~~ criteria (**Table 24**). Possible infective endocarditis requires one major criterion and one minor criterion, or three minor criteria. Infective endocarditis is excluded when there is a firm alternate diagnosis,

resolution of infective endocarditis syndrome with antibiotic therapy for 4 days or less, or no pathological evidence of infective endocarditis at surgery or autopsy with antibiotic therapy for 4 days or less.

Blood cultures are positive in 90% of infective endocarditis cases. In the remaining cases (that is, culture-negative infective endocarditis), serologic testing is required to identify the causative microorganism. For patients with infective endocarditis with a prosthetic valve, the syndrome is classified according to the time from surgery as early (within 60 days), intermediate (60–365 days), and late (>365 days). Early prosthetic valve endocarditis (PVE) is characterized by infection with hospital-acquired microbes, such as *Staphylococcus aureus*. Coagulase-negative staphylococci are the most common microbes in intermediate PVE. Although both *S. aureus* and coagulase-negative staphylococci remain important causes of late PVE, the microbes in late PVE more typically resemble those of native valve endocarditis.

TABLE 24.	Major and Minor Criteria Used in the Modified Duke Criteria
Major Criteria	
Blood culture positive for infective endocarditis	
Typical microorganisms consistent with infective endocarditis from two separate blood cultures: Viridans streptococci, *Streptococcus bovis*, HACEK group (*Haemophilus* spp., *Actinobacillus actinomycetemcomitans*, *Cardiobacterium hominis*, *Eikenella* spp., and *Kingella kingae*), *Staphylococcus aureus*; or community-acquired enterococci, in the absence of a primary focus; or	
Microorganisms consistent with infective endocarditis from persistently positive blood cultures, defined as follows:	
At least two positive cultures of blood samples drawn 12 h apart; or	
All of three or a majority of at least four separate cultures of blood (with first and last samples drawn at least 1 h apart)	
Single blood culture positive for *Coxiella burnetii* or antiphase I IgG antibody titer >1:800	
Evidence of endocardial involvement	
Echocardiogram positive for infective endocarditis (TEE recommended in patients with prosthetic valves, rated at least "possible infective endocarditis" by clinical criteria, or complicated infective endocarditis [paravalvular abscess]; TTE as first test in other patients), defined as follows:	
Oscillating intracardiac mass on valve or supporting structures, in the path of regurgitant jets, or on implanted material in the absence of an alternative anatomic explanation; or	
Abscess; or	
New partial dehiscence of prosthetic valve	
New valvular regurgitation (worsening or changing of pre-existing murmur not sufficient)	
Minor Criteria	
Predisposition, predisposing heart condition, or injection drug use	
Fever (temperature >38°C [100.4°F])	
Vascular phenomena: major arterial emboli, septic pulmonary infarcts, mycotic aneurysm, intracranial hemorrhage, conjunctival hemorrhages, and Janeway lesions	
Immunologic phenomena: glomerulonephritis, Osler nodes, Roth spots, and rheumatoid factor	
Microbiologic evidence: positive blood culture but does not meet a major criterion as noted above[a] or serologic evidence of active infection with organism consistent with infective endocarditis	

TEE = transesophageal echocardiography; TTE = transthoracic echocardiography.

[a]Excludes single culture positive for coagulase-negative staphylococci and organisms that do not cause endocarditis.

Reproduced with permission from Li JS, Sexton DJ, Mick N, Nettles R, Fowler VG Jr, Ryan T, et al. Proposed modifications to the Duke criteria for the diagnosis of infective endocarditis. Clin Infect Dis. 2000;30:637. [PMID: 10770721] Copyright 2000, Oxford University Press.

TTE is recommended to identify vegetations and associated hemodynamic derangements (for example, changes in LV function or pulmonary pressures). TEE is recommended in patients with intermediate or high suspicion for infective endocarditis when TTE is not diagnostic (such as with a prosthetic valve), intracardiac device leads are present, or complications such as abscess have developed or are suspected (conduction abnormalities on electrocardiogram or persistent bacteremia despite antibiotic therapy).

Appropriate antimicrobial therapy should be initiated once cultures have been obtained and guidance from sensitivity data and infectious disease consultants has been made available. Empiric antimicrobial therapy may be initiated in high-risk patients (such as those with septic shock) on the basis of patient characteristics, predisposing factors, and epidemiologic factors. For patients with VHD and unexplained fever, antimicrobials should not be administered before several blood cultures are drawn, and all efforts should be made to use targeted therapy when microbiologic results are available.

The decision to pursue surgery for treatment of infective endocarditis is complex and requires a multidisciplinary approach. Early surgery (during hospitalization and before completion of an antimicrobial course) is recommended for patients with (1) symptomatic heart failure and valvular dysfunction; (2) left-sided infective endocarditis caused by fungal infections or highly-resistant organisms; (3) associated complications, such as annular or aortic abscess, destructive penetrating lesions, or heart block; or (4) persistent bacteremia or fevers lasting more than 5 to 7 days despite appropriate antimicrobial therapy. Early surgery is reasonable in patients with recurrent emboli and persistent valve vegetations and may be considered in the presence of a large (>10-mm), left-sided vegetation. When infective endocarditis is associated with a pacemaker or defibrillator, the entire system (generator and leads) must be removed.

Infective endocarditis carries significant risk for morbidity and mortality, with high rates of in-hospital mortality (20%), 1-year mortality (40%), peripheral embolization (23%), stroke (17%), and need for cardiac surgery (48%).

Prophylaxis

Endocarditis prophylaxis is recommended in a specific group of patients before dental procedures that involve manipulation of gingival tissue or the periapical region of the teeth, or perforation of the oral mucosa (**Table 25**). Although endocarditis prophylaxis was previously advised for a broad population, current guidelines now recommend its use only for patients with (1) a history of endocarditis; (2) cardiac transplantation with valve regurgitation due to a structurally abnormal valve; (3) a prosthetic valve; (4) prosthetic material used for cardiac valve repair, including annuloplasty rings and chords; or (5) congenital heart disease, including unrepaired cyanotic disease, repaired lesions with residual defects at the site or adjacent to the site of a prosthetic patch or

TABLE 25. Prophylactic Infective Endocarditis Regimens for Adults at Highest Risk of an Adverse Outcome Before a Dental Procedure

Situation	Agent	Dosage[a]
Oral	Amoxicillin	2 g
Unable to take oral medication	Ampicillin	2 g IM or IV
	or	
	Cefazolin or ceftriaxone	1 g IM or IV
Allergic to penicillin or ampicillin - oral	Cephalexin[b,c]	2 g
	or	
	Clindamycin	600 mg
	or	
	Azithromycin or clarithromycin	500 mg
Allergic to penicillin or ampicillin and unable to take oral medication	Cefazolin or ceftriaxone	1 g IM or IV
	or	
	Clindamycin	600 mg IM or IV

IM = intramuscular; IV = intravenous.

[a]Regimen consists of a single dose 30 to 60 minutes before the dental procedure, or, if inadvertently not administered, drug may be given up to 2 hours after the procedure.

[b]Or other first- or second-generation oral cephalosporin in equivalent adult dosage.

[c]Cephalosporins should not be used in an individual with a history of anaphylaxis, angioedema, or urticaria with penicillins or ampicillin.

Information from Wilson W, Taubert KA, Gewitz M, Lockhart PB, Baddour LM, Levison M, et al; American Heart Association Rheumatic Fever, Endocarditis, and Kawasaki Disease Committee. Prevention of infective endocarditis: guidelines from the American Heart Association: a guideline from the American Heart Association Rheumatic Fever, Endocarditis, and Kawasaki Disease Committee, Council on Cardiovascular Disease in the Young, and the Council on Clinical Cardiology, Council on Cardiovascular Surgery and Anesthesia, and the Quality of Care and Outcomes Research Interdisciplinary Working Group. Circulation. 2007;116:1736-54. [PMID: 17446442].

prosthetic device, or disease that has been repaired with prosthetic material (surgical or catheter-based) within the previous 6 months.

KEY POINTS

- Risk factors for infective endocarditis include advanced age, diabetes mellitus, immunosuppression, injection drug use, congenital heart disease, and an implanted cardiovascular device.

- Early surgery is indicated for patients with acute infective endocarditis presenting with valve stenosis or regurgitation resulting in heart failure; left-sided infective endocarditis caused by fungal or other highly resistant organisms; infective endocarditis complicated by heart block, annular or aortic abscess, or destructive penetrating lesion; and infective endocarditis with persistent bacteremia or fever lasting longer than 5 to 7 days after starting antibiotic therapy.

Myocardial Disease

Hypertrophic Cardiomyopathy

Clinical Presentation

Hypertrophic cardiomyopathy (HCM) is a common autosomal dominant heritable disorder related to mutations in the genes that predominantly encode sarcomeric proteins. It is characterized by the presence of increased left ventricular (LV) wall thickness in the absence of loading conditions or other underlying causes. HCM affects approximately 1 in 500 persons. Most patients with HCM remain asymptomatic and have normal life expectancy; however, certain subsets of patients are more likely to develop symptomatic disease and are at risk for sudden cardiac death (SCD).

The diagnosis of HCM often results from the evaluation of a heart murmur or abnormal electrocardiogram. Symptomatic individuals usually present with signs and symptoms of heart failure or arrhythmias. HCM may be identified within all age groups. In the United States, most index cases present within the third to fourth decade of life.

Symptoms of heart failure may be associated with abnormal LV filling (diastolic dysfunction) or dynamic left ventricular outflow tract (LVOT) obstruction. Diastolic dysfunction is multifactorial, involving increased chamber stiffness related to hypertrophy, progressive fibrosis, and myocardial ischemia due to mismatch of coronary flow and LV mass. Dynamic LVOT obstruction, characterized by asymmetric LV hypertrophy with prominent interventricular septal thickening, is the most classic form of HCM. During ventricular systole, anterior motion of the mitral valve results in early to midsystolic obstruction of the LVOT and subsequent mitral regurgitation related to leaflet malcoaptation ("eject-obstruct-leak" triad). Patients with dynamic obstruction may develop dyspnea, presyncope, or syncope during periods of increased ventricular contractility (exercise) or with decreases in ventricular preload or afterload, all of which may worsen the degree of obstruction.

Arrhythmias may manifest as palpitations, syncope, atrial fibrillation, or SCD. Atrial fibrillation is common in patients with HCM, and risk increases with age. During atrial fibrillation with rapid ventricular response, diastolic filling periods shorten, worsening diastolic dysfunction; reduced LV filling may exacerbate the LVOT gradient. In some cases, SCD may be the initial presentation of HCM.

Evaluation

Physical examination may be normal in patients without LVOT obstruction. The most common finding related to LVOT obstruction is a cardiac murmur, and dynamic maneuvers during examination are helpful in differentiating HCM from fixed valvular obstruction (**Table 26**).

Twelve-lead electrocardiography (ECG) is useful in the evaluation of HCM and reveals abnormal findings in 75% to 95% of affected persons. The most common ECG abnormalities include increased QRS voltage, evidence of left atrial enlargement, LV conduction abnormalities, pathologic Q waves, and significant repolarization abnormalities (**Figure 26**); however, there is substantial interpersonal variability in the degree of abnormalities.

The clinical diagnosis of HCM is most commonly established by transthoracic echocardiography (TTE). Echocardiography demonstrates the magnitude and distribution of hypertrophy, reveals the presence and degree of dynamic LVOT obstruction and mitral regurgitation, and characterizes diastolic LV filling. Doppler echocardiography is the modality of choice for quantifying the LVOT gradient in patients suspected of having HCM. Increasingly, cardiac magnetic resonance (CMR) imaging has also been used for diagnosis, especially when the diagnosis is uncertain despite echocardiography (**Figure 27**). CMR imaging has higher resolution than echocardiography and better defines LV aneurysms and thrombi. When used with intravenous

TABLE 26. Physical Examination Findings of Dynamic Left Ventricular Outflow Tract Obstruction Versus Fixed Valvular Aortic Stenosis		
Finding or Maneuver	**Hypertrophic Cardiomyopathy with Dynamic LVOT Obstruction**	**Valvular Aortic Stenosis**
Characteristic of murmur	Ejection-quality murmur usually best heard at left lower sternal border; generally does not radiate to the carotid arteries	Ejection-quality murmur usually best heard at right second intercostal space with radiation to the carotid arteries
Carotid impulse	Brisk upstroke; may have two impulses for each ejection (bifid)	Upstroke is often diminished and delayed (parvus et tardus)
Valsalva maneuver	Increase in intensity of murmur during strain phase (+LR = 14)	No change or diminished murmur intensity during strain phase
Position	Increase in intensity of murmur with standing from squat or seated position (+LR = 6.0); decrease in murmur with elevation of legs when supine (+LR = 7.6)	No significant change in intensity of murmur with position
Peripheral pulse after PVC	No change or decrease in intensity of pulse	Increase in intensity of pulse

+LR = positive likelihood ratio; LVOT = left ventricular outflow tract; PVC = premature ventricular contraction.

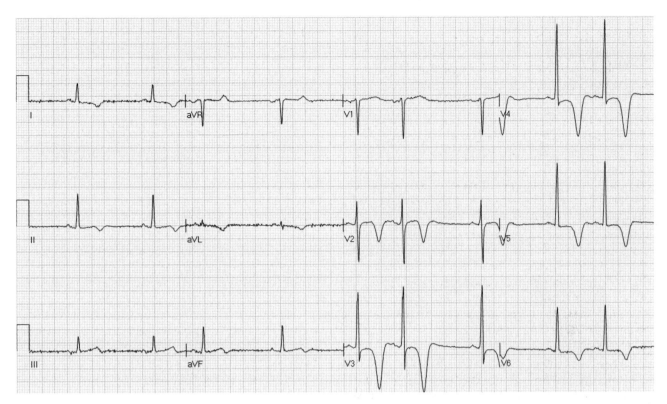

FIGURE 26. Electrocardiogram of a patient with apical hypertrophic cardiomyopathy. There are increased QRS voltage and marked repolarization abnormalities, especially in leads V_2 through V_5.

gadolinium contrast, CMR imaging has the added benefit of demonstrating the volume and distribution of late gadolinium enhancement (LGE), which reflects fibrosis. LGE has been associated with the presence of nonsustained ventricular tachycardia on ambulatory monitoring. Although studies have demonstrated a link between LGE, heart failure death, and cardiovascular death, current guidelines do not support the use of LGE for risk stratification. With more prospective data, the volume of LGE may emerge as a strong independent predictor of SCD.

Upon initial diagnosis of HCM, 24-hour ambulatory ECG monitoring should be performed to evaluate for arrhythmias. The presence of nonsustained ventricular tachycardia identifies patients at higher risk for SCD. Treadmill exercise stress testing is reasonable to determine functional status and to monitor blood pressure response to exercise. Two types of abnormal responses during exercise—a failure to increase systolic pressure more than 20 mm Hg or a drop of 20 mm Hg—may indicate independent risk for SCD. Exercise echocardiography may be useful to demonstrate the response of LVOT obstruction to exercise.

Evaluation for CAD is important in patients with HCM who develop chest discomfort. In patients with a low clinical likelihood of CAD, coronary CT angiography or nuclear myocardial perfusion imaging stress testing is reasonable for risk stratification. In patients at intermediate to high risk for CAD with chest discomfort, coronary angiography is indicated.

HCM must be differentiated from other conditions that may present with increased ventricular wall thickness (**Table 27**). Particularly challenging is the differentiation of HCM from hypertensive heart disease and from the normal and compensatory changes in LV wall thickness seen in competitive athletes. In patients with hypertension, the likelihood of concomitant HCM is increased if LV wall thickness is greater than 25 mm or if dynamic LVOT obstruction is present. In athletes, LV cavity dilatation and normal diastolic filling favor normal physiologic changes, whereas unusual or asymmetric patterns of hypertrophy on echocardiography favor HCM. A brief period of deconditioning demonstrating a decrease in wall thickness favors the athletic heart. When the diagnosis remains unclear, CMR imaging with gadolinium contrast may help with differentiation.

Risk Stratification

Patients with HCM have an annual incidence of cardiovascular death of 1% to 2%, predominantly related to fatal arrhythmia and heart failure. Most arrhythmic deaths are caused by ventricular fibrillation, and all patients with HCM, regardless of the presence of obstruction, should undergo risk stratification for SCD. Prevention with the use of an implantable cardioverter-defibrillator (ICD) is effective in appropriately selected high-risk patients. In patients with one or more established risk factors (**Table 28**), primary prevention with an ICD is indicated. Patients who have experienced SCD or

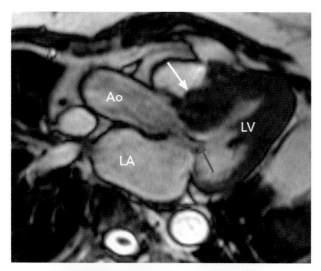

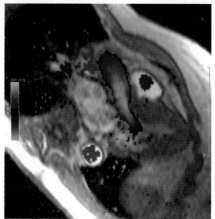

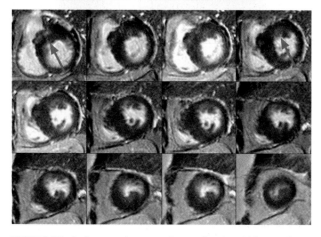

FIGURE 27. Cardiac magnetic resonance images of a patient with hypertrophic cardiomyopathy. *Top panel:* Long-axis image demonstrating marked asymmetric septal hypertrophy (*white arrow*) and systolic anterior motion of the mitral valve narrowing the left ventricular (LV) outflow tract (*red arrow*). *Middle panel:* Long-axis image with velocity flow mapping demonstrating increased flow velocity (lighter blue) originating within the LV outflow tract. *Bottom panel:* Short-axis images demonstrating patchy mid-myocardial late gadolinium enhancement (*red arrows*). Ao = aorta; LA = left atrium.

sustained ventricular tachycardia have an annual recurrent event rate of 10% and should receive an ICD for secondary prevention.

TABLE 27. Conditions with Increased Left Ventricular Wall Thickness	
Condition	**Clinical Features**
Hypertension	Elevated blood pressure
Athletic heart syndrome	No hypertension; normal or supranormal exercise capacity
Amyloidosis	Heart failure, low voltage on electrocardiography, possible neuropathy and/or nephropathy; usually older patients
Fabry disease	Male predominance (X-linked), neuropathic pain, kidney dysfunction, telangiectasias, angiokeratomas; typically young patients
Friedreich ataxia	Ataxia, scoliosis, pes cavus, visual and hearing impairment
Danon disease (*LAMP2* mutation)	Heart failure, mental retardation, skeletal myopathy; young patients

TABLE 28. Risk Factors for Sudden Cardiac Death in Patients with Hypertrophic Cardiomyopathy
Sudden death in a first-degree relative
Maximum left ventricular wall thickness ≥30 mm
Recent, unexplained syncope
Nonsustained ventricular tachycardia (≥3 beats)
Abnormal blood pressure response to exercise[a]
Sustained ventricular tachycardia or resuscitated sudden death event

[a]Defined as a failure to increase by at least 20 mm Hg or a drop of at least 20 mm Hg during effort.

Management

In addition to risk stratification for SCD and ICD therapy, management of HCM includes treatment of symptoms referable to LVOT obstruction, heart failure, and atrial fibrillation.

In patients with obstructive symptoms, such as dyspnea or syncope/near-syncope, lifestyle modification and medical therapy form the basis of management. Patients should be advised to avoid dehydration, excessive alcohol intake, and situational exposures that may result in vasodilation and decreased preload (for example, saunas, hot tubs) because these may provoke greater LVOT obstruction. Patients with probable or unequivocal clinical expression of HCM should not participate in most competitive or recreational sports, with the exception of low-intensity sports. Medical therapy should be initiated with nonvasodilating β-blockers titrated to maximum tolerance; carvedilol, labetalol, and nebivolol should be avoided. Verapamil or diltiazem may be used in patients in whom β-blockers are not tolerated or are contraindicated. Disopyramide, a class IA antiarrhythmic drug with potent negative inotropic activity, may be added if significant symptoms related to LVOT obstruction remain. Diuretics must be used cautiously and only if symptoms of dyspnea cannot be managed with other therapy. Because of their propensity to exacerbate LVOT obstruction, nitrates and phosphodiesterase type 5 inhibitors should not be used.

Invasive treatment of obstruction with open surgical septal myectomy or catheter-based alcohol septal ablation should be considered in patients who have moderate to severe symptoms of obstruction despite maximal medical therapy with a residual resting or provocable LVOT gradient of 50 mm Hg or greater, or in patients with recurrent syncope not related to arrhythmia. Although both surgical myectomy and alcohol septal ablation reduce the LVOT gradient and symptoms related to LVOT obstruction, appropriate patient selection for each procedure is controversial. Surgical myectomy is associated with a higher likelihood of complete symptom relief and lower rate for repeat procedures, and it may be associated with decreased risk for significant ventricular arrhythmias. Alcohol septal ablation carries a significant risk for atrioventricular block requiring pacemaker implantation, which is higher in older patients. Decisions regarding therapy must be individualized. Septal myectomy is favored in young patients, whereas alcohol septal ablation may be more appropriate for older patients with several comorbid conditions who have increased surgical risk. Outcomes with either procedure are best when the procedure is performed in a center with significant experience in the management of HCM. Surgical myectomy is associated with low operative mortality (0.4%) in such centers.

Atrial fibrillation should be managed with rate control and warfarin anticoagulation, irrespective of the patient's CHA_2DS_2-VASc score. Patients with HCM and atrial fibrillation often remain symptomatic despite rate control, and rhythm control in conjunction with anticoagulation should be considered early (see Arrhythmias). Digoxin should be avoided in patients with atrial fibrillation because the positive inotropic effects may worsen the LVOT gradient.

A small percentage of patients (<5%) will progress to end-stage HCM, manifesting as dilated cardiomyopathy with systolic dysfunction. These patients would appropriately be treated as would those with systolic heart failure (see Heart Failure).

Surveillance
ECG should be performed annually in asymptomatic patients with HCM to screen for changes in rhythm or conduction. Twenty-four–hour ambulatory ECG monitoring should be repeated every 1 to 2 years in asymptomatic patients and with the development of symptoms that suggest arrhythmia, such as palpitations or syncope.

Repeat TTE is recommended with any change in clinical status or new cardiac event. In asymptomatic patients, it is reasonable to repeat TTE every 1 to 2 years to assess for mitral regurgitation and changes in LV hypertrophy, function, and degree of obstruction. Although most patients with HCM demonstrate normal LV function, a decrease in LV systolic function is associated with worse outcomes, including death.

Role of Genetic Testing and Counseling
Patients known or suspected to have HCM should undergo an evaluation of familial inheritance and receive genetic counseling. Genetic testing is reasonable in patients who meet the clinical definition of HCM to aid screening of family members, but results must be interpreted carefully. A known sarcomeric mutation may be identified in up to 60% of patients with a family history of HCM; the incidence is lower (20%–30%) in isolated cases. The absence of an identified sarcomeric mutation in the index case does not exclude the diagnosis of HCM. Genetic testing is recommended in first-degree family members if a sarcomeric mutation is identified in the index case. Such testing may disclose genotype-positive persons who do not express clinical features of HCM, and these persons should be followed with clinical examination and serial echocardiography (Table 29). In the absence of a pathogenic mutation in the index case, first-degree family members should have ECG and echocardiographic screening for HCM. The use of genetic testing should not be used as the sole determinant for ICD placement for primary prevention.

TABLE 29. Proposed Clinical Screening Strategies with Echocardiography (and 12-Lead ECG) for Detection of HCM with Left Ventricular Hypertrophy in Families[a]

Age <12 y

  Optional unless:

    Malignant family history of premature death from HCM or other adverse complications

    Patient is competitive athlete in an intense training program

    Onset of symptoms

    Other clinical suspicion of early left ventricular hypertrophy

Age 12 to 18-21 y[b]

  Every 12-18 mo

Age >18-21 y

  At onset of symptoms or at least every 5 y. More frequent intervals are appropriate in families with a malignant clinical course or late-onset HCM

ECG = electrocardiography; HCM = hypertrophic cardiomyopathy.

[a]When pathologic mutations are not identified or genetic testing is either ambiguous or not performed.

[b]Age range takes into consideration individual variability in achieving physical maturity and in some patients may justify screening at an earlier age. Initial evaluation should occur no later than early pubescence.

Reproduced with permission from Gersh BJ, Maron BJ, Bonow RO, Dearani JA, Fifer MA, Link MS, et al; American College of Cardiology Foundation/American Heart Association Task Force on Practice Guidelines. 2011 ACCF/AHA guideline for the diagnosis and treatment of hypertrophic cardiomyopathy: a report of the American College of Cardiology Foundation/American Heart Association Task Force on Practice Guidelines. Developed in collaboration with the American Association for Thoracic Surgery, American Society of Echocardiography, American Society of Nuclear Cardiology, Heart Failure Society of America, Heart Rhythm Society, Society for Cardiovascular Angiography and Interventions, and Society of Thoracic Surgeons. J Am Coll Cardiol. 2011;58:e212-60. [PMID: 22075469] doi:10.1016/j.jacc.2011.06.011. Copyright 2011, Elsevier.

- Asymmetric septal hypertrophy with dynamic left ventricular outflow tract obstruction represents the classic form of hypertrophic cardiomyopathy.

- Doppler echocardiography is the modality of choice for quantification of the left ventricular outflow tract gradient in patients suspected of having hypertrophic cardiomyopathy.

- Patients with hypertrophic cardiomyopathy who have risk factors for sudden cardiac death should undergo implantable cardioverter-defibrillator placement.

- In patients with hypertrophic cardiomyopathy who have symptoms of left ventricular outflow tract obstruction, nonvasodilating β-blockers are first-line therapy.

- Transthoracic echocardiography should be performed every 1 to 2 years in asymptomatic patients with hypertrophic cardiomyopathy to assess for mitral regurgitation and changes in left ventricular hypertrophy, function, and degree of obstruction.

HVC
- Genetic testing is not indicated in first-degree relatives of patients with hypertrophic cardiomyopathy who do not have an identified sarcomeric mutation.

Restrictive Cardiomyopathy

Clinical Presentation and Evaluation

Restrictive cardiomyopathy (RCM) is a rare disorder characterized by abnormally stiff, noncompliant ventricles. RCM was once considered idiopathic; however, increasing evidence suggests that gene mutations in sarcomeric proteins and abnormalities in desmin, an intermediate filament that regulates sarcomere architecture, play an important role in familial and sporadic cases. The sarcomeric protein gene mutations of RCM are similar to or the same as those linked to HCM, raising the possibility that these disorders represent different phenotypic expressions of the same heritable defect.

RCM is characterized histologically by patchy interstitial fibrosis and myocyte disarray, which are also seen in HCM. With increasing interstitial fibrosis, the ventricles stiffen, resulting in increased pressure during normal diastolic filling. Patients may present at any age, usually with symptoms of dyspnea, peripheral edema, and exercise intolerance. Hepatomegaly and ascites may also be present late in the disease course.

The diagnosis of RCM should be suspected in patients when echocardiography demonstrates biatrial enlargement and severe diastolic dysfunction in the setting of normal ventricular size, wall thickness, and systolic function. There is usually evidence of significant pulmonary hypertension, and tricuspid and mitral valve regurgitation are commonly present. Patients with these findings should be referred to a cardiologist for further evaluation.

Primary RCM must be differentiated from other conditions that may present with restrictive physiology. These include fibrosis related to radiation and eosinophilic diseases as well as hemochromatosis, in which wall thickness is typically normal. A complete blood count with manual differential and transferrin saturation are reasonable as part of the evaluation. Infiltrative diseases with increased wall thickness may share restrictive physiology but are considered separate entities. When low ECG voltage accompanies increased wall thickness on echocardiogram, amyloidosis should be considered. Serum protein electrophoresis/urine protein electrophoresis and free light-chain analysis may help identify immunoglobulin light-chain amyloidosis, and technetium-99m cardiac imaging may help identify transthyretin amyloidosis. CMR imaging with gadolinium contrast may help identify and differentiate RCM from other myocardial diseases with restrictive physiology. When the diagnosis remains unclear, endomyocardial biopsy is reasonable to establish a diagnosis.

Differentiating Restrictive Cardiomyopathy from Constrictive Pericarditis

Patients with constrictive pericarditis and RCM present with similar symptoms and findings on echocardiography. Differentiating between these two disorders is essential because specific therapies, including surgical pericardiectomy, may relieve symptoms and prolong life in patients with constriction. In patients with previous cardiac surgery, pericarditis, or chest irradiation, constrictive pericarditis should be strongly considered.

On physical examination, patients with constriction and RCM both demonstrate increased jugular venous pressure. Increase in the height of the jugular waveform during inspiration (Kussmaul sign) has been associated more commonly with constriction. Both RCM and constrictive pericarditis may be associated with a diastolic sound. An S_3 gallop is often present in RCM, whereas a pericardial knock can be heard in constrictive pericarditis. Differentiating between these sounds may be very difficult (see Pericardial Disease).

A multimodality approach, including both noninvasive imaging and invasive hemodynamic evaluation, may be required to distinguish RCM from constrictive pericarditis. Clues to the presence of constrictive pericarditis include pericardial calcification on chest radiography or CT, pericardial thickening on CT or CMR imaging, or a B-type natriuretic peptide level below 100 pg/mL (100 ng/L) (usually ≥400 pg/mL [400 ng/L] in patients with RCM). A hallmark feature of constrictive pericarditis is ventricular interdependence, in which total cardiac volume is limited by the rigid pericardium. With ventricular interdependence, increased filling of the right or left ventricle can occur only with reciprocal decreased filling of the other ventricle. Ventricular interdependence may be demonstrated by Doppler echocardiography, CMR imaging, or invasive hemodynamic evaluation; it is not present in patients with RCM.

Management

There is no specific medical therapy for RCM. Loop diuretics are usually necessary for relief of congestive symptoms, especially in late-stage disease. However, patients with RCM require relatively high filling pressures to maintain cardiac output, and balancing relief of congestion with adequate cardiac output is often challenging. Even small changes in volume may lead to hypoperfusion of the kidneys; therefore, volume status should be monitored carefully.

Atrial fibrillation is a common complication due to left atrial dilatation and elevated pressure. It is poorly tolerated in patients with RCM because of increased heart rate and reduced ventricular filling. Anticoagulation and rate control are indicated, and rhythm control should be considered early in symptomatic patients. Digoxin should be used with caution because it indirectly increases intracellular calcium, which may affect diastolic relaxation.

Survival is poor in patients with RCM, with a 5-year mortality rate of 36% and a 10-year mortality rate of 63%. Cardiovascular mortality is predominantly related to progressive heart failure and arrhythmias. Cardiac transplantation may be considered in selected individuals who remain symptomatic despite maximal therapy. There is no accepted indication for ICD placement for primary prevention in patients with RCM who have preserved systolic function.

KEY POINTS

- Restrictive cardiomyopathy should be suspected in patients when echocardiography demonstrates biatrial enlargement and severe diastolic dysfunction in the setting of normal ventricular size, wall thickness, and systolic function.
- Restrictive cardiomyopathy must be differentiated from constrictive pericarditis because surgical pericardiectomy may relieve symptoms and prolong life in patients with constriction.

Cardiac Tumors

Most cardiac tumors are metastatic. Neoplasms with the highest metastatic potential are melanoma, malignant thymoma, and germ cell tumors. Common tumors with an intermediate risk for cardiac involvement include carcinoma of the lung, stomach, and colon. Therapy is directed at systemic treatment of the underlying neoplasm, with cardiac surgery reserved for patients with obstructive symptoms.

Primary cardiac tumors, which are exceedingly rare, are benign in two thirds of patients. Of the benign tumors, nearly 50% are atrial myxomas. Myxomas may occur in either atria but are most commonly attached to the fossa ovalis within the left atrium (**Figure 28**). Myxomas are usually solitary and discovered at a mean age of 50 years, often after a systemic embolic event. When tumors are multiple, recurrent, or discovered at a young age, they may indicate the Carney complex, which includes the LAMB (lentigines, atrial myxoma, blue nevi) syndrome and the NAME (nevi, atrial myxoma, myxoid neurofibromas, and ephelides) syndrome. The Carney complex is associated with mutations of the *PRKAR1A* gene, which may function as a tumor suppressor gene. Patients with a myxoma may present with constitutional symptoms related to interleukin production, embolic phenomena from tumor fragmentation, or symptoms referable to intracardiac obstruction (dyspnea, syncope). When mitral valvular obstruction is present, auscultatory findings are similar to those of mitral stenosis; however, findings may vary with position or be associated with an early diastolic sound, known as the tumor plop. Surgical removal is indicated to prevent embolic events, as is subsequent surveillance echocardiography for detection of recurrence.

Papillary fibroelastomas usually occur on the surface of the aortic and mitral valves and are commonly discovered in the eighth decade of life. Although most papillary fibroelastomas do not cause symptoms, they may be associated with stroke, transient ischemic attack, and, rarely, coronary embolization with

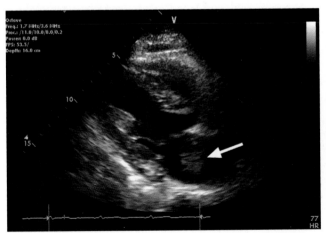 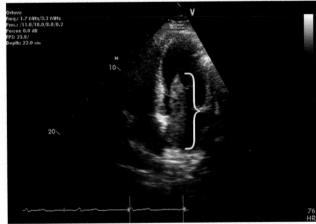

FIGURE 28. Transthoracic echocardiograms demonstrating a left atrial myxoma. *Left panel:* Parasternal long-axis view during ventricular systole showing a large left atrial soft tissue density (*arrow*). *Right panel:* Apical four-chamber view during diastole demonstrates attachment of the mass to the interatrial septum and prolapse of the mass across the mitral valve.

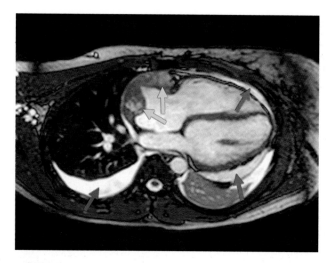

FIGURE 29. Cardiac magnetic resonance image of a patient with an angiosarcoma. A heterogeneous mass (*yellow arrows*) is infiltrating the right atrial wall. A pericardial effusion (*red arrows*) and pleural effusion (*blue arrow*) are also present.

TABLE 30.	Causes of Pericardial Disease
Category	**Cause**
Infectious	
Viral infection	Enterovirus, herpesvirus, adenovirus, parvovirus
Bacterial infection	*Mycobacterium tuberculosis*, *Pneumococcus* spp., *Staphylococcus* spp., *Coxiella burnetii*
Fungal infection	*Histoplasma, Aspergillus, Blastomyces, Candida* spp.
Noninfectious	
Autoimmune diseases	Systemic lupus erythematosus, rheumatoid arthritis, Sjögren syndrome, scleroderma, sarcoidosis, familial Mediterranean fever
Cancer	Metastatic lung cancer, breast cancer, and melanoma; lymphoma and leukemia
Metabolic conditions	Uremia, myxedema
Drug-related causes	Hydralazine, procainamide, minoxidil, all-*trans* retinoic acid
Iatrogenic causes	Cardiac surgery (postpericardiotomy syndrome), coronary perforation during percutaneous intervention, pacemaker lead penetration, radiofrequency ablation
Other	Radiation, aortic dissection, pulmonary arterial hypertension

infarction. On echocardiography, these tumors often have a heterogeneous globular shape or a mobile frond-like appearance. Patients with embolic symptoms are treated surgically. There are currently no randomized data comparing surgical therapy with antithrombotic or antiplatelet therapy to prevent embolic events.

Angiosarcomas are the most common primary malignant tumor. Angiosarcomas typically arise in the right atrium and are often associated with pericardial effusion (**Figure 29**). Dyspnea and chest pain are common presenting symptoms. Angiosarcomas are highly vascular tumors, and CT or CMR imaging with contrast may help differentiate an angiosarcoma from a right atrial myxoma. When complete surgical extirpation is possible, survival remains less than 2 years for most patients. With incomplete resection, survival is generally less than 10 months.

KEY POINT

- The primary treatment of atrial myxomas is surgical removal to prevent embolic events.

Pericardial Disease

Acute Pericarditis

Clinical Presentation and Evaluation

Pericarditis is defined as inflammation of the pericardium, the thin fibrous sac surrounding the heart. Pericarditis may be subclinical or present as sharp precordial pain of acute onset. Acute pericarditis has many causes (**Table 30**), but it is most often idiopathic or presumed to be viral in origin.

Acute pericarditis is diagnosed clinically by the presence of at least two of the following four criteria: chest pain typical for pericarditis, a pericardial friction rub, new electrocardiographic (ECG) changes, or a new pericardial effusion. The

chest pain of acute pericarditis is sharp and severe. It is not typically related to exertion and is not relieved with rest or nitroglycerin, unlike anginal pain. The pain is characteristically worse in the supine position and improves with sitting up and leaning forward. These pain features may be related to tension of the pericardium at its sternal and diaphragmatic attachments.

A pericardial friction rub is frequently present on auscultation. This harsh, scratchy sound classically has three components corresponding to the cardiac cycle during normal sinus rhythm: atrial systole, ventricular systole, and ventricular filling. The three phases of the pericardial friction rub differentiate it from a pleural friction rub, which has two components that are linked to respiration. The rub of pericarditis may also be monophasic or biphasic but is not affected by respiration. Auscultation should be performed during held end-expiration with the patient in the supine position or sitting upright.

The typical ECG feature of acute pericarditis is ST-segment elevation in multiple leads that does not correspond with a single coronary distribution. PR-segment depression in lead II or reciprocal PR-segment elevation in lead aVR may also be present (**Figure 30**). In contrast, ECG findings of acute myocardial infarction are hyperacute T waves, ST-segment elevation consistent with a single coronary distribution, reciprocal ST-segment depression, pathologic Q waves during the evolution of myocardial infarction, and lack of PR-segment change.

"knuckle sign"

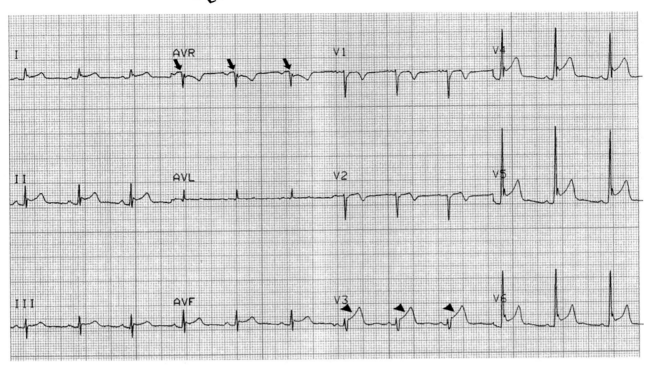

FIGURE 30. Electrocardiographic changes of acute pericarditis. Concave ST-segment elevation is present in most of the leads (*arrowheads*). The PR segment is depressed in all leads except aVR (*arrows*).

H
CONT.

Echocardiography should be used to detect a pericardial effusion, although an effusion is not found in all cases of acute pericarditis. When the diagnosis remains uncertain, cardiac magnetic resonance (CMR) imaging with gadolinium intravenous contrast may be used to identify evidence of pericardial inflammation, characterized by pericardial thickening and late gadolinium enhancement (**Figure 31**). Alternatively, gated cardiac CT may also demonstrate pericardial inflammation.

Additional findings that support acute pericarditis may include fever and serologic evidence of inflammation (leukocytosis and elevated erythrocyte sedimentation rate or C-reactive protein [CRP] level). Serum cardiac troponin levels in acute pericarditis are normal or may be slightly elevated if there is a component of myopericarditis.

Although most cases of acute pericarditis are idiopathic, a search for other causes is appropriate (see Table 30). Evaluation includes a thorough history and physical examination, with additional testing based on the suspected cause. Tuberculosis testing should be considered in hospital workers, patients who are incarcerated or residing in chronic care facilities, and patients who are from or have traveled to an endemic area. Treatment of tuberculosis may reduce the risk for reactive pericardial constriction from greater than 80% to less than 10%. Other causes include uremia, chest irradiation, and recent cardiac surgery. Cardiac surgery may be followed by postpericardiotomy syndrome, which is characterized by pericardial inflammation that is likely autoimmune in nature and usually follows a latent period of several weeks. The presentation and treatment of postpericardiotomy syndrome are similar to those of idiopathic pericarditis.

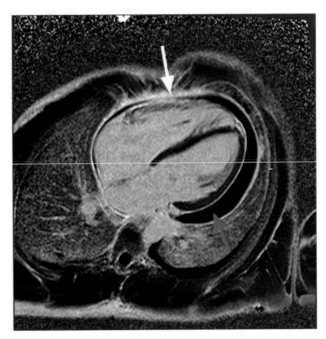

FIGURE 31. Cardiac magnetic resonance image obtained after intravenous administration of gadolinium. A pericardial effusion (*red arrow*) is present, and there is late gadolinium enhancement of the pericardium consistent with inflammation (*white arrow*).

Management

Most patients with acute pericarditis can be managed medically on an outpatient basis; however, patients with acute pericarditis accompanied by high-risk features may require hospitalization for treatment and monitoring. Predictors of poor prognosis include temperature higher than 38 °C (100.4 °F), subacute onset, a large pericardial effusion (>20-mm diastolic echo-free space) or tamponade at presentation, oral anticoagulation therapy, or lack of response (no improvement in symptoms and/or inflammatory markers) after 1 week of treatment.

First-line treatment for acute idiopathic pericarditis consists of aspirin (750-1000 mg) or NSAIDs (ibuprofen 600 mg) every 8 hours for 1 to 2 weeks. Colchicine (0.5 mg once or twice daily for 3 months) is recommended as adjunctive therapy to shorten the duration of symptoms and reduce the chances of treatment failure or recurrence. Patients who initially respond to therapy but develop recurrent pericarditis after treatment completion may benefit from a longer course of standard therapy with slow tapering. CRP may be useful as a marker of treatment response, with tapering initiated after the CRP level normalizes. Expert consensus opinion recommends that athletes not return to competitive exercise for 3 months from initial onset and that nonathletes restrict strenuous activity until symptoms resolve.

Some patients with acute pericarditis may develop incessant or chronic pericarditis. Incessant pericarditis has been defined as pericarditis lasting for longer than 4 to 6 weeks but less than 3 months without remission, whereas chronic pericarditis is defined as lasting longer than 3 months. Glucocorticoid therapy is reserved for patients with recurrent, incessant, or chronic pericarditis despite standard therapy (including patients with uremic pericarditis not responsive to intensive dialysis); patients with contraindications to NSAID therapy; and patients with autoimmune-mediated pericarditis. Prednisone should be initiated at a dosage of 0.25 mg/kg to 0.5 mg/kg and continue for 3 months. Tapering should not be initiated until after the first 2 to 4 weeks of therapy or until the CRP level normalizes.

Limited data suggest that the interleukin-1 receptor antagonist anakinra may be an effective therapy for idiopathic recurrent pericarditis that is refractory to standard treatment; however, its role in management is not established.

KEY POINTS

- Acute pericarditis is diagnosed by the presence of at least two of four criteria: chest pain typical for pericarditis, a pericardial friction rub, new electrocardiographic changes, or a new pericardial effusion.

- First-line treatment for acute idiopathic pericarditis is high-dose aspirin or NSAIDs and adjuvant colchicine therapy.

- Glucocorticoid therapy is reserved for patients with incessant, recurrent, or chronic pericarditis despite standard therapy; patients with contraindications to NSAID therapy; and patients with autoimmune-mediated pericarditis.

Pericardial Effusion and Cardiac Tamponade

Pericardial Effusion

Pericardial effusion is characterized by an increased amount of fluid in the pericardial cavity. Many patients with pericardial effusion are asymptomatic, and the effusion is discovered incidentally with chest radiography, CT, or echocardiography. In asymptomatic patients, most effusions are idiopathic; however, malignancy, infections, autoimmune disease, hypothyroidism, and iatrogenic causes (medications, anticoagulation therapy) should be considered (see Table 30). In countries where tuberculosis is endemic, more than 60% of effusions are caused by tuberculosis.

If cancer or bacterial infection is strongly suspected, pericardiocentesis should be considered for diagnostic purposes. In patients with a pericardial effusion of unknown cause and elevated inflammatory markers, empiric treatment of pericarditis may be reasonable. Drainage should be considered if large idiopathic effusions are present for more than 3 months because one in three patients progress to cardiac tamponade.

Cardiac Tamponade
Clinical Presentation and Evaluation

Cardiac tamponade occurs when fluid accumulation within the pericardial space compresses the heart and impedes diastolic filling. When fluid accumulates rapidly (such as with trauma, aortic dissection, or invasive cardiac procedures), tamponade may occur at relatively low pericardial volumes. Subacute or chronic processes, such as neoplastic disease or hypothyroidism, may be associated with much larger effusions (several hundred milliliters in volume).

Clinical signs of tamponade include tachycardia, hypotension, muffled heart sounds, and elevation of the jugular venous pulse. The y descent of the jugular venous pulse may be absent because passive filling of the ventricles is impeded by the intrapericardial pressure. This finding may be difficult to appreciate, especially in a patient with tachycardia. Pulsus paradoxus represents exaggerated ventricular interdependence and is a key clinical feature of cardiac tamponade. It is characterized by a fall in systolic pressure of greater than 10 mm Hg during inspiration. Pulsus paradoxus is not specific for tamponade and must be interpreted in conjunction with other clinical and echocardiographic features.

The ECG may demonstrate electrical alternans (related to a swinging motion of the heart within the pericardial fluid) or low voltage in patients with tamponade. If the accumulation of fluid has occurred slowly, the cardiac silhouette is typically enlarged on chest radiography.

Echocardiography is an essential tool in the diagnosis of cardiac tamponade because it defines the presence, distribution, and relative volume of pericardial fluid (**Figure 32**). Early diastolic collapse of the right ventricle, late diastolic collapse of the right atrium, and abnormal interventricular septal motion are features associated with cardiac tamponade. Additionally,

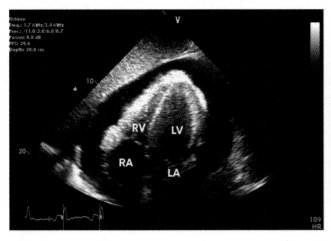
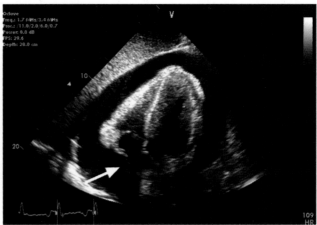

FIGURE 32. Apical four-chamber echocardiogram demonstrating a large circumferential pericardial effusion (*left panel*). Diastolic right atrial collapse (*arrow*) consistent with pericardial tamponade (*right panel*). LA = left atrium; LV = left ventricle; RA = right atrium; RV = right ventricle.

Doppler evaluation may demonstrate a decrease in mitral inflow velocity of more than 25% with inspiration, which is the echocardiographic equivalent of pulsus paradoxus (**Figure 33**).

Cardiac catheterization is rarely necessary for diagnosis. The hemodynamic hallmarks of tamponade include blunting or loss of the *y* descent within the right atrial pressure waveform and elevated and equalized diastolic pressures. The latter reflects the transmitted effect of the intrapericardial pressure. Invasive arterial pressure recordings also show pulsus paradoxus.

Management

Cardiac tamponade is life-threatening, and once a diagnosis is established, fluid removal is required. Drainage is most commonly accomplished with pericardiocentesis, with fluoroscopy or echocardiographic guidance. Surgical therapy via a subxiphoid approach is indicated to drain fluid when pericardiocentesis cannot be performed safely, to obtain pericardial tissue for diagnostic purposes, or to prevent recurrent pericardial effusion by creating a pericardial window (often used in cases of malignant pericardial effusion). In hemodynamically unstable patients, intravenous normal saline is used to stabilize the patient as a temporizing measure or as a bridge to definitive therapy.

After drainage of pericardial fluid, hemodynamic and clinical evaluation may occasionally disclose findings of underlying pericardial constriction, termed effusive constrictive pericarditis. If clinical evaluation and imaging techniques (such as CMR imaging) suggest an active inflammatory process, a course of medical therapy similar to that for acute pericarditis may be considered, and the patient should be re-evaluated before surgery is contemplated.

KEY POINTS

- Clinical signs of cardiac tamponade include tachycardia, hypotension, muffled heart sounds, elevation of the jugular venous pulse, and pulsus paradoxus.
- Patients with cardiac tamponade require drainage of pericardial fluid with pericardiocentesis; surgical drainage is indicated when pericardiocentesis cannot be performed safely, pericardial tissue is needed for diagnostic purposes, or a pericardial window is required to prevent recurrent pericardial effusion.

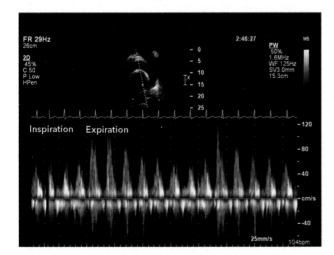

FIGURE 33. Pulsed-wave Doppler evaluation of mitral inflow velocity. A change in the flow between expiration and inspiration of greater than 25% is present, consistent with enhanced ventricular interdependence.

Constrictive Pericarditis

Clinical Presentation and Evaluation

Constrictive pericarditis is characterized by pericardial thickening, fibrosis, and sometimes calcification that impair diastolic filling and limit total cardiac volume. Within developed countries, most cases are viral or idiopathic in origin. Other causes include cardiac surgery, chest irradiation, autoimmune disease, and tuberculosis or other bacterial infection. Tuberculosis remains a major cause of constrictive pericarditis within developing countries.

CONT.

Patients with constrictive pericarditis most commonly present with indolent progression of right-sided heart failure symptoms, including peripheral edema, abdominal swelling, and fatigue. Dyspnea and fatigue limit exertion and are caused by increased diastolic pressures and limited ability to augment cardiac output due to the fixed stroke volume.

On physical examination, the jugular veins are distended, with prominent x and y descents. The height of the waveform does not fall or may increase during inspiration (Kussmaul sign), reflecting the fixed diastolic volume of the right heart. Early diastolic filling is unimpaired or even accentuated and is followed by sudden cessation when total acceptable volume is met, resulting in a high-frequency early diastolic sound (the pericardial knock). Characteristics that may be used to differentiate a pericardial knock from other diastolic sounds are listed in **Table 31**. Pulsus paradoxus is less frequent in constrictive pericarditis than in cardiac tamponade. Peripheral edema, ascites, hepatomegaly, and pleural effusions are common. Muscle wasting may be evident in advanced cases.

Constrictive pericarditis is diagnosed with imaging studies and hemodynamic evaluation. Chest radiography or CT may demonstrate partial or circumferential pericardial calcification, and CT or CMR imaging may demonstrate pericardial thickening (>3 mm). Importantly, constriction may exist in the absence of these findings. In one case series, 18% of cases of hemodynamically proven constrictive pericarditis occurred with normal pericardial thickness. CMR imaging may also demonstrate an inspiratory septal shift, a sign of ventricular interdependence.

Transthoracic echocardiography in constrictive pericarditis reveals normal right and left ventricular size and systolic function despite prominent symptoms and examination findings suggestive of heart failure. The echocardiographic finding of dilatation of the inferior vena cava reflects elevated right-sided filling (right atrial) pressure. Myocardial relaxation is impaired in myocardial disease, such as restrictive cardiomyopathy, but is unimpaired or even enhanced in constriction, in which early diastolic filling is rapid and unimpeded. Doppler echocardiography and tissue Doppler velocity are required to differentiate constrictive pericarditis from restrictive cardiomyopathy.

When constrictive pericarditis is suspected but not confirmed by echocardiography, cardiac catheterization can be performed. Invasive hemodynamic findings of constrictive pericarditis include a prominent y descent in the right atrial waveform, which corresponds with the dip of the right ventricular dip-and-plateau waveform ("square root sign"). The significant y descent and the right ventricular dip both represent unimpeded or rapid early diastolic ventricular filling. As inflow volume reaches the fixed pericardial constraint, pressure rises rapidly until maximum volume is achieved; pressure then remains constant, causing the plateau phase of the square root sign. A more specific finding is ventricular interdependence during simultaneous right and left ventricular systolic pressure measurement. During inspiration, right ventricular inflow is enhanced, and right ventricular systolic pressure rises; however, these changes occur with a concomitant decrease in left ventricular filling and reduction in left ventricular stroke volume and systolic pressure (**Figure 34**). The converse is seen during expiration.

Increased pericardial thickening and impaired distensibility may occur without fibrosis or calcification in the setting of acute or subacute inflammation. In these patients, constriction may be transient and resolve spontaneously. Patients with transient constrictive pericarditis present most commonly with symptoms of right-sided heart failure, although fever and chest pain may indicate the active inflammatory condition. Most cases are idiopathic; other causes include recent cardiac surgery, acute pericarditis, autoimmune disease, or chemotherapy. Systemic markers of inflammation (erythrocyte sedimentation rate and CRP) may be elevated in patients with transient constriction but are generally normal in patients with fixed constriction. Echocardiographic features are similar to those of fixed constriction; however, pericardial effusion is more likely to be present in patients with transient constrictive pericarditis.

Management

Treatment of transient constrictive pericarditis is the same as for acute pericarditis. Treatment with anti-inflammatory agents for 2 to 3 months is reasonable in hemodynamically stable patients before recommending surgical pericardiectomy. Response to therapy is monitored clinically,

TABLE 31. Characteristics of the Common Diastolic Heart Sounds		
Diastolic Heart Sound	**Condition**	**Characteristics**
Opening snap	Mitral stenosis	High frequency
		Heard best at the left lower sternal border and the apex
		Associated with a loud S_1, a loud P_2 with associated pulmonary hypertension, and a low-pitched diastolic rumble at the apex
Pericardial knock	Constrictive pericarditis	High frequency
		Heard throughout the precordium
		Earlier than an S_3
		Associated with deep x and y descents in the jugular venous pulse waveform
Tumor plop	Atrial myxoma	Low frequency
		Heard best at the apex
		May be positional
S_3	Heart failure	Low frequency
		Heard best at the apex and the left lateral decubitus position
		Displaced point of maximal impulse

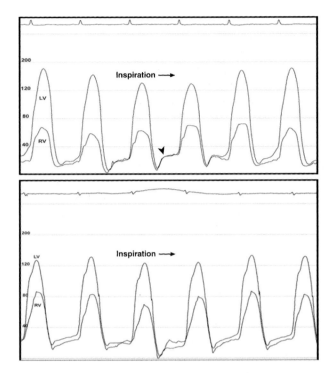

FIGURE 34. Comparison of hemodynamics of constrictive pericarditis versus restrictive cardiomyopathy. In constrictive pericarditis (*top panel*), there is significant enhancement of ventricular interdependence leading to discordance of the left ventricular and right ventricular pressures during respiration. Arrows indicate onset of inspiration and subsequent respective changes in left ventricular and right ventricular systolic pressures. In the top panel, note the diastolic dip and plateau (*arrowhead*), or "square root sign," characteristic of constrictive pericarditis. In restrictive cardiomyopathy (*bottom panel*), there is evidence of early rapid ventricular filling, but the ventricular pressures concordantly rise and fall during respiration. LV = left ventricle; RV = right ventricle.

echocardiographically, and, if initial inflammatory markers are elevated, serologically.

Patients with chronic pericardial constriction should be referred for surgical pericardial stripping (pericardiectomy performed via median sternotomy). In advanced cases, adequate resection of the pericardium may be difficult, leading to incomplete resolution of symptoms. Diuretic therapy to relieve symptoms of congestion may be useful in patients who are not deemed surgical candidates or in whom stripping was incomplete. **H**

KEY POINTS

- Constrictive pericarditis is characterized by pericardial thickening, fibrosis, and sometimes calcification that impair diastolic filling and limit total cardiac volume.

- Transthoracic echocardiography is the initial diagnostic test for evaluating constrictive pericarditis; however, additional imaging may be required to differentiate constrictive pericarditis from restrictive cardiomyopathy.

- Patients with chronic pericardial constriction should be referred for surgical pericardial stripping (pericardiectomy performed via median sternotomy).

Adult Congenital Heart Disease

Introduction

Medical and surgical advances have resulted in more adults living with congenital heart disease than children with these conditions in North America. All patients with repaired congenital cardiac defects require regular follow-up. In addition to a primary care provider, patients should have an adult congenital heart disease team. Regular care with specialists in adult congenital heart disease is critical for patients born with complex and cyanotic congenital cardiac disease, symptomatic patients, and patients who desire pregnancy. The frequency of follow-up depends on the underlying disorder and patient's status.

Patent Foramen Ovale

The foramen ovale is a passage in the superior portion of the fossa ovalis that allows oxygenated placental blood to transfer to the fetal circulation. It normally closes within the first weeks of life; however, in 25% to 30% of the population, it remains patent (**Figure 35**). A patent foramen ovale (PFO) is usually found incidentally on echocardiography or during evaluation for a cerebrovascular event.

A PFO is typically diagnosed by transesophageal echocardiography (TEE), less commonly by transthoracic echocardiography (TTE). Right-to-left shunting of blood across the PFO is demonstrated by color flow Doppler imaging or by using intravenously injected agitated saline and identifying subsequent transfer of the agitated saline through the PFO from the right atrium to the left atrium. No treatment or follow-up is needed in asymptomatic patients with an incidentally detected PFO.

Management of patients with a PFO and cryptogenic **H** stroke has been controversial. Antiplatelet therapy has traditionally been used as first-line therapy; however, three randomized trials have shown percutaneous PFO closure to be of benefit in the prevention of a second stroke in select patients. In two of the three trials, PFO closure was combined with

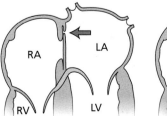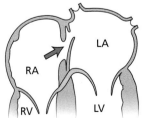

FIGURE 35. Patent foramen ovale. The arrows demonstrate the mechanism of right-to-left shunting through the patent foramen ovale. LA = left atrium; LV = left ventricle; RA = right atrium; RV = right ventricle.

Redrawn from original supplied courtesy of Dr. William D. Edwards, Department of Laboratory Medicine and Pathology, Mayo Clinic, Rochester, MN.

antiplatelet therapy. Results of these three trials demonstrated a small but statistically significant absolute risk reduction (approximately 1% per year) with closure of the PFO and a low rate of procedural complications (mainly transient atrial fibrillation). Therefore, PFO closure in addition to antiplatelet therapy can be considered in select patients after a thorough evaluation for alternative causes of stroke. Limited data support PFO closure in an effort to decrease the frequency of migraine. Asymptomatic patients require no treatment or follow-up.

Platypnea-orthodeoxia syndrome is a rare acquired disorder characterized by cyanosis and dyspnea in the upright position as a result of right-to-left shunting across a PFO or, less commonly, through an atrial septal defect. A transient increase in right atrial pressure or change in right atrial anatomy resulting from myocardial infarction, pulmonary embolism, tricuspid regurgitation, or acute right-sided heart failure may precipitate this syndrome. Device closure of the PFO may improve symptoms and oxygen saturation.

Atrial septal aneurysm is characterized by mobile, redundant atrial septal tissue that is often associated with a PFO. Atrial septal aneurysm with a PFO reportedly increases the risk for stroke compared with a PFO alone. Results of a randomized, open-label trial demonstrated that patients presenting with cryptogenic stroke in the setting of an atrial septal aneurysm with PFO had a lower rate of stroke recurrence when treated with PFO closure combined with antiplatelet therapy than with antiplatelet therapy alone. Rarely, surgical excision and defect closure is considered based on anatomic features.

KEY POINTS

HVC
- No treatment or follow-up is needed in asymptomatic patients with patent foramen ovale.
- Percutaneous closure of a patent foramen ovale can be considered in select patients with cryptogenic stroke after a thorough evaluation for alternative causes of stroke.

Atrial Septal Defect

Pathophysiology and Genetics

An atrial septal defect (ASD) is a flaw or hole in the atrial septum resulting in a left-to-right shunt with eventual right-sided cardiac chamber dilatation in most patients.

ASDs are generally classified by their location (**Figure 36**). Ostium secundum defects, the most common type of ASDs (75% of cases), are located in the mid portion of the atrial septum and are usually isolated anomalies. Located in the lowest portion of the atrial septum, ostium primum defects (15%-20% of ASDs) are a component of endocardial cushion defects. Associated abnormalities include mitral valve, ventricular septum, and subaortic anomalies. Sinus venosus defects (5%-10% of ASDs) are located near the superior vena cava or, rarely, the inferior vena cava; anomalous pulmonary venous connection

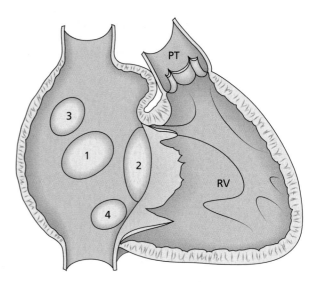

FIGURE 36. Positions of various atrial septal defects viewed from the right side of the heart. (1) Ostium secundum; (2) ostium primum; (3) sinus venosus; (4) coronary sinus. PT = pulmonary trunk; RV = right ventricle.

Redrawn from original supplied courtesy of Dr. William D. Edwards, Department of Laboratory Medicine and Pathology, Mayo Clinic, Rochester, MN.

(typically involving the right upper pulmonary vein) is present in more than 90% of patients with this defect. A coronary sinus ASD (<1% of cases) is a communication between the left atrium and the coronary sinus. These defects are commonly associated with a persistent left-sided superior vena cava or complex congenital heart lesions.

ASDs are rarely associated with genetic syndromes. The Holt-Oram syndrome involves bilateral upper extremity abnormalities and congenital heart defects, commonly an ASD. Familial ostium secundum ASDs may be autosomal dominant or linked to chromosome 5. Congenital heart defects are relatively common in patients with Down syndrome; the most frequent abnormalities reported are atrioventricular septal defects, including ostium primum ASD.

Clinical Presentation

ASDs may be suspected in patients with unexplained right heart enlargement or atrial arrhythmias. Atrial fibrillation is a common finding in adults with an ASD. The atrial fibrillation risk decreases but does not normalize after ASD closure. ASD size and associated defects influence the age of presentation; symptoms include fatigue, exertional dyspnea, arrhythmias, and paradoxical embolism. Rarely, patients with pulmonary hypertension (PH) are found to have isolated ASDs.

Clinical findings in patients with an ASD include a parasternal impulse, fixed splitting of the S_2, and a pulmonary outflow murmur. A diastolic flow rumble across the tricuspid valve can occur with a large left-to-right shunt.

Diagnostic Evaluation

The electrocardiographic and radiographic findings in patients with an ASD are presented in **Table 32**.

TABLE 32. Imaging Findings and Late Complications in Adult Congenital Heart Disease

Lesion	ECG and CXR Findings	Late Complications
Patent foramen ovale	Normal	Paradoxical embolism, platypnea-orthodeoxia syndrome
Ostium secundum ASD	ECG: Incomplete RBBB, RA enlargement, right axis deviation CXR: Right heart enlargement, prominent pulmonary artery, increased pulmonary vascularity	Right heart enlargement, atrial fibrillation, PH (rare) Post repair: residual shunt (rare)
Ostium primum ASD	ECG: Left axis deviation, first-degree atrioventricular block CXR: Right heart enlargement, prominent pulmonary artery, increased pulmonary vascularity	Right heart enlargement, atrial fibrillation, mitral regurgitation (from mitral valve cleft), PH (rare) Post repair: residual shunt (rare), mitral regurgitation (from mitral valve cleft), left ventricular outflow tract obstruction
Sinus venosus ASD	ECG: Abnormal P axis CXR: Right heart enlargement, prominent pulmonary artery, increased pulmonary vascularity	Right heart enlargement, atrial fibrillation, PH (rare) Post repair: residual shunt (rare), residual anomalous pulmonary venous connection
Small VSD	Normal	Endocarditis
Large VSD	ECG: RV or RV/LV hypertrophy CXR: RA and RV enlargement, increased pulmonary vascular markings; with PH: prominent central pulmonary arteries, reduced peripheral pulmonary vascular markings	PH with associated RA and RV enlargement, RV hypertrophy, Eisenmenger syndrome Post repair: residual VSD, residual shunt (rare)
Small PDA	Normal	Endocarditis
Large PDA	ECG: LA enlargement, LV hypertrophy; with PH: RV hypertrophy CXR: Cardiomegaly, increased pulmonary vascular markings; calcification of PDA (occasional); with PH: prominent central pulmonary arteries, reduced peripheral pulmonary vascular markings	Endocarditis, right heart failure, PH, Eisenmenger syndrome Post repair: residual shunt (rare)
Pulmonary valve stenosis	ECG: Normal when RV systolic pressure <60 mm Hg; if RV systolic pressure >60 mm Hg: RA enlargement, right axis deviation, RV hypertrophy CXR: Pulmonary artery dilatation, calcification of pulmonary valve (rare); RA enlargement may be noted	Post repair: Severe pulmonary valve regurgitation after pulmonary valvotomy or valvuloplasty
Aortic coarctation	ECG: LV hypertrophy and ST-T wave abnormalities CXR: Dilated ascending aorta, "figure 3 sign" beneath aortic arch, rib notching from collateral vessels	Hypertension (75% of cases), bicuspid aortic valve (>50% of cases), increased risk for aortic aneurysm (ascending or at repair site) and intracranial aneurysm Post repair: Recoarctation, hypertension, aortic aneurysm
Repaired tetralogy of Fallot	ECG: RBBB, increased QRS duration (QRS duration reflects degree of RV dilatation) CXR: Cardiomegaly with pulmonary or tricuspid valve regurgitation; right aortic arch in 25% of cases	Post repair: Increased atrial and ventricular arrhythmia risk, pulmonary valve regurgitation or stenosis; tricuspid regurgitation QRS >180 ms increases risk for ventricular tachycardia and sudden death
Eisenmenger syndrome	ECG: Right axis deviation, RA enlargement, RV hypertrophy CXR: RV dilatation, prominent pulmonary artery, reduced pulmonary vascularity	Right heart failure, hemoptysis, stroke

ASD = atrial septal defect; CXR = chest radiography; ECG = electrocardiography; LA = left atrial; LV = left ventricular; PH = pulmonary hypertension; PDA = patent ductus arteriosus; RA = right atrial; RBBB = right bundle branch block; RV = right ventricular; VSD = ventricular septal defect.

TTE is the preferred imaging modality for identification of ostium secundum and primum ASDs. TTE also measures associated features, such as right-sided cardiac chamber enlargement, tricuspid regurgitation related to annular dilatation, and right ventricular pressure elevation. Agitated saline contrast injection (microcavitation study) in a peripheral vein during TTE may help identify an atrial-level shunt. Sinus venosus and coronary sinus ASDs are less readily diagnosed by TTE in adults and often require other imaging modalities, such as TEE, cardiac magnetic resonance (CMR) imaging, or CT. CMR imaging and CT are rarely used as the primary imaging modality when an ASD is suspected but can identify anomalous pulmonary veins and quantify right ventricular volume and ejection fraction.

Cardiac catheterization is the only method for accurately calculating pulmonary-to-systemic blood flow ratio (Qp:Qs) but is rarely required for uncomplicated ASDs. Cardiac catheterization may be recommended in patients with an ASD and PH when ASD closure is being considered.

Treatment

The main indications for ASD closure include right-sided cardiac chamber enlargement or symptoms of dyspnea; closure is reasonable for orthodeoxia-platypnea syndrome and also before pacemaker placement because of the increased risk for systemic thromboembolism. In asymptomatic patients with a small ASD and no right heart enlargement, periodic clinical monitoring and echocardiographic imaging are recommended.

Percutaneous device closure is an option for patients with an isolated ostium secundum ASD. Surgical ASD closure is indicated for nonsecundum ASDs, large secundum ASDs, unfavorable anatomy for device closure, and coexistent cardiovascular disease that requires operative intervention, such as coronary artery disease or tricuspid regurgitation.

Patients with an ASD and PH require specialty care; ASD closure may be considered for persistent left-to-right shunting without fixed PH. Medical therapy targeted at PH should also be considered.

Patients with an isolated anomalous pulmonary venous connection may present with clinical findings and TTE features similar to an ASD. Surgical redirection of the pulmonary vein is the only feasible treatment and requires surgical expertise in congenital heart disease.

Patients with small ASDs do not require physical activity limitation. Large left-to-right shunts result in self-limited exercise restriction. Patients with severe PH are advised to avoid isometric or competitive exercise.

Pregnancy is generally well tolerated in patients with an ASD in the absence of PH. The risk for congenital heart disease transmission with a sporadic ASD is estimated to be around 5%. Holt-Oram syndrome is inherited in an autosomal dominant fashion, and other genetic syndromes have variable inheritance; genetic counseling is suggested if a syndrome is suspected.

Follow-up After Atrial Septal Defect Closure

Follow-up is recommended for patients after surgical or percutaneous ASD closure. TTE and clinical assessment are recommended within the first year after closure and then periodically after that. Atrial fibrillation risk persists after closure, and frequency increases related to age at the time of ASD closure. Rare complications after device closure include device

migration, erosion into the pericardium or aorta, and sudden death.

KEY POINTS

- Clinical findings in patients with atrial septal defect include a parasternal impulse, fixed splitting of the S_2, and a pulmonary outflow murmur.

- Cardiac catheterization is the only method for accurately calculating pulmonary-to-systemic blood flow ratio but is rarely required for diagnostic purposes other than in patients with an atrial septal defect (ASD) and pulmonary hypertension when ASD closure is being considered.

- The main indications for atrial septal defect (ASD) closure include right-sided cardiac chamber enlargement, symptoms of dyspnea, or atrial arrhythmias; asymptomatic, small ASDs without right heart enlargement can simply be monitored with clinical and echocardiographic surveillance.

Ventricular Septal Defect

Pathophysiology

Ventricular septal defects (VSDs) are defined by their location on the ventricular septum (**Figure 37**). They are common at birth, but many small VSDs close spontaneously, resulting in lower prevalence by adulthood. Perimembranous VSDs are most common (80% of cases) and are usually isolated abnormalities. Muscular VSDs (10% of cases) can be located anywhere in the ventricular septum and often close spontaneously. Subpulmonary VSDs (also called outlet or supracristal

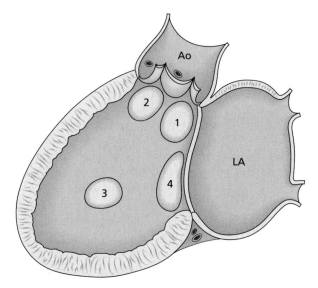

FIGURE 37. Positions of various ventricular septal defects viewed from the left side of the heart. (1) Perimembranous; (2) subpulmonary; (3) muscular; (4) inlet. Ao = aorta; LA = left atrium.

Redrawn from original supplied courtesy of Dr. William D. Edwards, Department of Laboratory Medicine and Pathology, Mayo Clinic, Rochester, MN.

VSDs) account for approximately 6% of defects in non-Asians and 33% in Asians and are associated with aortic regurgitation caused by aortic cusp distortion. Inlet VSDs (4% of cases) occur in the superior-posterior portion of the ventricular septum adjacent to the tricuspid valve. They occur as part of the atrioventricular septal defect complex, characteristically seen in patients with Down syndrome.

Clinical Presentation

The presentation of an isolated VSD depends on the VSD size and pulmonary vascular resistance. A small VSD without PH presents with a loud (often palpable) holosystolic murmur located at the left sternal border that may obliterate the S_2. Small VSDs do not cause left heart enlargement or PH.

A VSD with a moderate left-to-right shunt may cause left ventricular volume overload and PH. Patients are asymptomatic for many years but eventually present with heart failure symptoms. A displaced left ventricular apical impulse suggests volume overload. A holosystolic murmur at the left sternal border is noted; the pressure gradient between the ventricles determines the murmur quality and duration. Progressive PH results in shortening of the murmur.

VSDs associated with large left-to-right shunts are usually detected by the presence of a murmur, heart failure, and failure to thrive in infancy. Failure to close the defect early in life usually causes fixed PH within several years with subsequent development of Eisenmenger syndrome (see later discussion) and shunt reversal.

Diagnostic Evaluation

The electrocardiographic and radiographic findings in patients with a VSD are presented in Table 32.

TTE is the imaging modality of choice for identification of VSD location, size, and hemodynamic impact. Rarely, TEE, CMR imaging, or CT is needed to delineate cardiac anatomy when TTE is unsatisfactory. Cardiac catheterization is primarily performed to delineate the Qp:Qs ratio and pulmonary pressures.

Treatment

VSD closure is indicated when the Qp:Qs ratio is 2.0 or greater with evidence of left ventricular volume overload or a history of endocarditis. Most patients are treated surgically, but percutaneous device closure is an option for select VSDs.

VSD closure is not indicated for patients with a small left-to-right shunt and no chamber enlargement or valve disease, but periodic clinical evaluation and imaging are recommended. Large VSDs with shunt reversal (right-to-left shunting) and PH (Eisenmenger syndrome) should not be closed because this causes clinical deterioration owing to reduced cardiac output.

Patients with small VSDs do not require activity restrictions. If the pulmonary artery pressure is greater than 50% of systolic blood pressure, isometric or competitive exercise is discouraged.

Pregnancy in women with VSDs is generally well tolerated in the absence of PH; women with VSDs and associated fixed PH should be counseled to avoid pregnancy.

Follow-up After Ventricular Septal Defect Closure

Residual or recurrent VSD, arrhythmias, PH, endocarditis, and valve regurgitation are recognized complications following VSD closure. Clinical assessment and TTE are recommended within 1 year of VSD closure. Subsequent follow-up frequency depends on clinical and cardiac status.

> **KEY POINTS**
> - A small ventricular septal defect without pulmonary hypertension presents with a loud (often palpable) holosystolic murmur located at the left sternal border that may obliterate the S_2.
> - Ventricular septal defect closure is indicated when the Qp:Qs ratio is 2.0 or greater with evidence of left ventricular volume overload or in patients with a history of endocarditis.

Patent Ductus Arteriosus

Pathophysiology

A patent ductus arteriosus (PDA) is a persistent fetal connection between the aorta and the pulmonary artery. Prematurity and maternal rubella predispose to a PDA. It may be an isolated abnormality or associated with other congenital cardiac defects.

Clinical Presentation

The typical murmur of a PDA is a continuous "machinery" murmur that envelops the S_2, making it inaudible; the murmur is heard beneath the left clavicle. A tiny PDA is generally asymptomatic and inaudible. Patients with a moderate-sized PDA may present with bounding pulses, a wide pulse pressure, left-heart enlargement and dysfunction, and, rarely, clinical heart failure.

A large unrepaired PDA may cause PH with eventual shunt reversal (Eisenmenger syndrome); characteristic features of an Eisenmenger PDA are clubbing and oxygen desaturation affecting the feet but not the hands, owing to desaturated blood reaching the lower extremities preferentially (differential cyanosis).

Diagnostic Evaluation

The electrocardiographic and radiographic findings in patients with a PDA are presented in Table 32.

TTE is the imaging modality of choice for identification of a PDA. The PDA may be difficult to visualize in patients with severe PH owing to equalization of pressures between the aorta and pulmonary artery. In patients with a PDA and PH, cardiac catheterization is used to determine shunt size and reversibility of PH. Angiography confirms PDA morphology and helps determine whether percutaneous closure is feasible. TEE, CT, and CMR imaging may identify a PDA but are not the primary diagnostic techniques.

Treatment

PDA closure is indicated for left-sided cardiac chamber enlargement in the absence of severe PH. Percutaneous or surgical closure may be performed; referral to a congenital cardiac center for consideration of closure options is recommended.

A tiny PDA requires no intervention. PDA closure is reasonable for small PDAs with previous endocarditis. Moderate-sized PDAs are generally closed percutaneously. Large PDAs with severe PH and shunt reversal should be observed; closure may be detrimental, but medical therapy for PH should be considered.

Patients with a small PDA without PH do not require physical activity restrictions, and women should be able to tolerate pregnancy.

KEY POINTS

- A continuous "machinery" murmur heard beneath the left clavicle that makes the S_2 inaudible is typical for a patent ductus arteriosus.

- Angiography can determine patent ductus arteriosus morphology and whether percutaneous closure is feasible.

- The size of a patent ductus arteriosus (PDA) determines management; a tiny PDA requires no intervention.

- A large patent ductus arteriosus with severe pulmonary hypertension (PH) and shunt reversal should be observed; closure may be detrimental, but medical therapy for PH should be considered.

Pulmonary Valve Stenosis

Pathophysiology

Pulmonary valve stenosis (PS), an autosomal dominant disorder, causes obstruction to right ventricular outflow and is usually an isolated valve lesion. Isolated PS is associated with Noonan syndrome, which includes short stature, variable intellectual capacity, neck webbing, and ocular hypertelorism (abnormally increased distance between the orbits).

Clinical Presentation

Mild and moderate PS is generally asymptomatic. On physical examination, mild PS is characterized by a normal jugular venous waveform and precordial impulse.

Severe PS can cause exertional dyspnea. Right ventricular hypertrophy caused by pressure overload results in a prominent *a wave* on the jugular venous pressure waveform and a palpable right ventricular lift.

Auscultatory findings in PS include a systolic ejection click immediately after the S_1 (which is the only right-sided heart sound to decrease during inspiration), followed by a crescendo-decrescendo murmur. In severe PS, the ejection systolic murmur at the left sternal border increases in intensity and duration, and the pulmonary valve component of S_2 is delayed (splitting of S_2) and eventually disappears. A right ventricular S_4 is often heard in severe PS.

Diagnostic Evaluation

The electrocardiographic and radiographic findings in patients with PS are presented in Table 32.

TTE is the imaging modality of choice for identification of PS. Severe PS is present when the peak gradient is 50 mm Hg or greater. Treatment options depend on valve mobility, calcification, and the effects of obstruction on the right ventricle. PS causes right ventricular hypertrophy. Right ventricular dilatation should prompt a search for an associated lesion, such as pulmonary valve regurgitation or an ASD. TEE, CMR imaging, and CT are not routinely used in patients with PS. Cardiac catheterization is performed when percutaneous intervention for PS is considered.

Treatment

Pulmonary balloon valvuloplasty is the preferred treatment for valvular PS. It is indicated for asymptomatic patients with appropriate pulmonary valve morphology who have a peak Doppler gradient of at least 60 mm Hg or a mean gradient greater than 40 mm Hg and pulmonary valve regurgitation that is less than moderate. Balloon valvuloplasty is also recommended for symptomatic patients with appropriate valve morphology who have a peak Doppler gradient of greater than 50 mm Hg or a mean gradient greater than 30 mm Hg. Surgical intervention is recommended for PS associated with a small annulus, more than moderate pulmonary valve regurgitation, severe subvalvar or supravalvar PS, or another cardiac lesion that requires operative intervention.

Patients with mild and moderate PS (peak gradient <50 mm Hg) do not require exercise restriction. Patients with severe PS should participate only in low-intensity sports.

Pregnancy is generally well tolerated with PS; percutaneous valvotomy has been performed during pregnancy for severe symptomatic PS. Sporadic congenital heart disease recurrence in offspring is rare. Noonan syndrome should be suspected with PS recurrence in offspring.

Follow-up After Pulmonary Valve Stenosis Repair

Patients with previous PS intervention (balloon or surgical) often have severe pulmonary valve regurgitation; thus, long-term clinical and TTE follow-up is recommended. The frequency of follow-up depends on regurgitation severity and impact on the heart.

- Auscultation findings in pulmonary valve stenosis include a systolic ejection click immediately after S_1, followed by a crescendo-decrescendo murmur.

- Surgical intervention is recommended for pulmonary valve stenosis (PS) associated with a small annulus, more than moderate pulmonary valve regurgitation, severe subvalvar or supravalvar PS, or another cardiac lesion that requires operative intervention.

Aortic Coarctation

Pathophysiology

Aortic coarctation is a discrete narrowing of the aorta, usually located just beyond the left subclavian artery, causing hypertension proximal and hypotension distal to the narrowing.

Clinical Presentation

Patients with aortic coarctation may present with heart failure early in life. Adults are usually asymptomatic, but exertional leg fatigue or headaches may occur. Upper extremity hypertension and reduced blood pressure and pulse amplitude in the lower extremities cause a radial artery–to–femoral artery pulse delay. A systolic or continuous murmur is heard in the left infraclavicular region or over the back. A murmur from collateral intercostal vessels may also be audible and palpable over the chest wall. Fifty percent of patients with aortic coarctation have a bicuspid aortic valve. Auscultation of the heart may reveal an ejection click, a systolic murmur at the cardiac base, or, sometimes, an S_4.

Turner syndrome, a chromosomal abnormality secondary to partial or total loss of chromosome X, is often associated with congenital cardiac disease, including coarctation. Turner syndrome is characterized by short stature, webbed neck, broad chest, and widely spaced nipples. Aortic coarctation is also associated with aortic and subaortic stenosis, parachute mitral valve (Shone syndrome), ventricular septal defect, and cerebral aneurysms.

Diagnostic Evaluation

The electrocardiographic and radiographic findings in patients with aortic coarctation are presented in Table 32.

The characteristic radiographic features of aortic coarctation include the "figure 3 sign" (**Figure 38**), which is caused by dilatation of the aorta above and below the area of coarctation. Dilatation of intercostal collateral arteries as a result of aortic obstruction may lead to the radiographic appearance of rib notching.

TTE is often the initial diagnostic test in patients suspected of having aortic coarctation; it usually identifies the coarctation and associated features, such as bicuspid aortic valve and left ventricular hypertrophy. CMR imaging and CT are recommended to identify the anatomy, severity, and location of the coarctation; the presence of collateral vessels; and

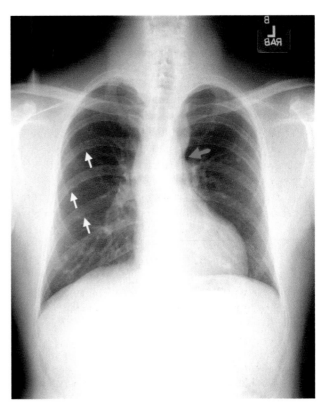

FIGURE 38. Chest radiograph of a patient with aortic coarctation exhibiting the "figure 3 sign," caused by dilatation of the aorta above and below the area of coarctation (*blue arrow*), and rib notching (*white arrows*).

associated abnormalities, such as aortic aneurysm. Cardiac catheterization is primarily used in patients in whom percutaneous intervention is being considered.

Treatment

Severe aortic coarctation is associated with excess morbidity and mortality, including hypertension, coronary artery disease, stroke, aortic dissection, and heart failure. Age at the time of coarctation repair is the most important predictor of long-term survival.

Indications for intervention in patients with coarctation include a systolic peak (peak-to-peak) pressure gradient of 20 mm Hg or greater or radiologic evidence of severe coarctation with collateral flow. Percutaneous or surgical intervention options are available; selection depends on the length, location, and severity of coarctation and the presence of associated cardiovascular lesions.

Physical activity restriction is recommended for patients with severe postintervention residual or unrepaired coarctation, aortic stenosis, or a dilated aorta; these patients should avoid contact sports and isometric exercise.

A comprehensive preconception evaluation is warranted in all patients with coarctation who are considering pregnancy. Pregnancy is reasonable in women with repaired aortic coarctation without significant residua. Women with mild or moderate residua or unoperated coarctation will generally tolerate pregnancy well but should undergo blood pressure monitoring and cardiovascular evaluation during pregnancy. Pregnancy should be avoided by patients with severe unrepaired coarctation.

Follow-up After Aortic Coarctation Repair

Following coarctation repair, hypertension occurs in up to 75% of patients and should be treated. Additional intervention following repair may be required for bicuspid aortic valve, aortic aneurysm or dissection, recoarctation, coronary artery disease, systolic or diastolic heart failure, or intracranial aneurysm. Regular follow-up should include TTE, periodic aortic imaging, and evaluation by a cardiologist specializing in congenital heart disease.

KEY POINTS

- In patients with aortic coarctation, findings may include upper extremity hypertension and reduced blood pressure and pulse amplitude in the lower extremities, causing a radial artery–to–femoral artery pulse delay.
- The "figure 3 sign" is a characteristic radiographic feature of aortic coarctation.
- Indications for intervention in patients with aortic coarctation include a systolic peak (peak-to-peak) pressure gradient of 20 mm Hg or greater or radiologic evidence of severe coarctation with collateral flow.

Tetralogy of Fallot

Tetralogy of Fallot (TOF) is characterized by a large subaortic VSD, infundibular or valvular PS, aortic override, and right ventricular hypertrophy (**Figure 39**). It is the most common cyanotic congenital cardiac lesion. Repair is usually performed early in life; adults who have not undergone an operation are rarely encountered.

Genetic screening is recommended for all patients with TOF who are planning reproduction. Approximately 15% of patients with TOF have the 22q11.2 chromosome microdeletion (DiGeorge syndrome). When present, congenital heart disease inheritance is approximately 50%, compared with 5% in unaffected patients. TOF is common in persons with Down syndrome.

TOF repair involves VSD patch closure and relief of PS/right ventricular outflow tract obstruction by transannular patch placement; the transannular patch disrupts integrity of the pulmonary valve, causing severe pulmonary valve regurgitation. Severe long-standing pulmonary valve regurgitation causes right heart enlargement, tricuspid regurgitation, exercise limitation, and arrhythmias and is the most common reason for reoperation after TOF repair. Annual congenital cardiology follow-up is recommended for patients with repaired TOF to determine optimal timing for intervention.

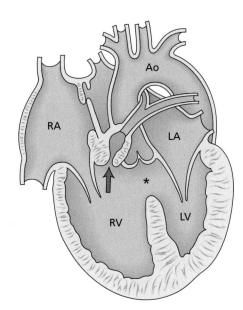

FIGURE 39. Tetralogy of Fallot. A subarterial ventricular septal defect (*asterisk*) and pulmonary stenosis (*arrow*) are associated with secondary aortic override and right ventricular hypertrophy. Ao = aorta; LA = left atrium; LV = left ventricle; RA = right atrium; RV = right ventricle.

Redrawn from original supplied courtesy of Dr. William D. Edwards, Department of Laboratory Medicine and Pathology, Mayo Clinic, Rochester, MN.

Diagnostic Evaluation after Repair of Tetralogy of Fallot

The electrocardiographic and radiographic findings in patients with repaired TOF are presented in Table 32.

Symptoms, arrhythmias, or right heart chamber enlargement should prompt a search for severe pulmonary valve regurgitation. Prolongation of the QRS complex reflects the degree of right ventricular dilatation; QRS duration of 180 milliseconds or longer and nonsustained ventricular tachycardia are risk factors for sudden cardiac death.

TTE is the imaging modality of choice for identifying valve dysfunction, residual VSD, left ventricular dysfunction, and aortic dilatation. CMR imaging or CT is preferred for assessment of right ventricular size and function, which helps determine appropriate timing for pulmonary valve replacement. Cardiac catheterization may be required to assess hemodynamics and residual shunts and to delineate coronary artery and pulmonary artery anatomy.

Treatment of Tetralogy of Fallot Residua

Indications for pulmonary valve replacement in patients with repaired TOF and severe pulmonary valve regurgitation include symptoms, decreased exercise tolerance, more than moderate right heart enlargement or dysfunction, arrhythmias, and development of tricuspid regurgitation. Tricuspid valve repair may also be needed. Percutaneous pulmonary valve replacement is possible in select patients with previous TOF surgery.

Physical activity restriction is recommended for patients with repaired TOF and residual sequelae; contact sports and heavy isometric exercise should be avoided.

- Genetic screening is recommended for all patients with tetralogy of Fallot who are planning reproduction because the presence of the 22q11.2 chromosome microdeletion (15% of patients) results in congenital heart disease inheritance of approximately 50%.

- Indications for pulmonary valve replacement in patients with repaired tetralogy of Fallot and severe pulmonary valve regurgitation include symptoms, decreased exercise tolerance, more than moderate right heart enlargement or dysfunction, arrhythmias, and development of tricuspid regurgitation.

Adults with Cyanotic Congenital Heart Disease

General Management

Right-to-left cardiac shunts, such as palliated or unrepaired TOF and Eisenmenger syndrome, result in hypoxemia, erythrocytosis, and cyanosis. An increased erythrocyte mass is a compensatory response to improve oxygen transport.

Physical features include digital clubbing and central cyanosis. These patients are predisposed to arthropathy, scoliosis, gallstones, pulmonary hemorrhage or thrombus, paradoxical cerebral emboli or abscess, kidney dysfunction, pheochromocytoma/paraganglioma, and hemostatic problems. Patients with cyanotic congenital heart disease should be evaluated annually by a congenital cardiac specialist.

Perioperative complications are common in patients with cyanosis, so elective procedures and operations should be performed at specialized multidisciplinary care centers; a congenital cardiac specialist should be consulted when patients are hospitalized. Additional considerations in these patients include antimicrobial prophylaxis for nonsterile procedures; placement of intravenous line filters to prevent paradoxical air embolism; and early ambulation, pneumatic compression devices, and anticoagulation to prevent venous stasis, venous thrombosis, and paradoxical embolism. Venous thromboembolism prophylaxis is especially important in these patients because of the risk for paradoxical embolism if a venous thromboembolism were to occur. ◨

Most patients with cyanosis have compensated, stable erythrocytosis. Phlebotomy is recommended for patients with symptomatic hyperviscosity (headaches and reduced concentration) with a hemoglobin level greater than 20 g/dL (200 g/L) and hematocrit greater than 65% in the absence of dehydration. Phlebotomy should be performed no more than three times each year and should be followed by fluid administration. Repeated phlebotomies deplete iron stores and cause iron-deficient erythrocytes or microcytosis, increasing the risk for stroke. Short-term iron therapy is administered for iron deficiency in patients with destabilized erythropoiesis.

Maternal and fetal morbidity and mortality increase related to the degree of cyanosis and pulmonary pressures; thus, pregnancy in patients with cyanosis is considered high risk.

Eisenmenger Syndrome

Eisenmenger syndrome is severe PH with cardiac shunt reversal (right-to-left shunting) caused by a long-standing, unrepaired VSD, PDA, or ASD. TTE evaluation and appropriate intervention has decreased the frequency of Eisenmenger syndrome, but PH related to complex congenital heart disease is increasingly identified.

Conservative medical measures for patients with Eisenmenger syndrome include avoiding iron deficiency, dehydration, acute exposure to excess heat, and moderate or severe strenuous or isometric exercise. Phlebotomy is rarely performed. Additionally, long-term altitude exposure should be avoided or limited because it results in a reduced partial pressure of oxygen. Air travel should be undertaken in pressurized aircrafts; supplemental oxygen may be beneficial with prolonged air travel.

All patients with Eisenmenger syndrome should undergo annual evaluation by a congenital cardiac specialist. Noncardiac surgery should be performed at centers with expertise in the care of patients with complex congenital cardiac disease. Patients with progressive cardiovascular symptoms may benefit from pulmonary vasodilator therapy or, in rare cases, heart and lung transplantation.

Women with Eisenmenger syndrome should be cautioned to avoid pregnancy because of the high risk for maternal mortality.

- Phlebotomy is recommended for patients with cyanotic congenital heart disease who have symptomatic hyperviscosity with a hemoglobin level greater than 20 g/dL (200 g/L) and hematocrit greater than 65% in the absence of dehydration; iron deficiency should be avoided.

- Patients with cyanotic congenital heart disease who are undergoing surgery or elective procedures require additional care considerations, including antimicrobial prophylaxis for nonsterile procedures; intravenous line filters to prevent paradoxical air embolism; and early ambulation, pneumatic compression devices, and anticoagulation to prevent venous stasis, venous thrombosis, and paradoxical embolism.

- In patients with Eisenmenger syndrome, air travel should be undertaken in pressurized aircrafts, with supplemental oxygen for prolonged air travel.

Diseases of the Aorta

Introduction

Diseases of the aorta include chronic conditions, such as thoracic and abdominal aortic aneurysms and aortic atheromas, and potentially life-threatening acute conditions, such as aortic dissection and aneurysm rupture. Once chronic aortic diseases are diagnosed, surveillance and treatment are critical to prevent disease progression, complications, and mortality.

Thoracic Aortic Aneurysm

Thoracic aortic aneurysm (TAA) is defined as an increase in the thoracic aortic diameter of greater than 50% relative to the expected or normal aortic dimension. TAAs may occur at the level of the aortic root, ascending aorta, aortic arch, or descending aorta. They most commonly involve the aortic root and ascending aorta, often forming at the site of aortic atherosclerosis. TAAs are usually the result of cystic medial degeneration and weakening of the aortic wall due to loss of smooth muscle fibers and elastic fiber degeneration.

Common causes of TAA are summarized in **Table 33**. TAAs that occur in patients younger than 50 years are often caused by connective tissue disorders, such as Marfan or Ehlers-Danlos syndrome. Bicuspid aortic valve morphology is also an important risk factor for TAA formation; TAAs occur in approximately 50% of patients with a bicuspid aortic valve. Other risk factors for TAA include age and hypertension.

TAAs are often asymptomatic and are commonly detected by echocardiography during an evaluation of left ventricular function or murmurs. Infrequently, symptoms of hoarseness and dysphagia occur when an aneurysm compresses surrounding structures. Physical examination findings, such as a diastolic heart murmur or wide pulse pressure, are found in the setting of aortic regurgitation, which often occurs in combination with TAA. If the aneurysm ruptures, patients present with severe chest or back pain, sudden shortness of breath, or sudden cardiac death.

Screening and Surveillance

Screening for abnormalities of the thoracic aorta with aortic imaging is indicated in asymptomatic patients with genetic conditions (such as Marfan or Ehlers-Danlos syndrome), a bicuspid aortic valve, or a family history of TAA or aortic dissection. Screening is not recommended in other asymptomatic persons.

After TAA is detected, noninvasive imaging is indicated to determine aortic cross-sectional area (**Table 34**). Aortic diameter measurement often varies substantially depending on the type of imaging study used. Care must be taken to measure the dimension perpendicular to the long axis of the aorta because oblique measurements may overestimate the true aortic diameter. The maximum aortic diameter at the site of an aneurysm (measured in cm) is generally used in the criteria for surveillance and treatment.

Because the leading cause of death in patients with TAA is rupture, surveillance and treatment depend on the aneurysm size and risk for rupture. Once the diameter of the aneurysm has grown larger than 5.0 cm, the average growth rate is 0.1 cm/year, and risk for rupture increases. Additional independent risk factors for rupture are a rapid rate of expansion (>0.5 cm/year), the presence of an aneurysm during pregnancy, and previous aortic dissection. Annual surveillance is appropriate in patients with a first-degree relative with a history of familial thoracic aortic aneurysm and aortic dissection.

Transthoracic echocardiography is most commonly used for annual surveillance of TAAs smaller than 5.0 cm in diameter. In patients with previous rapid rate of expansion or in patients with a TAA of 5.0 cm in diameter or larger, more frequent surveillance is often warranted. Patients with rapid expansion of the TAA or aortic dimension of 5.5 cm should undergo additional imaging with CT angiography (CTA) or magnetic resonance angiography (MRA).

In patients with a TAA and a genetic condition (Marfan or Ehlers-Danlos syndrome) or bicuspid aortic valve, it is recommended that repeat assessment occur 6 months after diagnosis to determine the rate of enlargement. Thereafter, annual imaging is recommended if the aortic diameter has been stable and smaller than 4.5 cm. If the aortic diameter is 4.5 cm or larger or the rate of enlargement exceeds 0.5 cm/year, imaging should be performed every 6 months.

Treatment

TAAs with a diameter smaller than 5.0 cm can usually be managed with medical therapy and active surveillance (see Table 34). Medical therapy includes aggressive blood pressure control with a goal blood pressure below 130/80 mm Hg. β-Blockers are the preferred antihypertensive agents in patients with

TABLE 33.	Causes of Thoracic Aortic Aneurysm
Category	**Syndrome**
Atherosclerosis	
Connective tissue disorders	Marfan syndrome
	Ehlers-Danlos syndrome type IV
	Loeys-Dietz syndrome
Other genetic and/or congenital conditions	Familial thoracic aortic aneurysm and aortic dissection syndrome
	Bicuspid aortic valve
	Turner syndrome
Vasculitis	Takayasu arteritis
	Giant cell arteritis
	Nonspecific (idiopathic) aortitis
	Other autoimmune conditions (Behçet syndrome, systemic lupus erythematosus)
Infectious	Septic embolism
	Direct bacterial inoculation
	Bacterial seeding
	Contiguous infection
	Syphilis
Aortic injury	Prior acute aortic syndrome
	Chest trauma

TABLE 34. Comparison of Thoracic Aortic Imaging Modalities

Modality	Advantages	Disadvantages
Transthoracic echocardiography (TTE)	Good visualization of aortic root/proximal ascending aorta No exposure to radiation or contrast dye Allows definition of valvular pathology, myocardial function, pericardial disease Bedside diagnosis	Requires experienced operator Limited visualization of the distal ascending aorta and aortic arch and branches of the great vessels A negative TTE result does not rule out aortic dissection, and other imaging techniques must be considered
Transesophageal echocardiography (TEE)	TEE has superior imaging quality compared with TTE Excellent visualization of the aorta from its root to the descending aorta No exposure to radiation or contrast dye Allows definition of valvular pathology, myocardial function, pericardial disease Bedside diagnosis	Requires experienced operator Invasive procedure
CT angiography	Visualization of entire aorta and side branches Rapid imaging Multiplanar reconstruction	Exposes patient to radiation, iodinated contrast dye
Magnetic resonance angiography	Visualization of entire aorta and side branches No exposure to radiation or iodinated contrast dye	For acute disease, prolonged image acquisition away from acute care area Contraindicated in patients with implanted pacemaker or defibrillator Gadolinium contrast dye contraindicated in patients with kidney disease
Aortography	Visualization of aortic lumen, side branches, and collaterals Provides exact information on aorta size and shape and any anomalies	Diseases of the aortic wall and thrombus-filled discrete aortic aneurysms may be missed Invasive procedure that requires power injection within the aorta Requires dye load and may be nephrotoxic

TAA. In patients with Marfan syndrome, β-blockers and losartan have been associated with a reduced rate of aneurysm growth.

Once ascending aortic aneurysm size exceeds 5.5 cm in diameter, repair is warranted to prevent the morbidity and mortality associated with aneurysm rupture. In patients with an ascending aorta or aortic root greater than 4.5 cm in diameter who require coronary artery bypass grafting or surgery to repair valve pathology, aortic repair should be performed at the time of cardiac surgery. Current guidelines recommend that all patients with a bicuspid aortic valve and ascending aortic aneurysm undergo aortic repair when the aneurysm exceeds 5.5 cm in diameter, unless there is an indication to repair concomitant coronary artery disease or aortic valve pathology. In patients with Marfan or Ehlers-Danlos syndrome, the American College of Cardiology/American Heart Association guidelines recommend that patients undergo aortic repair at a lower threshold (4.5–5.0 cm).

The aneurysm location, associated aortic valve pathology, and presence of concomitant coronary artery disease all dictate the type of thoracic aortic repair performed. Open surgical repair is indicated for TAAs that involve the aortic root, ascending aorta, and aortic arch. Thoracic endovascular aortic repair (TEVAR) with stent grafting should be used when a descending aortic aneurysm has a diameter greater than 6.0 cm, has exhibited rapid growth (>0.5 cm/year), or has caused end-organ damage, owing to a lower morbidity and shorter hospital stay relative to open repair. TEVAR has the advantage of avoiding an open surgical operation, although complications (stroke, spinal ischemia, aortic graft endoleaks) can occur.

KEY POINTS

- Asymptomatic patients with Marfan or Ehlers-Danlos syndrome, a bicuspid aortic valve, or a family history of thoracic aortic aneurysm or aortic dissection should undergo screening for abnormalities of the thoracic aorta.

- Patients with a thoracic aortic aneurysm smaller than 5.0 cm in diameter should undergo annual echocardiography to monitor aortic aneurysm growth.

(Continued)

- In patients with an ascending aortic diameter exceeding 5.5 cm, elective aortic repair is warranted to prevent the morbidity and mortality associated with aneurysm rupture; patients with Marfan or Ehlers-Danlos syndrome should undergo aortic repair at 4.5 to 5.0 cm.

- Thoracic endovascular aortic repair is recommended in patients with a descending aortic aneurysm when the diameter is greater than 6.0 cm, has exhibited rapid growth (>0.5 cm/year), or has caused end-organ damage.

Abdominal Aortic Aneurysm

Abdominal aortic aneurysm (AAA) is defined as an abnormal dilatation of the aorta with an anteroposterior diameter greater than 3.0 cm. Risk factors include male sex (6:1 male-to-female incidence ratio), advanced age, smoking, atherosclerosis, hypertension, and a family history of AAA.

Screening and Surveillance

AAA is most commonly diagnosed incidentally by CTA or abdominal ultrasonography. Approximately 75% of patients with AAA are asymptomatic at the time of diagnosis. Because of the high mortality rate associated with aneurysm rupture, the U.S. Preventive Services Task Force recommends one-time screening with duplex ultrasonography in all men aged 65 to 75 years who have smoked at least 100 cigarettes in their lifetime and selective screening in men in this age group who have never smoked (see MKSAP 18 General Internal Medicine).

Estimated annual risk for aortic rupture according to AAA dimension is shown in **Table 35**. In patients with an AAA diameter of 4.0 cm or less, surveillance with duplex ultrasonography every 2 to 3 years is warranted. In patients with an AAA diameter of 4.1 to 5.4 cm, surveillance with CTA or duplex ultrasonography should be performed every 6 to 12 months. Once the aortic diameter meets the threshold for aortic repair, anatomic imaging tests, such as CTA or MRA, are indicated to determine the exact location of the AAA (suprarenal, juxtarenal, or infrarenal) in planning for repair.

Treatment

Medical treatment of AAA involves risk factor reduction to reduce the risk for rupture, cardiovascular morbidity, and overall mortality. Aortic repair should be performed in patients with an AAA diameter of 5.5 cm or larger, in those with rapid expansion in AAA size (>0.5 cm/year), and in patients presenting with symptoms resulting from AAA (abdominal or back pain/tenderness). In patients with an indication for aortic repair, the choice between open surgical repair and endovascular aneurysm repair (EVAR) is driven by the location of the AAA and involvement of the renal and mesenteric arteries. Suprarenal and juxtarenal aneurysms most often necessitate open surgical repair. Patient age, comorbid conditions, and ability to tolerate open surgical repair determine which procedure should be performed in patients with an infrarenal AAA. EVAR is associated with lower short-term (30-day) morbidity and mortality but no significant differences in long-term mortality. Additionally, EVAR is associated with increased need for repeat intervention and significantly higher rates of endoleak, device failure, and postimplantation syndrome (fever, leukocytosis, elevated serum C-reactive protein). These complications necessitate diligent follow-up with noninvasive imaging tests (CTA or ultrasonography) to evaluate the stent graft.

- Risk factors for abdominal aortic aneurysm include male sex, increased age, smoking, and family history.

- Aortic repair should be performed in patients with an abdominal aortic aneurysm (AAA) diameter of 5.5 cm or larger, in those with rapid expansion in AAA size, and in patients presenting with symptoms resulting from AAA (abdominal or back pain/tenderness).

Aortic Atheroma

Aortic atherosclerotic plaques commonly occur in patients with evidence of atherosclerosis in other vascular beds. The most frequent complication of aortic atheromas is systemic embolism and stroke. Aortic atheromas greater than 4 mm in diameter or with a mobile component are more likely to be associated with thromboembolism compared with smaller atheromas.

Aortic atheromas are most frequently detected as an incidental finding on imaging studies. The presence of an aortic atheroma represents a coronary artery disease risk equivalent, and patients should be considered for antiplatelet and statin therapies in addition to other risk factor interventions.

- Patients with an aortic atheroma should be treated with antiplatelet and statin therapies to reduce cardiovascular risk.

TABLE 35. Annual Rupture Risk of Abdominal Aortic Aneurysm by Diameter

Aneurysm Diameter	Annual Rupture Risk
<4.0 cm	<0.5%
4.0-4.9 cm	0.5%-5%
5.0-5.9 cm	3%-15%
6.0-6.9 cm	10%-20%
7.0-7.9 cm	20%-40%
≥8.0 cm	30%-50%

Reproduced with permission from Brewster DC, Cronenwett JL, Hallett JW Jr, Johnston KW, Krupski WC, Matsumura JS; Joint Council of the American Association for Vascular Surgery and Society for Vascular Surgery. Guidelines for the treatment of abdominal aortic aneurysms. Report of a subcommittee of the Joint Council of the American Association for Vascular Surgery and Society for Vascular Surgery. J Vasc Surg. 2003;37:1106-17. [PMID: 12756363] Copyright 2003, Elsevier.

Acute Aortic Syndromes

The most common and life-threatening acute aortic syndromes include acute aortic dissection and aortic aneurysm rupture. Additional acute aortic syndromes include intramural aortic hematoma and penetrating atherosclerotic ulcer.

Pathophysiology

Acute aortic dissection involves tearing of the aortic intima, leading to passage of blood from the true lumen of the aorta into a false lumen (**Figure 40**). Dissection of the aorta can propagate in an antegrade or retrograde fashion, mainly due to shear forces. Propagation of the dissection can result in cardiac

Acute aortic dissection

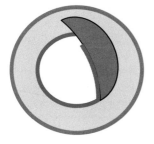

Acute intramural hematoma

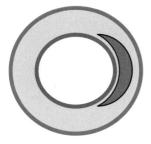

Penetrating atherosclerotic ulcer

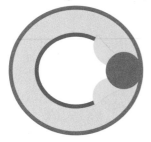

FIGURE 40. Cross-sectional representation of acute aortic syndromes. Acute aortic dissection: interruption of intima (*blue*) with creation of an intimal flap and false lumen formation within the media (*red*). Color flow by Doppler echocardiography or intravenous (IV) contrast by CT is present within the false lumen in the acute phase. Acute intramural hematoma: crescent-shaped hematoma contained within the media without interruption of the intima (*blue*). No color flow by Doppler echocardiography or IV contrast by CT within crescent. Penetrating atherosclerotic ulcer: atheroma (*yellow*) with plaque rupture disrupting intimal integrity; blood pool contained within intima-medial layer (pseudoaneurysm). Color flow by Doppler echocardiography or IV contrast by CT enters the ulcer crater.

tamponade; acute aortic regurgitation; compromise of arterial side branches (carotid, mesenteric, renal, or iliac arteries); and underperfusion of organs such as the brain, intestines, or kidneys. Aortic dissections are categorized according to their location of origin by use of the Stanford classification, which describes type A dissections as originating within the ascending aorta or arch and type B dissections as originating distal to the left subclavian artery. Type A aortic dissections require surgical intervention due to risk for rupture and death, whereas type B aortic dissections can often be initially managed with medical stabilization and blood pressure control.

Intramural aortic hematomas result from microtears in the aortic intima and rupture of the vasa vasorum (**Figure 41**). Penetrating atherosclerotic ulcers are caused by erosion of the internal elastic membrane at the site of aortic atherosclerotic plaque, leading to a blood-filled false space within the wall of the aorta (**Figure 42**). Both intramural hematomas and penetrating atherosclerotic ulcers are more common in type B dissections.

Diagnosis and Evaluation

Acute aortic dissection is a medical emergency, and a high index of suspicion is needed for immediate diagnosis and treatment. It classically presents with the sudden onset of chest or back pain that has a tearing or ripping quality; however, not all patients will have this symptom. Patients may present with hypertension, syncope, a murmur of aortic regurgitation, or heart failure in the setting of sudden aortic insufficiency. The findings of asymmetric blood pressures in the upper extremities, asymmetric pulses, or pulsus paradoxus should all raise suspicion for acute aortic dissection.

Abnormalities may be present on chest radiography (widened mediastinum) and electrocardiography (ST-segment depression), but these findings are not diagnostic for acute aortic dissection. In patients with a high likelihood of acute aortic dissection, diagnostic imaging tests should not be delayed based on the results of chest radiography, electrocardiography, or laboratory testing.

Transesophageal echocardiography, CTA, and MRA have similar sensitivity and specificity in patients with acute thoracic aortic disease. Transthoracic echocardiography is often used but is limited by the inability to image the distal ascending aorta, transverse aortic arch, and descending aorta. Compared with CTA or MRA, the primary advantages of transesophageal echocardiography in patients suspected of having aortic dissection include its portability for an unstable patient and the lack of iodinated contrast. With the increased availability of CTA, it has become the primary diagnostic test for acute thoracic aortic disease. Invasive aortography is rarely indicated for the diagnosis of acute disease; however, it is indicated at the time of endovascular repair or when noninvasive testing is contraindicated or cannot be performed.

Treatment

Patients with acute aortic dissection without evidence of cardiogenic shock should be treated with medical therapy to

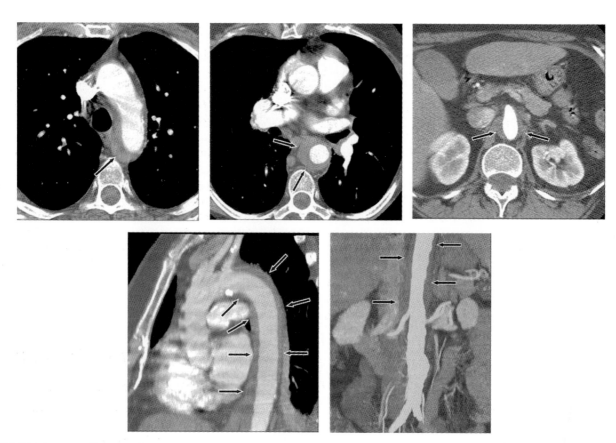

FIGURE 41. Intramural hematoma demonstrated as a low-attenuation band of hematoma (*arrows*) in the aortic wall on CT images. Axial images at the level of the aortic arch (*top left*), through the mid thorax (*top middle*), and at the level of the superior mesenteric artery with narrowing of the aortic lumen (*top right*). Oblique sagittal reformatted image through the thorax (note band artifact evident without the use of electrocardiographic gating) (*bottom left*). Coronal reformatted image through the abdomen demonstrates the length of the hematoma and an incidental infrarenal aortic aneurysm (*bottom right*).

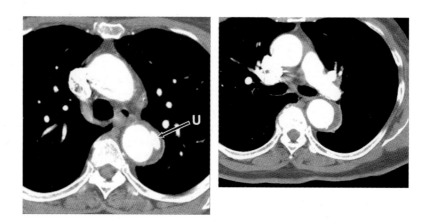

FIGURE 42. Penetrating atherosclerotic ulcer of the proximal descending thoracic aorta. Axial CT images at the level of the aortopulmonary window (*left*) and at the level of the left pulmonary artery (*right*) demonstrate a small penetrating ulcer (*arrow*) that extends beyond the expected confines of the aortic lumen with adjacent intramural hematoma both at the level of the ulcer itself and that extends a few centimeters caudally in the wall of the descending thoracic aorta. U = penetrating ulcer.

control heart rate and reduce blood pressure. Current guidelines recommend reducing systolic blood pressure to 120 mm Hg or less in the first hour in patients with aortic dissection. Intravenous β-blockers are first-line treatment; for hypertension that does not completely respond to β-blockers, intravenous vasodilators (nitroprusside, nicardipine) should be administered. Pain control is often necessary and is best accomplished with intravenous opioids.

An algorithm for the management of acute ascending aortic dissections is shown in **Figure 43**. Referral for emergency surgery should be considered in all patients with acute aortic dissection and cardiogenic shock, patients with type A aortic dissection, and patients with type A intramural hematoma, given the very high mortality rate associated with these conditions. Decisions regarding concomitant aortic arch reconstruction, aortic valve replacement, branch vessel repair, and/or coronary artery bypass graft surgery or coronary artery reimplantation depend on the anatomy of the aortic dissection, involvement of the aortic valve or branch vessels, and various other patient characteristics.

Patients who present with uncomplicated type B aortic syndromes may be treated with medical therapy initially. TEVAR, when compared with medical therapy, is associated with similar clinical outcomes and improved survival and disease progression measures at 2 years. Patients with type B aortic dissection and refractory chest/back pain or hypertension, rapid aortic expansion, or organ malperfusion should undergo aortic repair.

In patients with an intramural aortic hematoma or penetrating aortic ulcer, treatment choices depend on the location of the hematoma or ulcer, progression to aortic dissection, and evidence of aortic enlargement. Immediate aortic repair is indicated in patients with an ascending aortic intramural hematoma or penetrating aortic ulcer and in those with enlargement or progression of disease after detection. **H**

KEY POINTS

- Acute aortic dissection classically presents with the sudden onset of ripping or tearing pain in the chest, back, or abdomen.

- Clinical examination findings that increase the index of suspicion for an acute aortic syndrome include pulsus paradoxus, asymmetric blood pressures in the upper extremities, and asymmetric pulses.

- CT angiography is the primary diagnostic test in patients in whom acute thoracic aortic disease is suspected.

- Intravenous β-blockers are first-line treatment to reduce heart rate and control blood pressure in patients with acute aortic dissection without cardiogenic shock.

- Emergency surgery should be considered in all patients with acute aortic dissection and cardiogenic shock, type A aortic dissection, and type A intramural hematoma.

Role of Genetic Testing and Family Screening

Genetic conditions that predispose patients to thoracic aortic aneurysm syndromes include Marfan, Ehlers-Danlos, and Loeys-Dietz syndromes (see Table 33). Clinical findings and a family history of connective tissue disease often lead to genetic testing, for either diagnostic confirmation or screening of family members. Noninvasive imaging of the aorta should be performed if a pathogenic genetic mutation is found, and routine surveillance (initially at 6 months and then annually, if findings are stable) should follow to ensure that the aorta is not rapidly enlarging.

In first-degree relatives of patients with TAA and/or dissection, noninvasive imaging of the aorta should be performed to identify those with asymptomatic disease. In first-degree relatives of patients with a mutant gene (*FBN1, TGFBR1, TGFBR2, COL3A1, MYH11*) and aortic aneurysm and/or dissection, genetic counseling and testing should be performed. Relatives with the genetic mutation should then undergo noninvasive imaging of the aorta.

Peripheral Artery Disease
Epidemiology and Screening

Peripheral artery disease (PAD) is most commonly characterized by narrowing of the aortic bifurcation and arteries of the lower extremities, including the iliac, femoral, popliteal, and tibial arteries. Stenosis in the upper extremity arteries, typically at the origin of the subclavian arteries or at branch points of other major vessels, can also occur. Atherosclerosis is the most common cause. Risk factors for PAD include smoking (current or past), diabetes mellitus, and increasing age. PAD occurs at a later age in women than in men, and because women have a longer lifespan, the overall prevalence of PAD is higher in women. The incidence of PAD begins to increase around age 40 years and rises to approximately 10% at age 70 years.

PAD is considered a coronary heart disease risk equivalent, and both asymptomatic and symptomatic patients with PAD are at increased risk for ischemic events, including myocardial infarction, stroke, and cardiovascular death. Patients with atherosclerotic risk factors (smoking, diabetes, hypertension, dyslipidemia, advanced age) who have atypical limb symptoms (leg weakness, paresthesias), exertional leg discomfort, and/or nonhealing ulcers should undergo initial testing with ankle-brachial index (ABI) measurement. According to guidelines from the American Heart Association and American College of Cardiology, a screening ABI is reasonable in asymptomatic persons with one of the following characteristics that signify increased risk: (1) age 65 years and older, (2) age 50 to 64 years with risk factors for atherosclerosis or family history of PAD, (3) age younger than 50 years with diabetes and one additional risk factor for atherosclerosis, or (4) known atherosclerotic disease in another vascular bed (coronary, carotid, subclavian, renal, or mesenteric artery stenosis, or abdominal aortic aneurysm). The U.S. Preventive Services Task Force

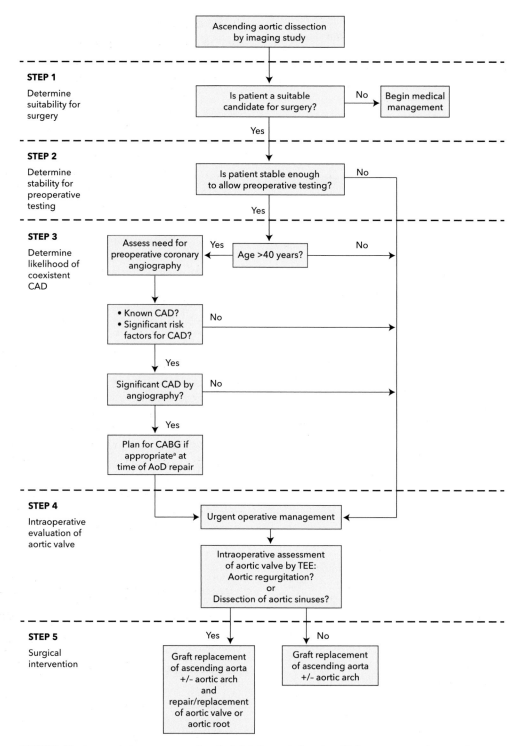

FIGURE 43. Acute surgical management pathway for AoD. AoD = aortic dissection; CABG = coronary artery bypass graft surgery; CAD = coronary artery disease; TEE = transesophageal echocardiography.

[a]Addition of "if appropriate" based on Patel MR, Dehmer GJ, Hirshfeld JW, Smith PK, Spertus JA; American College of Cardiology Foundation Appropriateness Criteria Task Force. ACCF/SCAI/STS/AATS/AHA/ASNC 2009 appropriateness criteria for coronary revascularization: a report by the American College of Cardiology Foundation Appropriateness Criteria Task Force, Society for Cardiovascular Angiography and Interventions, Society of Thoracic Surgeons, American Association for Thoracic Surgery, American Heart Association, and the American Society of Nuclear Cardiology Endorsed by the American Society of Echocardiography, the Heart Failure Society of America, and the Society of Cardiovascular Computed Tomography. J Am Coll Cardiol. 2009;53:530-53. [PMID: 19195618] doi:10.1016/j.jacc.2008.10.005.

Reproduced with permission from Hiratzka LF, Bakris GL, Beckman JA, Bersin RM, Carr VF, Casey DE Jr, et al; American College of Cardiology Foundation/American Heart Association Task Force on Practice Guidelines. 2010 ACCF/AHA/AATS/ACR/ASA/SCA/SCAI/SIR/STS/SVM guidelines for the diagnosis and management of patients with thoracic aortic disease. A report of the American College of Cardiology Foundation/American Heart Association Task Force on Practice Guidelines, American Association for Thoracic Surgery, American College of Radiology, American Stroke Association, Society of Cardiovascular Anesthesiologists, Society for Cardiovascular Angiography and Interventions, Society of Interventional Radiology, Society of Thoracic Surgeons, and Society for Vascular Medicine. J Am Coll Cardiol. 2010;55:e27-e129. [PMID: 20359588] doi:10.1016/j.jacc.2010.02.015. Copyright 2010, Elsevier.

concluded that there is insufficient evidence to support screening for lower extremity PAD with an ABI in all patients, especially those without risk factors for atherosclerotic vascular disease. Measurement of bilateral arm pressures is indicated in asymptomatic and symptomatic patients with atherosclerotic risk factors to assess for upper extremity PAD.

Clinical Presentation

Because lower extremity PAD is defined by an abnormal ABI value rather than by symptoms, there is a wide spectrum of clinical manifestations. Patients may present with exertional leg pain relieved by rest (intermittent claudication), atypical exertional leg pain, rest pain, nonhealing wounds, ischemic ulcers, or gangrene. Approximately 25% to 30% of patients with lower extremity PAD present with intermittent claudication, and less than 5% of patients present with critical limb ischemia. Most patients with upper extremity PAD have no symptoms, although patients may present with arm claudication, arm ischemia, or dizziness with arm activity (subclavian steal syndrome).

Patients with intermittent claudication often have reduced exercise capacity and functional status compared with age- and sex-matched controls. Their annual risk for myocardial infarction, stroke, or cardiovascular death is approximately 5% to 7%. Most patients with intermittent claudication have stable symptoms; however, symptoms worsen in approximately 25% of patients, and 10% to 20% of patients will undergo lower extremity revascularization procedures over a period of 5 years.

Critical limb ischemia, the most severe form of PAD, manifests as ischemic rest pain, tissue ulceration, and gangrene. Patients with critical limb ischemia often have reduced exercise capacity and functional status, and these patients have a 30% rate of major amputation and 20% mortality rate within 1 year of diagnosis.

Evaluation

History and Physical Examination

A detailed history, review of symptoms, and physical examination are critical in the evaluation of patients suspected of having vascular disease. Patients should be asked about walking impairment, atypical limb symptoms, intermittent claudication, and ischemic rest pain. In patients with exertional leg symptoms, intermittent claudication should be differentiated from pseudoclaudication (symptoms that arise from spinal stenosis) (**Table 36**). Patients should be questioned about skin breakdown and foot ulcers, and clinicians should educate patients on the importance of foot protection and wearing shoes (specifically, hard-soled shoes) when walking outside the home.

Elements of the physical examination of patients suspected of having PAD are listed in **Table 37**. Vascular examination of patients suspected of having lower extremity PAD should include comprehensive pulse examination, auscultation for bruits, and inspection of the feet for skin and toenail changes. Patients with PAD may exhibit diminished, absent, or asymmetric pulses, and bruits may be heard at or near sites of arterial stenosis. Patients with critical limb ischemia may have decreased temperature or lack of hair growth in the affected extremity, as well as evidence of poor wound healing or active ulceration (typically involving the digits, plantar aspect of the foot, or heel). Clinicians should distinguish between signs of chronic venous disease (leg edema; pigmented, brawny induration of the gaiter zone; ulceration of the shin or ankle) and critical limb ischemia when evaluating patients with leg ulcers because venous leg ulcers are treated differently than ulcerations in patients with critical limb ischemia (see MKSAP 18 Dermatology).

In patients with upper extremity PAD, a characteristic finding on physical examination is a difference in systolic

TABLE 36.	Discriminating Claudication from Pseudoclaudication	
Characteristic	**Claudication**	**Pseudoclaudication**
Nature of discomfort	Cramping, tightness, aching, fatigue	Same as for claudication plus tingling, burning, numbness, weakness
Location of discomfort	Buttock, hip, thigh, calf, foot	Same as for claudication; most often bilateral
Exercise-induced	Yes	Variable
Walking distance at onset of symptoms	Consistent	Variable
Discomfort occurs with standing still	No	Yes
Action for relief	Stand or sit	Sit, flexion at the waist
Time to relief	<5 min	≤30 min

TABLE 37. Physical Examination of Patients for Peripheral Artery Disease

Measure blood pressure in both arms (systolic blood pressure difference >15 mm Hg suggests subclavian stenosis)

Auscultate for presence of arterial bruits (e.g., femoral artery)

Palpate for presence of abdominal aortic aneurysm

Palpate and record pulses (radial, brachial, carotid, femoral, popliteal, posterior tibial, dorsalis pedis)

Evaluate for elevation pallor and dependent rubor

Inspect feet for ulcers, fissures, calluses, tinea, and tendinous xanthoma; evaluate overall skin care

blood pressures between the arms, typically more than 15 mm Hg.

Diagnostic Testing

The most frequently used diagnostic modality to identify lower extremity PAD is measurement of the ABI, which is the ratio of lower extremity to upper extremity systolic blood pressures. ABI measurement is simple, inexpensive, and noninvasive, with a sensitivity and specificity approaching 90%. When undergoing ABI testing, patients should rest for 10 minutes in a supine position before the clinician measures the ankle pressures and brachial pressures with a Doppler machine. Blood pressures should be measured in both arms and in both legs at the dorsalis pedis and posterior tibial ankle locations. To calculate the ABI for each leg, the higher ankle pressure in each leg is divided by the higher brachial artery pressure. In healthy persons, the ankle pressure should be the same as or slightly higher than the brachial pressure; therefore, a normal resting ABI is between 1.00 and 1.40 (**Table 38**). In the presence of atherosclerotic narrowing of the limb arteries, the downstream blood pressure and concomitant ABI value is lower. A resting ABI of 0.90 or less is diagnostic for PAD and correlates with abnormalities seen on imaging of the arterial tree. A resting ABI greater than 1.40 indicates the presence of noncompressible, calcified arteries in the lower extremities and is considered uninterpretable. In patients with an ABI greater than 1.40, a toe-brachial index is used for diagnosis. A toe-brachial index less than 0.70 is diagnostic for PAD.

TABLE 38. Interpretation of the Ankle-Brachial Index

Ankle-Brachial Index	Interpretation
>1.40	Noncompressible (calcified) vessel (uninterpretable result)
1.00-1.40	Normal
0.91-0.99	Borderline
0.41-0.90	Mild to moderate PAD
0.00-0.40	Severe PAD

PAD = peripheral artery disease.

An exercise ABI test is useful when resting ABI values are between 0.91 and 1.40 and the pretest probability of PAD is high. It requires ABI measurements at rest and after treadmill walking or plantar flexion exercises. The American Heart Association has proposed a postexercise ankle pressure decrease of more than 30 mm Hg or a postexercise ABI decrease of more than 20% as a diagnostic criterion for PAD. Other organizations have proposed a postexercise ABI of less than 0.90 and/or a 30-mm Hg drop in ankle pressure after exercise.

Segmental pressure measurements may be performed in a vascular laboratory to localize diseased vessels. This procedure involves pulse volume recordings (measurement of the magnitude and contour of blood pulse volume in the lower extremities) and blood pressure measurements at several locations in the lower extremities (high thigh, low thigh, calf, posterior tibial artery, and dorsalis pedis artery) (**Figure 44**).

Hemodynamic measurements (ABI, toe-brachial index, exercise ABI, and segmental pressure measurements) remain the most commonly used diagnostic tests for patients suspected of having lower extremity PAD. The ABI does not correlate with the patient's perception of symptom severity or functional limitations; however, lower ABI values are associated with higher rates of myocardial infarction, stroke, and death.

Other imaging tests used to delineate the anatomic location and severity of lower extremity PAD include arterial duplex ultrasonography, CT angiography, and magnetic resonance angiography (**Table 39**). These imaging modalities are most often used to plan for endovascular or surgical revascularization procedures. Invasive angiography is often preferred because endovascular revascularization procedures can be performed concurrently.

TABLE 39. Comparison of Imaging Modalities for the Diagnosis of Peripheral Artery Disease

Imaging Modality	Advantages	Limitations
Arterial duplex ultrasonography	Widely available Does not require administration of contrast dye Inexpensive	Limited ability to detect stenoses in the pelvis and in patients with severe calcifications Poor utility for infrapopliteal stenosis
CT angiography	Widely available Useful in defining the severity of PAD Very expensive	Risk for contrast-induced nephropathy
Magnetic resonance angiography	Useful in defining the severity of PAD Very expensive	Contraindicated in patients with implanted pacemakers and defibrillators Risk for nephrogenic systemic fibrosis in patients with severe kidney disease

PAD = peripheral artery disease.

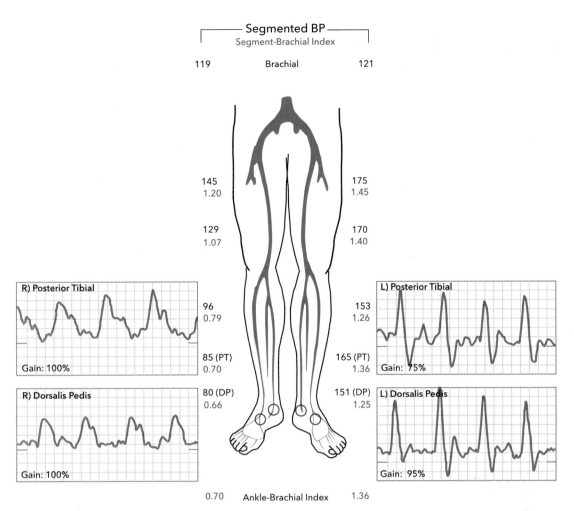

FIGURE 44. A pulse volume recording demonstrating decreased perfusion in the patient's right side. An ankle-brachial index value of 0.70 on the right side is consistent with the diagnosis of mild to moderate peripheral artery disease (ankle-brachial index <0.90). The normal pulse volume recording on the patient's left side has a sharp systolic upstroke and downstroke (the width of the waveform is much narrower compared with the waveform on the right side). When the amplitude of the waveform is significantly blunted and the width is broader, it suggests moderate to severe disease. BP = blood pressure; DP = dorsalis pedis; PT = posterior tibial.

Duplex ultrasonography, CT angiography, and magnetic resonance angiography are also appropriate in patients with upper extremity PAD to confirm the diagnosis and plan for intervention, such as revascularization.

KEY POINTS

- An ankle-brachial index of 0.90 or less indicates peripheral artery disease.

- An ankle-brachial index greater than 1.40 indicates the presence of noncompressible arteries in the lower extremities and is considered uninterpretable; a toe-brachial index is used for diagnosis of peripheral artery disease in these patients.

- Imaging with CT angiography or magnetic resonance angiography is useful to identify the location of stenosis and severity of peripheral artery disease in planning for endovascular or surgical revascularization procedures.

Medical Therapy

Treatment of PAD focuses on reducing cardiovascular risk; improving functional status, quality of life, and claudication symptoms; and preventing tissue loss and amputation.

Cardiovascular Risk Reduction

Cigarette smoking is the most important modifiable risk factor for the development of PAD. Smoking cessation is associated with decreased risk for major amputation, improved patency rates following revascularization, and less disease progression. Smoking cessation is imperative to lower the risk for myocardial infarction and stroke and improve overall survival in patients with PAD.

Diabetes is also a strong risk factor for PAD; however, intensive glucose control has not been demonstrated to reduce macrovascular complications, including myocardial infarction, stroke, or amputation. Regardless, patients with PAD and diabetes should adhere to American Diabetes Association recommendations on diabetes management, with particular attention to foot care.

Dyslipidemia has a mild effect on the development of PAD. Patients with symptomatic PAD should be treated with high-intensity statin therapy, and patients with PAD who are older than 75 years or intolerant of high-intensity statins should be treated with moderate-intensity statin therapy (see MKSAP 18 General Internal Medicine).

Hypertension also has a mild effect on the development of PAD, and control of blood pressure has been associated with reduction of cardiovascular events in patients with PAD. The 2017 high blood pressure guideline from the American College of Cardiology, the American Heart Association, and nine other organizations recommends a blood pressure target of less than 130/80 mm Hg in patients with PAD. There is no consensus on the antihypertensive therapy of choice in patients with PAD; therefore, thiazide diuretics, ACE inhibitors or angiotensin receptor blockers, and calcium channel blockers remain first-line agents in patients with PAD and hypertension. In patients at high risk for cardiovascular events or with comorbid conditions (such as diabetes), ACE inhibitors are effective in reducing cardiovascular morbidity and mortality.

Antithrombotic Therapy

Current guidelines recommend antiplatelet monotherapy in patients with PAD to reduce risk for myocardial infarction, stroke, and peripheral arterial events. Despite little supporting evidence, aspirin has been recommended by experts as the primary antiplatelet agent in patients with PAD. In patients who are aspirin intolerant, clopidogrel is recommended as an acceptable alternative. There is no compelling evidence for the use of dual antiplatelet therapy with aspirin plus clopidogrel in patients with PAD alone. In the CHARISMA trial, patients with PAD who were treated with aspirin plus clopidogrel had a reduced rate of hospitalization for myocardial infarction and ischemic events, which was mitigated by a higher rate of bleeding.

Evidence from the TRA 2P-TIMI 50 trial demonstrated that vorapaxar, a thrombin receptor antagonist, was associated with improved limb endpoints (specifically, hospitalization for acute limb ischemia) when compared with placebo in patients with PAD. However, most patients in the TRA 2P-TIMI 50 trial were treated with aspirin, and 30% of patients were treated with aspirin plus clopidogrel. Vorapaxar was also associated with an increased risk for moderate or severe bleeding, including intracranial hemorrhage.

In a large secondary prevention study of patients with prior myocardial infarction receiving aspirin therapy, ticagrelor was superior to placebo in reducing the composite endpoint of cardiovascular death, myocardial infarction, or stroke and major adverse limb events in the subset of patients with PAD. Major bleeding was increased in patients randomly assigned to ticagrelor. However, the absolute risk for major bleeding in patients with PAD was lower than in patients without PAD.

There is no evidence that oral anticoagulation with vitamin K antagonists (such as warfarin) is more effective than antiplatelet monotherapy in patients with PAD, and anticoagulant therapy is associated with an increased risk for major bleeding. There is also no evidence that non–vitamin K antagonist oral anticoagulants are superior to antiplatelet agents in patients with PAD.

Symptom Relief

Improving functional status and improving quality of life are critical goals for patients with PAD. In patients who can exercise, supervised exercise training has been associated with improved functional performance and is recommended for patients with intermittent claudication. Systematic reviews comparing supervised exercise with home exercise have reported improvements in maximal walking distance and initial claudication distance that favor supervised exercise; however, no statistically significant differences in quality of life were observed. Despite its effectiveness and safety, supervised exercise training is limited by lack of insurance coverage and unavailability of these programs for patients with claudication.

Medical therapy for patients with intermittent claudication consists of cilostazol, a phosphodiesterase inhibitor with antiplatelet and vasodilator activity. Cilostazol has demonstrated increases in pain-free walking distance and overall walking distance in patients with claudication, and clinical guidelines recommend that patients with claudication be considered for a therapeutic trial of cilostazol. As with other oral phosphodiesterase inhibitors (for example, inotropes such as milrinone), the FDA has placed a black box warning on the use of cilostazol in patients with heart failure. There is no approved pharmacotherapy for patients with critical limb ischemia.

KEY POINTS

- Smoking cessation is essential to reduce cardiovascular risk in patients with peripheral artery disease.
- Antiplatelet monotherapy with aspirin is recommended for patients with peripheral artery disease to reduce the risk for myocardial infarction, stroke, and peripheral arterial events.
- Supervised exercise training is the most effective treatment for improvement of functional status in patients with peripheral artery disease.
- Cilostazol is recommended for patients with intermittent claudication.

Interventional Therapy

Endovascular or surgical revascularization procedures are effective in improving symptoms, increasing functional capacity, and improving wound healing in patients with intermittent claudication or critical limb ischemia. Referral for revascularization is indicated in patients with lifestyle-limiting claudication, rest pain, ulceration, or gangrene, especially if there has been an inadequate response to exercise training, cilostazol, and/or wound treatment. Patients with critical limb ischemia (ABI <0.40, a flat waveform on pulse volume recording, and low or absent pedal flow on duplex ultrasonography) should be considered for urgent revascularization. Endovascular or surgical revascularization should also be considered in patients with a favorable risk-benefit ratio, which is determined by patient factors (age, frailty, comorbid conditions), anatomic factors (severity and burden of atherosclerotic disease, location of disease in lower extremities), operator expertise, and type of procedure. Revascularization is not recommended in asymptomatic patients. **H**

Endovascular revascularization has dramatically increased in recent years because the procedure is minimally invasive and confers a lower risk for perioperative adverse events compared with surgical revascularization. Endovascular revascularization procedures include balloon angioplasty (standard, cutting, drug-coated), stenting (nitinol [nickel-titanium] bare metal and drug eluting), and atherectomy (laser, orbital, rotational, directional). In patients with isolated iliac disease, endovascular revascularization is favored over surgical revascularization owing to lower morbidity and mortality, high procedural success, and high patency rates over time. Most patients undergo balloon angioplasty and stenting of the iliac arteries, given the significantly higher long-term success rate with stenting compared with angioplasty alone.

In patients with femoral, popliteal, or tibial artery (infrainguinal) disease, the patency rates of endovascular revascularization are not as high as in the iliac arteries. Although infrainguinal disease was traditionally treated with angioplasty alone, the advent of atherectomy devices and nitinol stents has changed management. Recently, FDA-approved drug-coated angioplasty balloons and drug-eluting stents have demonstrated superior efficacy compared with standard angioplasty balloons in these patients.

The use of surgical revascularization has declined in the United States; however, patients with complex anatomy that may limit percutaneous procedural success and long-term patency (for example, long chronic total occlusions, multisegment disease) should still be referred for surgical revascularization. The two most common techniques of surgical revascularization are endarterectomy and surgical bypass.

Hybrid revascularization is the concomitant performance of surgical revascularization and endovascular revascularization in a single setting or finite time frame. Hybrid revascularization has increased in conjunction with the rise in endovascular revascularization; however, there are currently no clinical guideline recommendations for hybrid revascularization.

KEY POINTS

- In patients with life-limiting claudication who have had an inadequate response to exercise or pharmacologic therapy, endovascular or surgical revascularization is indicated.

- Patients with critical limb ischemia should be considered for urgent revascularization.

Acute Limb Ischemia

Acute limb ischemia is an infrequent but life-threatening manifestation of PAD. Classically, patients present with at least one of the "6 Ps": paresthesia, pain, pallor, pulselessness, poikilothermia (coolness), and paralysis. Acute limb ischemia is most commonly caused by acute thrombosis of a lower extremity artery, stent, or bypass graft. Other causes include thromboembolism, vessel dissection (usually occurring periprocedurally), or trauma. The presentation of acute limb ischemia represents a true medical emergency; 10% to 15% of patients undergo amputation during initial hospitalization, and 20% of patients die within 1 year.

Anticoagulation, typically with unfractionated heparin, should be initiated as soon as the diagnosis is suspected. Specialists with expertise in revascularization should be consulted, and diagnostic angiography should be performed immediately to define the anatomic level of occlusion. In addition to surgical and endovascular revascularization options, catheter-directed thrombolysis improves outcomes in patients with acute limb ischemia.

Careful monitoring is required after limb reperfusion because of frequent reocclusion, limb edema, and the possibility of compartment syndrome. Signs and symptoms of compartment syndrome include severe pain, hypoesthesia, and leg weakness. If compartment syndrome occurs, surgical fasciotomy is indicated to prevent irreversible neurologic and soft-tissue damage. **H**

KEY POINTS

- Acute limb ischemia is characterized by at least one of the "6 Ps": paresthesia, pain, pallor, pulselessness, poikilothermia (coolness), and paralysis.

- Patients with acute limb ischemia should receive immediate anticoagulation therapy and diagnostic angiography in preparation for emergent endovascular or surgical revascularization.

- Careful monitoring after limb reperfusion is required because of frequent reocclusion, limb edema, and the possibility of compartment syndrome.

Cardiovascular Disease in Cancer Survivors

Cardiotoxicity of Radiation Therapy to the Thorax

Radiation therapy improves survival in patients with Hodgkin lymphoma, early-stage breast cancer, and other thoracic malignancies. With higher survival rates, cardiovascular disease has emerged as the most common nonmalignant cause of death in patients treated with chest radiation therapy, accounting for 25% of deaths in survivors of Hodgkin lymphoma.

Radiation therapy causes a wide spectrum of cardiac diseases (**Table 40**). Thoracic irradiation damages all cells, including those of the pericardium, myocardium, valves, coronary vasculature, and conduction system, with clinical disease usually presenting two to three decades after treatment. The risk for radiation-induced cardiac injury is further increased in patients who are concomitantly taking anthracyclines or trastuzumab. Recognition of the cardiovascular complications associated with radiation therapy has led to techniques that limit total dosage and field size.

Acute pericarditis is the most common early manifestation of radiotoxicity; however, it is now less common (incidence of 2.5%) because of changes in shielding, divided dosing, and lower cumulative doses. The presentation, diagnosis, and treatment are similar to those of idiopathic acute pericarditis. Chronic or constrictive pericarditis develops in up to 10% to 20% of patients at 5 to 10 years after radiation therapy. Pericardial calcification is not always present radiographically (**Figure 45**). Late constriction can occur in those who have not experienced acute pericarditis.

Radiation therapy also damages the microvasculature, causing endothelial dysfunction and ischemia that result in myocardial fibrosis, diastolic dysfunction, and restrictive physiology. Radiation-induced cardiomyopathy presents similarly to primary restrictive cardiomyopathy. Differentiating cardiomyopathy due to myocardial fibrosis from pericardial constriction is essential because the conditions have different treatments and outcomes.

Although all cardiac valves may be affected by radiation therapy, left-sided involvement predominates. Valvular insufficiency due to tissue retraction is the most common valvular lesion in the first two decades after therapy, with later fibrosis and calcification leading to mixed regurgitation and stenosis.

Radiation therapy results in fibrosis of the conduction system and may lead to sinus node dysfunction, fascicular and bundle branch blocks, and complete heart block. The need for a permanent pacemaker is more common after valve replacement surgery in patients who have received radiation therapy.

Coronary artery disease (CAD) occurs earlier and with increased incidence in patients treated with radiation therapy. Coronary artery lesions are typically ostial, long, smooth,

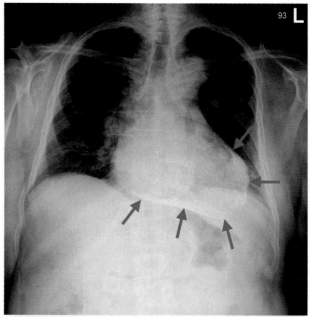

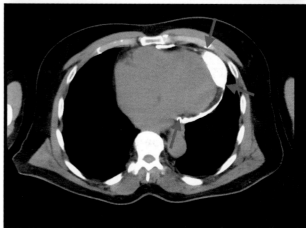

FIGURE 45. Chest radiograph (*top panel*) and chest CT (*bottom panel*) demonstrating pericardial calcification in a patient who received chest radiation therapy for esophageal cancer. Pericardial calcification most often occurs as a circumferential rim but may be incomplete or heterogeneous (*arrows*).

and concentric and have a higher fibrotic content than typical atherosclerotic lesions. The incidence of CAD is increased by traditional risk factors (such as smoking, dyslipidemia, and hypertension), and therapy to address these risk factors is indicated. In-stent restenosis rates with bare metal stents are significantly higher in patients with radiation-induced CAD. There are no data on the outcomes with drug-eluting stents. In patients with radiation-induced CAD, native vessels, including the left internal mammary artery, may be rendered unusable for bypass. The postoperative course may be complicated by radiation-induced lung injury (pleural effusion, prolonged ventilation) and a higher incidence of atrial fibrillation. Limited data are available on outcomes in patients undergoing cardiac surgery for radiation-related valvular or coronary disease.

TABLE 40. Cardiovascular Diseases Related to Radiation Therapy
Cardiomyopathy
Conduction defects (atrioventricular block, bundle branch block)
Coronary artery disease
Coronary microvascular injury
Pericardial disease (acute pericarditis, chronic constrictive pericarditis, pericardial effusion)
Peripheral artery disease
Valvular disease

There is no consensus on cardiac testing in asymptomatic patients after chest radiation. Baseline cardiac evaluation that includes echocardiography is reasonable, and several organizations have recommended starting stress echocardiography at 5 to 10 years after completion of therapy or at age 30 years, whichever comes first. The role of serum biomarkers in surveillance is unclear, and their use is not recommended. Routine screening with nuclear medicine testing or coronary CT should be avoided.

Although effective for risk factor reduction, statins, ACE inhibitors, and aldosterone inhibitors have not been proved to prevent radiation-induced cardiovascular disease.

KEY POINTS

- Thoracic irradiation damages all cells, including those of the pericardium, myocardium, valves, coronary vasculature, and conduction system, with clinical disease usually presenting two to three decades after treatment.

- Traditional cardiovascular risk factors, such as smoking, dyslipidemia, and hypertension, should be aggressively managed because of the increased risk for coronary artery disease in patients with a history of chest radiation therapy.

Cardiotoxicity of Chemotherapy

Chemotherapy may result in many types of cardiovascular toxicity (**Table 41**). Two broad categories of chemotherapeutic

cardiac injury have been defined based on severity: type I, which is marked by dose-dependent cardiac dysfunction with irreversible ultrastructural necrosis, and type II, which is not dose dependent and is often reversible.

Type I injury is associated with the use of anthracyclines, such as doxorubicin, daunorubicin, and epirubicin. Acute anthracycline toxicity, which can present as heart block, arrhythmias, heart failure, myocarditis, and pericarditis, occurs in less than 1% of patients and may be reversible. Chronic progressive anthracycline toxicity usually presents as dilated cardiomyopathy and is most closely linked with the use of doxorubicin. Chronic progressive toxicity has an early onset (within 1 year of treatment) in 1.6% to 2% of patients and a late onset (after 1 year) in up to 5% of patients. Late-onset chronic progressive toxicity is related to total cumulative dose. In patients with a cumulative anthracycline dose of 550 mg/m^2, the incidence of heart failure is up to 26%, and toxicity may not become clinically evident until 10 to 20 years after treatment. Factors associated with increased risk for anthracycline toxicity include concomitant use of cyclophosphamide, trastuzumab, or paclitaxel; previous chest irradiation; and female sex. Lower risk for cardiotoxicity is associated with epirubicin and idarubicin compared with doxorubicin. Concomitant dexrazoxane reduces the risk for doxorubicin toxicity. Limited data from small studies have shown the angiotensin receptor blocker valsartan may protect against some of the cardiotoxicity of anthracyclines.

TABLE 41.	Cardiovascular Toxicities Associated with Chemotherapy	
Toxicity	**Class**	**Drug**
Left ventricular dysfunction	Anthracyclines	Doxorubicin, epirubicin, idarubicin
	Alkylating agents	Cyclophosphamide, ifosfamide
	Antimicrotubular agents	Paclitaxel, docetaxel
	Monoclonal antibody	Trastuzumab
	Tyrosine kinase inhibitor	Sunitinib
	Proteasome inhibitor	Bortezomib
Ischemia	Antimetabolites	5-Fluorouracil, capecitabine
	Antimicrotubular agents	Paclitaxel, docetaxel
	Monoclonal antibody	Bevacizumab
	Tyrosine kinase inhibitors	Erlotinib, sorafenib
Hypertension	Monoclonal antibody	Bevacizumab
	Tyrosine kinase inhibitors	Sorafenib, sunitinib
Venous thromboembolism	Alkylating agent	Cisplatin
	Angiogenesis inhibitor	Thalidomide
	Tyrosine kinase inhibitor	Erlotinib
Bradycardia	Angiogenesis inhibitor	Thalidomide
	Antimicrotubular agent	Paclitaxel
QT prolongation	Tyrosine kinase inhibitor	Dasatinib
	Histone deacetylase inhibitor	Vorinostat
	Miscellaneous	Arsenic

Type II injury is more commonly associated with molecularly targeted therapy, such as trastuzumab. Trastuzumab toxicity results in left ventricular systolic dysfunction, with symptoms of heart failure in 3% to 7% of patients. It is more common in patients older than 50 years or with concomitant anthracycline use. Patients who demonstrate normalization of left ventricular function after discontinuation of trastuzumab may receive additional therapy.

Multitargeted tyrosine kinase inhibitors and anti–vascular endothelial growth factor antibodies are increasingly being used as targeted molecular therapy. Of the tyrosine kinase inhibitors, sunitinib has been most frequently associated with cardiotoxicity, with up to a 50% incidence of new or worsened hypertension and up to a 15% incidence of decreased left ventricular ejection fraction (LVEF). These effects may be reversible with early recognition. Surveillance with baseline N-terminal proB-type natriuretic peptide measurement and LVEF assessment at baseline, 1 month, and every 3 months thereafter has been advocated for patients taking sunitinib. Not all tyrosine kinase inhibitors carry the same risk for cardiotoxicity. The anti–vascular endothelial growth factor antibody bevacizumab is associated with significant but reversible hypertension.

In patients preparing to receive chemotherapy associated with known cardiotoxicity, an electrocardiogram should be obtained at baseline. Baseline evaluation of LVEF (with echocardiography or multigated acquisition scanning) is important if the associated cardiotoxicity includes left ventricular dysfunction and heart failure. It is reasonable to repeat echocardiography at a total cumulative anthracycline dose of 300 mg/m² and before each dose in patients with pre-existent left ventricular dysfunction or those receiving higher cumulative doses. European guidelines suggest that patients receiving trastuzumab should undergo repeat echocardiography every 3 months. In general, cardiovascular consultation should be obtained in asymptomatic patients who demonstrate a decline in LVEF of 10% or more or in patients with symptoms of heart failure associated with a decline in LVEF of 5% or more to a level below 55%. Three-dimensional echocardiographic evaluation of left ventricular volumes may be more accurate in detecting small changes.

In patients with clinical signs or symptoms of cardiac dysfunction, cardiac biomarkers (such as troponin and N-terminal proB-type natriuretic peptide) along with imaging techniques (such as echocardiographically derived global longitudinal strain) may be helpful in identifying early toxicity and guiding individual therapy. At present, treatment of patients with chemotherapy-induced heart failure follows standard paradigms.

KEY POINTS

- Chronic anthracycline toxicity usually presents as irreversible dilated cardiomyopathy.
- Cardiotoxicity from trastuzumab manifests as reversible left ventricular systolic dysfunction.

Pregnancy and Cardiovascular Disease
Cardiovascular Changes During Pregnancy

Knowledge of the cardiovascular changes of pregnancy is necessary to distinguish between normal and pathologic signs and symptoms in the pregnant patient (**Table 42**). During a normal pregnancy, patients develop a relative anemia due to increases in plasma volume and, to a lesser degree, erythrocyte mass. Mean arterial pressure slightly decreases in the setting of reduced systemic vascular resistance and increased heart rate and cardiac output. By the 32nd week of pregnancy, maternal cardiac output peaks at approximately 40% above the prepregnancy level. During delivery, the cardiac output may increase to as much as 80% above the prepregnancy level owing to increased heart rate and blood pressure.

Prepregnancy Evaluation

All women with cardiovascular disease who are anticipating pregnancy should undergo specialized prepregnancy cardiovascular evaluation, high-risk obstetrics consultation, obstetric anesthesia consultation, and, if appropriate, genetic counseling

TABLE 42. Normal Versus Pathologic Signs and Symptoms in Pregnancy

Type of Sign or Symptom	Normal	Pathologic
Pulmonary	Mild dyspnea, dyspnea with exertion	Orthopnea, paroxysmal nocturnal dyspnea, cough, pulmonary edema
Cardiac	No symptoms	Chest pressure, heaviness, or pain
Edema	Mild peripheral edema	More than mild edema
Heart rhythm	Atrial and ventricular premature beats	Atrial fibrillation or flutter, ventricular tachycardia
Heart rate	Heart rate increased by 20%-30%	Heart rate >100/min
Blood pressure	Blood pressure typically is modestly decreased (~10 mm Hg)	Low blood pressure associated with symptoms, high blood pressure (≥140 mm Hg systolic or ≥90 mm Hg diastolic)
Auscultatory	Basal systolic murmur grade 1/6 or 2/6 present in 80% of pregnant women, S₃	Systolic murmur grade ≥3/6, any diastolic murmur, S₄

to evaluate the risks of pregnancy and develop a management plan for labor and the postpartum period. Prepregnancy risk assessment tools include the CARPREG index (**Table 43**), ZAHARA risk score (**Table 44**), and the modified World Health Organization pregnancy risk classification (**Table 45**). All of these tools are used to estimate risk for complications during pregnancy in women with cardiovascular disease.

Pregnancy is contraindicated in patients with ventricular outflow tract obstruction (for example, aortic stenosis or coarctation of aorta) and those with left ventricular systolic dysfunction (ejection fraction <40%) accompanied by New York Heart Association functional class III or IV heart failure symptoms because these conditions confer a high risk for maternal and fetal complications. Women with severe pulmonary hypertension are at high risk for maternal death, with a mortality rate of up to 30%.

KEY POINTS

- Women with cardiovascular disease who are anticipating pregnancy should undergo prepregnancy evaluation with a cardiologist, obstetrician, and anesthesiologist as well as genetic counseling, if appropriate.

- Pregnancy is contraindicated in patients with ventricular outflow tract obstruction and those with left ventricular systolic dysfunction (ejection fraction <40%) accompanied by New York Heart Association functional class III or IV heart failure symptoms.

- Women with severe pulmonary hypertension are at high risk for maternal mortality.

Management of Cardiovascular Disease During Pregnancy

Women with obstructive cardiac lesions may experience symptoms during pregnancy as a result of the increases in blood volume and cardiac output. These patients should be evaluated to determine whether cardiac intervention should be considered before pregnancy. Women with regurgitant valve lesions tend to tolerate pregnancy well.

Vaginal delivery is generally preferred for patients with cardiovascular disease because it results in less blood loss, quicker recovery, and lower risk for thrombosis than does cesarean delivery. Cesarean delivery is recommended for obstetric reasons in women with severe decompensated cardiovascular disease or a markedly dilated aorta. In women receiving warfarin therapy, cesarean delivery is indicated to reduce the risk for fetal intracranial hemorrhage because the fetus is fully anticoagulated.

Peripartum Cardiomyopathy

Peripartum cardiomyopathy is left ventricular systolic dysfunction recognized toward the end of pregnancy or in the months following delivery in the absence of another identifiable cause. Risk factors for peripartum cardiomyopathy include multiparity, age older than 30 years, African descent, multifetal pregnancy, gestational hypertension, preeclampsia, a previous episode of peripartum cardiomyopathy, and therapy with a tocolytic agent.

Death in women with peripartum cardiomyopathy is caused by heart failure, thromboembolic events, and arrhythmias. Most

TABLE 43. Predictors of Maternal Cardiac Events in Women with Congenital or Acquired Cardiac Disease (CARPREG Index)	
Risk Factor (Predictor)	**Operational Definition**
Previous cardiac event or arrhythmia	Heart failure, transient ischemic attack, stroke, arrhythmia
Baseline NYHA functional class III or IV or cyanosis	Mild symptoms (mild shortness of breath and/or angina) and slight limitation during ordinary activity
Left-sided heart obstruction	Mitral valve area <2 cm²; aortic valve area <1.5 cm² or resting peak left ventricular outflow tract gradient >30 mm Hg
Reduced systemic ventricular systolic function	Ejection fraction <40%

Estimated Risk for Cardiac Events[a]		
No. of Predictors	**Estimated Risk (%)**	**Recommendation**
0	4	Consider preconception cardiac intervention for specific lesions; increase frequency of follow-up; delivery at community hospital
1	31	Consider preconception cardiac intervention for specific lesions; refer to regional center for ongoing care
>1	69	Consider preconception cardiac intervention for specific lesions; refer to regional center for ongoing care

NYHA = New York Heart Association.

[a]Cardiac events include pulmonary edema, tachyarrhythmia, embolic stroke, and cardiac death.

Data and recommendations from Siu SC, Sermer M, Colman JM, Alvarez AN, Mercier LA, Morton BC, et al; Cardiac Disease in Pregnancy (CARPREG) Investigators. Prospective multicenter study of pregnancy outcomes in women with heart disease. Circulation. 2001;104:515-21. [PMID: 11479246]

TABLE 44.	ZAHARA Risk Score Used to Predict Adverse Maternal Cardiac Events
Risk Factor (Predictor)	**Risk Score (Points)**
Mechanical heart valve	4.25
Severe left heart obstruction (mean gradient >50 mm Hg or aortic valve area <1.0 cm^2)	2.5
History of arrhythmias	1.5
History of cardiac medication use before pregnancy	1.5
History of cyanotic heart disease (uncorrected or corrected)	1.0
Moderate to severe pulmonary or systemic atrioventricular valve regurgitation	0.75
Symptomatic heart failure before pregnancy (NYHA functional class ≥II)	0.75

Estimated Risk for Maternal Cardiac Complications[a]	
Points	**Estimated Risk (%)**
0-0.5	2.9
0.51-1.50	7.5
1.51-2.50	17.5
2.51-3.50	43.1
≥3.51	70.0

NYHA = New York Heart Association; ZAHARA = Zwangerschap bij Aangeboren HARtAfwijkingen.

[a]Cardiac complications include clinically significant episodes of arrhythmia or heart failure (episodes requiring treatment with at least a drug prescription), cardiovascular complications (thromboembolic complications, myocardial infarction, and/or cerebrovascular accidents), and endocarditis (including in the first 6 months postpartum).

Data and recommendations from Drenthen W, Boersma E, Balci A, Moons P, Roos-Hesselink JW, Mulder BJ, et al; ZAHARA Investigators. Predictors of pregnancy complications in women with congenital heart disease. Eur Heart J. 2010;31:2124-32. [PMID: 20584777] doi:10.1093/eurheartj/ehq200

women who develop peripartum cardiomyopathy recover fully, as measured by improvement in ejection fraction; however, 13% have major cardiovascular events or persistent severe cardiomyopathy. Studies suggest that the time frame for recovery is 6 months. Prognostic factors that portend a worse outcome include severe left ventricular dysfunction/dilatation or black race.

Women with peripartum cardiomyopathy should be promptly treated with medical therapy, which may include β-blockers, digoxin, hydralazine, nitrates, or diuretics. ACE inhibitors, angiotensin receptor blockers, and aldosterone antagonists are teratogenic and should be avoided until after delivery. Owing to the risk for thromboembolism associated with peripartum cardiomyopathy, anticoagulation is recommended for women with left ventricular ejection fraction below 35%. The choice of anticoagulant (heparin or warfarin) depends on whether the patient is still pregnant and the time since delivery; the decision should be made in consultation with a cardiologist. Duration of anticoagulation is at least 8 weeks, although therapy can be discontinued sooner if the ejection fraction normalizes.

Women with severe refractory heart failure due to peripartum cardiomyopathy should be referred for further evaluation and treatment, including ventricular assist device placement or heart transplantation. Limited evidence from small studies suggests that bromocriptine, which blocks prolactin secretion, improves left ventricular ejection fraction and clinical outcomes when added to peripartum-related heart failure therapy; however, its use is considered investigational.

Because subsequent pregnancy is often associated with recurrent or further reduction of left ventricular function, potentially resulting in clinical deterioration or death, women with a previous episode of peripartum cardiomyopathy with persistent left ventricular dysfunction should be advised to avoid future pregnancy.

Other Cardiovascular Disorders

Women with Marfan syndrome have an increased risk for pregnancy-related aortic dissection. Aortic repair is recommended before pregnancy in women with Marfan syndrome and an aortic diameter of 4.5 cm or greater. Risk factors for dissection during pregnancy in patients with Marfan syndrome with an aortic diameter of less than 4.5 cm include rapid dilatation of the aorta or a personal or family history of aortic dissection. These patients should be counseled to have aortic replacement before pregnancy.

Spontaneous coronary artery dissections may occur during pregnancy or in the postpartum period. Conservative, noninterventional therapy is preferred for most patients. A high index of suspicion is required, as patients presenting with spontaneous coronary artery dissection are generally considered at low risk for acute coronary syndromes.

Cardiovascular Medication Use During Pregnancy

Guidelines for the use of select cardiovascular drugs during pregnancy are outlined in **Table 46**. The FDA formerly used a letter system to categorize drugs by their fetal effects during pregnancy; however, with the implementation of a new pregnancy and lactation labeling rule in 2015, more information is now provided on drug effects in pregnant women, lactating women, and women and men of reproductive potential (see MKSAP 18 General Internal Medicine). Most cardiovascular drugs are not FDA approved for use during pregnancy because of limited safety data. Cardiovascular medications should be used only when needed and at the lowest possible dosage, and the desired therapeutic effect should outweigh the risk.

β-Blocker use during pregnancy or lactation requires periodic fetal and newborn heart rate monitoring because β-blockers cross the placenta and are present in human breast milk. Labetalol is the preferred β-blocker in this setting. Atenolol has been linked to premature delivery and small-for-gestational-age babies; therefore, it is usually avoided during pregnancy.

Adenosine is the drug of choice for treatment of acute symptomatic supraventricular tachycardia during pregnancy. Recurrent episodes of tachycardia are often treated with β-blockers and

TABLE 45. Modified WHO Classification of Pregnancy Risk in Women with Heart Disease

Class	Estimated Risk	Conditions
I	No detectable increased risk for maternal mortality and no/mild increase in morbidity	Uncomplicated small patent ductus arteriosus, mild pulmonary valve stenosis, or mitral valve prolapse
		Successfully repaired simple lesions (atrial or ventricular septal defect, patent ductus arteriosus, or anomalous pulmonary venous drainage)
		Isolated atrial or ventricular ectopic beats
II	Small increased risk for maternal mortality	Unrepaired atrial or ventricular septal defect
		Repaired tetralogy of Fallot
		Most arrhythmias
II-III	Moderate increase in morbidity	Mild left ventricular impairment
		Hypertrophic cardiomyopathy
		Native or bioprosthetic valvular heart disease not considered WHO class I or IV
		Repaired coarctation
		Marfan syndrome with aortic dimension <40 mm without aortic dissection
		Bicuspid aortic valve with ascending aortic diameter <45 mm
III	Significantly increased risk for maternal mortality or severe morbidity	Mechanical valve
		Systemic right ventricle
		Fontan circulation[a]
		Cyanotic heart disease (unrepaired)
		Other complex congenital heart disease
		Bicuspid aortic valve with ascending aortic diameter of 45-50 mm
		Marfan syndrome with aortic diameter of 40-45 mm
IV	Extremely high risk for maternal mortality or severe morbidity; pregnancy is contraindicated	Severe mitral stenosis
		Symptomatic severe aortic stenosis
		Bicuspid aortic valve with ascending aortic diameter >50 mm
		Marfan syndrome with aortic diameter >45 mm
		Severe systemic ventricular systolic dysfunction (left ventricular ejection fraction <30%, NYHA functional class III-IV)
		Native severe coarctation
		Significant pulmonary arterial hypertension of any cause (i.e., pulmonary artery systolic pressure >25 mm Hg at rest or >30 mm Hg with exercise)

NYHA = New York Heart Association; WHO = World Health Organization.

[a]Fontan circulation is a palliative surgical procedure performed for patients with complex congenital heart disease with one functional ventricular chamber. The procedure redirects venous blood directly to the lungs without a pumping chamber in the circulation.

Information from Thorne S, MacGregor A, Nelson-Piercy C. Risks of contraception and pregnancy in heart disease. Heart. 2006;92:1520-5. [PMID: 16973809]

digoxin; sotalol and flecainide have also been safely used. Because of toxicity concerns, amiodarone is rarely used.

ACE inhibitors, angiotensin receptor blockers, and aldosterone antagonists should be avoided during pregnancy because of their associated teratogenicity, although some ACE inhibitors are safe to use while breastfeeding. There is inconclusive evidence on the safety of angiotensin receptor blockers while breastfeeding; thus, these drugs are generally avoided during lactation. Spironolactone is considered compatible with breastfeeding.

The LactMed database (toxnet.nlm.nih.gov/newtoxnet/lactmed.htm) provides information on drugs to which breastfeeding mothers may be exposed, including potential adverse effects and suggested therapeutic alternatives.

Anticoagulation Therapy During Pregnancy

Pregnancy is associated with hypercoagulability, and anticoagulation is often indicated in pregnant patients. **Table 47** lists the indications, recommended regimens, and monitoring parameters for therapy. Prepregnancy counseling is recommended for all women requiring long-term anticoagulation to enable them to make informed decisions regarding anticoagulant preference and to understand the maternal and fetal risks.

TABLE 46. Drugs for Cardiac Disorders in Pregnancy

Drug	Use in Pregnancy	Compatibility with Breastfeeding	Comments
ACE inhibitors			
Captopril, enalapril	No	Yes	Teratogenic in first trimester; cause fetal/neonatal kidney failure with second- or third-trimester exposure; scleroderma renal crisis is only indication
Lisinopril	No	?	Same as above
ARBs	No	?	Teratogenic in first trimester; cause fetal/neonatal kidney failure with second- or third-trimester exposure
Adenosine	Yes	?	No change in fetal heart rate when used for supraventricular tachycardia
Amiodarone	No	No	Fetal hypothyroidism, prematurity
Antiplatelet and anticoagulant agents			
Dipyridamole, clopidogrel	Yes	?	Second-line agent; no evidence of harm in animal clopidogrel studies; no human data
Aspirin (≤81 mg)	Yes	Yes	
NOACs (apixaban, dabigatran, rivaroxaban, edoxaban)	?	?	Pregnancy and lactation should be avoided in NOAC-treated patients; available data do not suggest a high risk for NOAC embryopathy or neonatal complications
β-Blockers			
Atenolol	Yes	No	Second-line agent; low birth weight, intrauterine growth restriction
Esmolol	Yes	?	Second-line agent; more pronounced bradycardia
Labetalol	Yes	Yes	Preferred drug in class
Metoprolol	Yes	Yes	Shortened half-life
Propranolol	Yes	Yes	Second-line agent; intrauterine growth restriction
Sotalol	Yes	?	Second-line agent; insufficient data; reserve use for arrhythmia not responding to alternative agent
Calcium channel blockers			
Diltiazem, verapamil	Yes	Yes	Second-line agent; maternal hypotension with rapid intravenous infusion; used for fetal supraventricular tachycardia
Digoxin	Yes	Yes	Second-line agent; shortened half-life
Disopyramide	Yes	Yes	Second-line agent; case reports of preterm labor
Diuretics	Yes	Yes	Second-line agent; use when needed for maternal volume overload only
Flecainide	Yes	?	Second-line agent; inadequate data but used for fetal arrhythmia; case report of fetal hyperbilirubinemia
Hydralazine	Yes	Yes	Vasodilator of choice
Lidocaine	Yes	Yes	Treatment of choice for ventricular arrhythmias
Sodium nitroprusside	No	No	Potential fetal thiocyanate toxicity
Organic nitrates	Yes	?	No apparent increased risk
Phenytoin	No	Yes	Known teratogenicity and bleeding risk; last resort for arrhythmia
Procainamide	Yes	Yes	Used for fetal arrhythmia
Propafenone	Yes	?	Second-line agent; used for fetal arrhythmia
Quinidine	Yes	Yes	Preferred drug in class; increases digoxin levels

? = unknown; ARB = angiotensin receptor blocker; NOAC = non–vitamin K antagonist oral anticoagulant.

Adapted with permission from Rosene-Montella K, Keely EJ, Lee RV, Barbour LA. Medical Care of the Pregnant Patient. 2nd Edition. Philadelphia, PA: American College of Physicians; 2008. pp 356-357. Copyright 2008, American College of Physicians.

TABLE 47. Anticoagulation Regimens During Pregnancy

Weeks of Gestation	Recommended Regimen
Venous Thromboembolism	
Weeks 6-12	Warfarin (if dose to attain INR 2-3 is ≤5 mg)
	UFH (IV or SQ; aPTT 2 × control)
	Weight-based LMWH
Weeks 13-37	UFH (SQ; aPTT 2 × control)
	Weight-based LMWH
	Warfarin (INR 2-3)
Weeks 37 to term	UFH (IV; aPTT 2 × control)
Atrial Fibrillation	
Weeks 6-12	Warfarin (if dose to attain INR 2-3 is ≤5 mg)
	UFH (IV or SQ; aPTT 2 × control)
	Weight-based LMWH
Weeks 13-37	UFH (SQ; aPTT 2 × control)
	Weight-based LMWH
	Warfarin (INR 2-3)
Weeks 37 to term	UFH (IV; aPTT 2 × control)
Mechanical Valve Prosthesis	
Weeks 6-12	Warfarin dose ≤5 mg for therapeutic INR
	Continue warfarin (class IIa recommendation)
	UFH: IV; aPTT 2 × control (class IIb recommendation)
	Anti–factor Xa adjusted LMWH (class IIb recommendation)
	Warfarin dose >5 mg for therapeutic INR
	UFH: IV; aPTT 2 × control (class IIa recommendation)
	Anti–factor Xa adjusted LMWH (class IIa recommendation)
Weeks 13-37	Warfarin (therapeutic INR)
Weeks 37 to term	UFH (IV; aPTT 2 × control)

aPTT = activated partial thromboplastin time; IV = intravenous; LMWH = low-molecular-weight heparin; SQ = subcutaneous; UFH = unfractionated heparin.

Recommendations from Nishimura RA, Otto CM, Bonow RO, Carabello BA, Erwin JP 3rd, Guyton RA, et al; American College of Cardiology/American Heart Association Task Force on Practice Guidelines. 2014 AHA/ACC guideline for the management of patients with valvular heart disease: executive summary: a report of the American College of Cardiology/American Heart Association Task Force on Practice Guidelines. J Am Coll Cardiol. 2014;63:2438-88. [PMID: 24603192] doi:10.1016/j.jacc.2014.02.537 and Bates SM, Greer IA, Middeldorp S, Veenstra DL, Prabulos AM, Vandvik PO. VTE, thrombophilia, antithrombotic therapy, and pregnancy: antithrombotic therapy and prevention of thrombosis, 9th ed: American College of Chest Physicians evidence-based clinical practice guidelines. Chest. 2012;141:e691S-e736S. [PMID: 22315276] doi:10.1378/chest.11-2300 and Furie KL, Kasner SE, Adams RJ, Albers GW, Bush RL, Fagan SC, et al; American Heart Association Stroke Council, Council on Cardiovascular Nursing, Council on Clinical Cardiology, and Interdisciplinary Council on Quality of Care and Outcomes Research. Guidelines for the prevention of stroke in patients with stroke or transient ischemic attack: a guideline for healthcare professionals from the American Heart Association/American Stroke Association. Stroke. 2011;42:227-76. [PMID: 20966421] doi:10.1161/STR.0b013e3181f7d043

Warfarin, unfractionated heparin, and low-molecular-weight heparin can all be used during pregnancy. Careful monitoring and dosage adjustment are indicated for all anticoagulation regimens. It is important to note that warfarin use during the first trimester can cause warfarin embryopathy when the daily dose is greater than 5 mg. Warfarin is stopped before delivery owing to the risk for fetal intracranial hemorrhage if spontaneous labor and vaginal delivery occur while the mother (and thus the fetus) is anticoagulated with warfarin.

Pregnant women with a mechanical valve prosthesis represent a high-risk subset of patients; concerns include valve thrombosis with its associated maternal risks, bleeding, and fetal morbidity and mortality. Warfarin appears to be the safest agent to prevent maternal prosthetic valve thrombosis; however, warfarin poses an increased fetal risk, with possible teratogenicity, miscarriage, and fetal loss due to intracranial hemorrhage. Data suggest that low-molecular-weight heparin and unfractionated heparin are safer for the fetus than warfarin is, but these therapies appear to increase the risk for maternal prosthetic valve thrombosis.

Guidelines from the American College of Cardiology/American Heart Association on the management of anticoagulation during pregnancy in the setting of mechanical valve prosthesis recommend warfarin during the first trimester if the daily dose is 5 mg or less at the time of conception. Intravenous unfractionated heparin or dose-adjusted low-molecular-weight heparin is preferred if the warfarin dose is more than 5 mg daily. During the second and early third trimesters, warfarin therapy is preferred. Intravenous unfractionated heparin is preferred for anticoagulation around the time of delivery in patients with a mechanical valve prosthesis. Weekly monitoring of the anticoagulation level is recommended during pregnancy irrespective of the regimen used, with dosage adjustment as indicated.

Limited data do not suggest a high risk for embryopathy or neonatal complications with exposure to non–vitamin K antagonist oral anticoagulants. However, owing to small case numbers, it is recommended that pregnancy and lactation be avoided in patients receiving non–vitamin K antagonist oral anticoagulants.

KEY POINTS

- Women with peripartum cardiomyopathy should be initially treated with medical therapy, which may include β-blockers, digoxin, hydralazine, nitrates, or diuretics.

- ACE inhibitors, angiotensin receptor blockers, and aldosterone antagonists should be avoided during pregnancy because of their associated teratogenicity.

- In pregnant patients with a mechanical valve prosthesis, warfarin anticoagulation is preferred during the first trimester if the daily dose is 5 mg or less at the time of conception; intravenous unfractionated heparin or dose-adjusted low-molecular-weight heparin is preferred if the warfarin dose is more than 5 mg daily.

Bibliography

Epidemiology and Risk Factors

Centers for Disease Control and Prevention. National Center for Chronic Disease Prevention and Health Promotion. Division of Nutrition, Physical Activity, and Obesity. Data, trends and maps [online]. [Accessed Jan 13, 2017]. URL: https://nccd.cdc.gov/NPAO_DTM/LocationSummary.aspx?statecode=94.

Garcia M, Mulvagh SL, Merz CN, Buring JE, Manson JE. Cardiovascular disease in women: clinical perspectives. Circ Res. 2016;118:1273-93. [PMID: 27081110] doi:10.1161/CIRCRESAHA.116.307547

Goff DC Jr, Lloyd-Jones DM, Bennett G, Coady S, D'Agostino RB Sr, Gibbons R, et al; American College of Cardiology/American Heart Association Task Force on Practice Guidelines. 2013 ACC/AHA guideline on the assessment of cardiovascular risk: a report of the American College of Cardiology/American Heart Association Task Force on Practice Guidelines. J Am Coll Cardiol. 2014;63:2935-59. [PMID: 24239921] doi:10.1016/j.jacc.2013.11.005

McSweeney JC, Rosenfeld AG, Abel WM, Braun LT, Burke LE, Daugherty SL, et al; American Heart Association Council on Cardiovascular and Stroke Nursing, Council on Clinical Cardiology, Council on Epidemiology and Prevention, Council on Hypertension, Council on Lifestyle and Cardiometabolic Health, and Council on Quality of Care and Outcomes Research. Preventing and experiencing ischemic heart disease as a woman: state of the science: a scientific statement from the American Heart Association. Circulation. 2016;133:1302-31. [PMID: 26927362] doi:10.1161/CIR.0000000000000381

Mehta LS, Beckie TM, DeVon HA, Grines CL, Krumholz HM, Johnson MN, et al; American Heart Association Cardiovascular Disease in Women and Special Populations Committee of the Council on Clinical Cardiology, Council on Epidemiology and Prevention, Council on Cardiovascular and Stroke Nursing, and Council on Quality of Care and Outcomes Research. Acute myocardial infarction in women: a scientific statement from the American Heart Association. Circulation. 2016;133:916-47. [PMID: 26811316] doi:10.1161/CIR.0000000000000351

Mozaffarian D, Benjamin EJ, Go AS, Arnett DK, Blaha MJ, Cushman M, et al; Writing Group Members. Heart disease and stroke statistics-2016 update: a report from the American Heart Association. Circulation. 2016;133:e38-360. [PMID: 26673558] doi:10.1161/CIR.0000000000000350

Stein JH, Hsue PY. Inflammation, immune activation, and CVD risk in individuals with HIV infection [Editorial]. JAMA. 2012;308:405-6. [PMID: 22820794] doi:10.1001/jama.2012.8488

Whelton PK, Carey RM, Aronow WS, Casey DE Jr, Collins KJ, Dennison Himmelfarb C, et al. 2017 ACC/AHA/AAPA/ABC/ACPM/AGS/APhA/ASH/ASPC/NMA/PCNA guideline for the prevention, detection, evaluation, and management of high blood pressure in adults: a report of the American College of Cardiology/American Heart Association Task Force on Clinical Practice Guidelines. J Am Coll Cardiol. 2017. [PMID: 29146535] doi:10.1016/j.jacc.2017.11.006

Yusuf S, Hawken S, Ounpuu S, Dans T, Avezum A, Lanas F, et al; INTERHEART Study Investigators. Effect of potentially modifiable risk factors associated with myocardial infarction in 52 countries (the INTERHEART study): case-control study. Lancet. 2004;364:937-52. [PMID: 15364185]

Diagnostic Testing in Cardiology

Douglas PS, Garcia MJ, Haines DE, Lai WW, Manning WJ, Patel AR, et al; American College of Cardiology Foundation Appropriate Use Criteria Task Force. ACCF/ASE/AHA/ASNC/HFSA/HRS/SCAI/SCCM/SCCT/SCMR 2011 appropriate use criteria for echocardiography. a report of the American College of Cardiology Foundation Appropriate Use Criteria Task Force, American Society of Echocardiography, American Heart Association, American Society of Nuclear Cardiology, Heart Failure Society of America, Heart Rhythm Society, Society for Cardiovascular Angiography and Interventions, Society of Critical Care Medicine, Society of Cardiovascular Computed Tomography, and Society for Cardiovascular Magnetic Resonance Endorsed by the American College of Chest Physicians. J Am Coll Cardiol. 2011;57:1126-66. [PMID: 21349406] doi:10.1016/j.jacc.2010.11.002

Douglas PS, Hoffmann U, Patel MR, Mark DB, Al-Khalidi HR, Cavanaugh B, et al; PROMISE Investigators. Outcomes of anatomical versus functional testing for coronary artery disease. N Engl J Med. 2015;372:1291-300. [PMID: 25773919] doi:10.1056/NEJMoa1415516

Fihn SD, Blankenship JC, Alexander KP, Bittl JA, Byrne JG, Fletcher BJ, et al. 2014 ACC/AHA/AATS/PCNA/SCAI/STS focused update of the guideline for the diagnosis and management of patients with stable ischemic heart disease: a report of the American College of Cardiology/American Heart Association Task Force on Practice Guidelines, and the American Association for Thoracic Surgery, Preventive Cardiovascular Nurses Association, Society for Cardiovascular Angiography and Interventions, and Society of Thoracic Surgeons. Circulation. 2014;130:1749-67. [PMID: 25070666] doi:10.1161/CIR.0000000000000095

Goff DC Jr, Lloyd-Jones DM, Bennett G, Coady S, D'Agostino RB Sr, Gibbons R, et al; American College of Cardiology/American Heart Association Task Force on Practice Guidelines. 2013 ACC/AHA guideline on the assessment of cardiovascular risk: a report of the American College of Cardiology/American Heart Association Task Force on Practice Guidelines. J Am Coll Cardiol. 2014;63:2935-59. [PMID: 24239921] doi:10.1016/j.jacc.2013.11.005

Hendel RC, Berman DS, Di Carli MF, Heidenreich PA, Henkin RE, Pellikka PA, et al; American College of Cardiology Foundation Appropriate Use Criteria Task Force. ACCF/ASNC/ACR/AHA/ASE/SCCT/SCMR/SNM 2009 appropriate use criteria for cardiac radionuclide imaging: a report of the American College of Cardiology Foundation Appropriate Use Criteria Task Force, the American Society of Nuclear Cardiology, the American College of Radiology, the American Heart Association, the American Society of Echocardiography, the Society of Cardiovascular Computed Tomography, the Society for Cardiovascular Magnetic Resonance, and the Society of Nuclear Medicine. J Am Coll Cardiol. 2009;53:2201-29. [PMID: 19497454] doi:10.1016/j.jacc.2009.02.013

Mark DB, Berman DS, Budoff MJ, Carr JJ, Gerber TC, Hecht HS, et al; American College of Cardiology Foundation Task Force on Expert Consensus Documents. ACCF/ACR/AHA/NASCI/SAIP/SCAI/SCCT 2010 expert consensus document on coronary computed tomographic angiography: a report of the American College of Cardiology Foundation Task Force on Expert Consensus Documents. J Am Coll Cardiol. 2010;55:2663-99. [PMID: 20513611] doi:10.1016/j.jacc.2009.11.013

Rybicki FJ, Udelson JE, Peacock WF, Goldhaber SZ, Isselbacher EM, Kazerooni E, et al. 2015 ACR/ACC/AHA/AATS/ACEP/ASNC/NASCI/SAEM/SCCT/SCMR/SCPC/SNMMI/STR/STS appropriate utilization of cardiovascular imaging in emergency department patients with chest pain: a joint document of the American College of Radiology Appropriateness Criteria Committee and the American College of Cardiology Appropriate Use Criteria Task Force. J Am Coll Cardiol. 2016;67:853-79. [PMID: 26809772] doi:10.1016/j.jacc.2015.09.011

Coronary Artery Disease

Amsterdam EA, Wenger NK, Brindis RG, Casey DE Jr, Ganiats TG, Holmes DR Jr, et al; ACC/AHA Task Force Members. 2014 AHA/ACC guideline for the management of patients with non-ST-elevation acute coronary syndromes: a report of the American College of Cardiology/American Heart Association Task Force on Practice Guidelines. Circulation. 2014;130:e344-426. [PMID: 25249585] doi:10.1161/CIR.0000000000000134

Boden WE, O'Rourke RA, Teo KK, Hartigan PM, Maron DJ, Kostuk WJ, et al; COURAGE Trial Research Group. Optimal medical therapy with or without PCI for stable coronary disease. N Engl J Med. 2007;356:1503-16. [PMID: 17387127]

Bonaca MP, Bhatt DL, Cohen M, Steg PG, Storey RF, Jensen EC, et al; PEGASUS-TIMI 54 Steering Committee and Investigators. Long-term use of ticagrelor in patients with prior myocardial infarction. N Engl J Med. 2015;372:1791-800. [PMID: 25773268] doi:10.1056/NEJMoa1500857

Fihn SD, Gardin JM, Abrams J, Berra K, Blankenship JC, Dallas AP, et al; American College of Cardiology Foundation. 2012 ACCF/AHA/ACP/AATS/PCNA/SCAI/STS guideline for the diagnosis and management of patients with stable ischemic heart disease: a report of the American College of Cardiology Foundation/American Heart Association Task Force on Practice Guidelines, and the American College of Physicians, American Association for Thoracic Surgery, Preventive Cardiovascular Nurses Association, Society for Cardiovascular Angiography and Interventions, and Society of Thoracic Surgeons. J Am Coll Cardiol. 2012;60:e44-e164. [PMID: 23182125] doi:10.1016/j.jacc.2012.07.013

Fox CS, Golden SH, Anderson C, Bray GA, Burke LE, de Boer IH, et al; American Heart Association Diabetes Committee of the Council on Lifestyle and Cardiometabolic Health, Council on Clinical Cardiology, Council on Cardiovascular and Stroke Nursing, Council on Cardiovascular Surgery and Anesthesia, Council on Quality of Care and Outcomes Research, and the American Diabetes Association. Update on prevention of cardiovascular disease in adults with type 2 diabetes mellitus in light of recent evidence: a scientific statement from the American Heart Association and the American Diabetes Association. Circulation. 2015;132:691-718. [PMID: 26246173] doi:10.1161/CIR.0000000000000230

Levine GN, Bates ER, Bittl JA, Brindis RG, Fihn SD, Fleisher LA, et al. 2016 ACC/AHA guideline focused update on duration of dual antiplatelet therapy in patients with coronary artery disease: A report of the American College of Cardiology/American Heart Association Task Force on Clinical Practice Guidelines. J Thorac Cardiovasc Surg. 2016;152:1243-1275. [PMID: 27751237] doi:10.1016/j.jtcvs.2016.07.044

Levine GN, Bates ER, Blankenship JC, Bailey SR, Bittl JA, Cercek B, et al. 2015 ACC/AHA/SCAI focused update on primary percutaneous coronary intervention for patients with ST-elevation myocardial infarction: an update of the 2011 ACCF/AHA/SCAI guideline for percutaneous coronary intervention and the 2013 ACCF/AHA guideline for the management of st-elevation myocardial infarction: a report of the American College of Cardiology/American Heart Association Task Force on Clinical Practice Guidelines and the Society for Cardiovascular Angiography and Interventions. Circulation. 2016;133:1135-47. [PMID: 26490017] doi:10.1161/CIR.0000000000000336

Marso SP, Daniels GH, Brown-Frandsen K, Kristensen P, Mann JF, Nauck MA, et al; LEADER Steering Committee. Liraglutide and cardiovascular outcomes in type 2 diabetes. N Engl J Med. 2016;375:311-22. [PMID: 27295427] doi:10.1056/NEJMoa1603827

Pasupathy S, Air T, Dreyer RP, Tavella R, Beltrame JF. Systematic review of patients presenting with suspected myocardial infarction and nonobstructive coronary arteries. Circulation. 2015;131:861-70. [PMID: 25587100] doi:10.1161/CIRCULATIONAHA.114.011201

Rodriguez F, Mahaffey KW. Management of patients with NSTE-ACS: a comparison of the recent AHA/ACC and ESC guidelines. J Am Coll Cardiol. 2016;68:313-21. [PMID: 27417010] doi:10.1016/j.jacc.2016.03.599

Stergiopoulos K, Boden WE, Hartigan P, Möbius-Winkler S, Hambrecht R, Hueb W, et al. Percutaneous coronary intervention outcomes in patients with stable obstructive coronary artery disease and myocardial ischemia: a collaborative meta-analysis of contemporary randomized clinical trials. JAMA Intern Med. 2014;174:232-40. [PMID: 24296791] doi:10.1001/jamainternmed.2013.12855

Velazquez EJ, Lee KL, Jones RH, Al-Khalidi HR, Hill JA, Panza JA, et al; STICHES Investigators. Coronary-artery bypass surgery in patients with ischemic cardiomyopathy. N Engl J Med. 2016;374:1511-20. [PMID: 27040723] doi:10.1056/NEJMoa1602001

Wallentin L, Becker RC, Budaj A, Cannon CP, Emanuelsson H, Held C, et al; PLATO Investigators. Ticagrelor versus clopidogrel in patients with acute coronary syndromes. N Engl J Med. 2009;361:1045-57. [PMID: 19717846] doi:10.1056/NEJMoa0904327

Whelton PK, Carey RM, Aronow WS, Casey DE Jr, Collins KJ, Dennison Himmelfarb C, et al. 2017 ACC/AHA/AAPA/ABC/ACPM/AGS/APhA/ASH/ASPC/NMA/PCNA guideline for the prevention, detection, evaluation, and management of high blood pressure in adults: A Report of the American College of Cardiology/American Heart Association Task Force on Clinical Practice Guidelines. J Am Coll Cardiol. 2017. [PMID: 29146535] doi:10.1016/j.jacc.2017.11.006

Heart Failure

Ponikowski P, Voors AA, Anker SD, Bueno H, Cleland JG, Coats AJ, et al; Authors/Task Force Members. 2016 ESC guidelines for the diagnosis and treatment of acute and chronic heart failure: the task force for the diagnosis and treatment of acute and chronic heart failure of the European Society of Cardiology (ESC). Developed with the special contribution of the Heart Failure Association (HFA) of the ESC. Eur Heart J. 2016;37:2129-200. [PMID: 27206819] doi:10.1093/eurheartj/ehw128

Redfield MM. Heart failure with preserved ejection fraction. N Engl J Med. 2016;375:1868-1877. [PMID: 27959663]

Thiele H, Ohman EM, Desch S, Eitel I, de Waha S. Management of cardiogenic shock. Eur Heart J. 2015;36:1223-30. [PMID: 25732762] doi:10.1093/eurheartj/ehv051

Whelton PK, Carey RM, Aronow WS, Casey DE Jr, Collins KJ, Dennison Himmelfarb C, et al. 2017 ACC/AHA/AAPA/ABC/ACPM/AGS/APhA/ASH/ASPC/NMA/PCNA guideline for the prevention, detection, evaluation, and management of high blood pressure in adults: a report of the American College of Cardiology/American Heart Association Task Force on Clinical Practice Guidelines. J Am Coll Cardiol. 2017. [PMID: 29146535] doi:10.1016/j.jacc.2017.11.006

Yancy CW, Jessup M, Bozkurt B, Butler J, Casey DE Jr, Drazner MH, et al; American College of Cardiology Foundation. 2013 ACCF/AHA guideline for the management of heart failure: a report of the American College of Cardiology Foundation/American Heart Association Task Force on Practice Guidelines. J Am Coll Cardiol. 2013;62:e147-239. [PMID: 23747642] doi:10.1016/j.jacc.2013.05.019

Yancy CW, Jessup M, Bozkurt B, Butler J, Casey DE Jr, Colvin MM, et al. 2017 ACC/AHA/HFSA focused update of the 2013 ACCF/AHA guideline for the management of heart failure: a report of the American College of Cardiology/American Heart Association Task Force on Clinical Practice Guidelines and the Heart Failure Society of America. Circulation. 2017 Aug 8;136(6):e137-e161. [PMID: 28455343] doi:10.1161/CIR.0000000000000509

Arrhythmias

Conen D, Adam M, Roche F, Barthelemy JC, Felber Dietrich D, Imboden M, et al. Premature atrial contractions in the general population: frequency and risk factors. Circulation. 2012;126:2302-8. [PMID: 23048073] doi:10.1161/CIRCULATIONAHA.112.112300

Cheng S, Keyes MJ, Larson MG, McCabe EL, Newton-Cheh C, Levy D, et al. Long-term outcomes in individuals with prolonged PR interval or first-degree atrioventricular block. JAMA. 2009;301:2571-7. [PMID: 19549974] doi:10.1001/jama.2009.888

Delacrétaz E. Clinical practice. Supraventricular tachycardia. N Engl J Med. 2006;354:1039-51. [PMID: 16525141]

Epstein AE, DiMarco JP, Ellenbogen KA, Estes NA 3rd, Freedman RA, Gettes LS, et al; American College of Cardiology Foundation. 2012 ACCF/AHA/HRS focused update incorporated into the ACCF/AHA/HRS 2008 guidelines for device-based therapy of cardiac rhythm abnormalities: a report of the American College of Cardiology Foundation/American Heart Association Task Force on Practice Guidelines and the Heart Rhythm Society. Circulation. 2013;127:e283-352. [PMID: 23255456] doi:10.1161/CIR.0b013e318276ce9b

Epstein AE, DiMarco JP, Ellenbogen KA, Estes NA 3rd, Freedman RA, Gettes LS, et al; American College of Cardiology/American Heart Association Task Force on Practice Guidelines (Writing Committee to Revise the ACC/AHA/NASPE 2002 Guideline Update for Implantation of Cardiac Pacemakers and Antiarrhythmia Devices). ACC/AHA/HRS 2008 guidelines for device-based therapy of cardiac rhythm abnormalities: a report of the American College of Cardiology/American Heart Association Task Force on Practice Guidelines (Writing Committee to Revise the ACC/AHA/NASPE 2002 Guideline Update for Implantation of Cardiac Pacemakers and Antiarrhythmia Devices): developed in collaboration with the American Association for Thoracic Surgery and Society of Thoracic Surgeons. Circulation. 2008;117:e350-408. [PMID: 18483207] doi:10.1161/CIRCUALTIONAHA.108.189742

Fuster V, Rydén LE, Cannom DS, Crijns HJ, Curtis AB, Ellenbogen KA, et al; American College of Cardiology. ACC/AHA/ESC 2006 guidelines for the management of patients with atrial fibrillation: full text: a report of the American College of Cardiology/American Heart Association Task Force on practice guidelines and the European Society of Cardiology Committee for Practice Guidelines (Writing Committee to Revise the 2001 guidelines for the management of patients with atrial fibrillation) developed in collaboration with the European Heart Rhythm Association and the Heart Rhythm Society. Europace. 2006;8:651-745. [PMID: 16987906]

January CT, Wann LS, Alpert JS, Calkins H, Cigarroa JE, Cleveland JC Jr, et al; American College of Cardiology/American Heart Association Task Force on Practice Guidelines. 2014 AHA/ACC/HRS guideline for the management of patients with atrial fibrillation: a report of the American College of Cardiology/American Heart Association Task Force on Practice Guidelines and the Heart Rhythm Society. J Am Coll Cardiol. 2014;64:e1-76. [PMID: 24685669] doi:10.1016/j.jacc.2014.03.022

Link MS, Berkow LC, Kudenchuk PJ, Halperin HR, Hess EP, Moitra VK, et al. Part 7: Adult Advanced Cardiovascular Life Support: 2015 American Heart Association Guidelines Update for Cardiopulmonary Resuscitation and Emergency Cardiovascular Care. Circulation. 2015;132:S444-64. [PMID: 26472995] doi:10.1161/CIR.0000000000000261

Page RL, Joglar JA, Caldwell MA, Calkins H, Conti JB, Deal BJ, et al. 2015 ACC/AHA/HRS guideline for the management of adult patients with supraventricular tachycardia: a report of the American College of Cardiology/American Heart Association Task Force on Clinical Practice Guidelines and the Heart Rhythm Society. J Am Coll Cardiol. 2016;67:e27-e115. [PMID: 26409259] doi:10.1016/j.jacc.2015.08.856

Piccini JP, Fauchier L. Rhythm control in atrial fibrillation. Lancet. 2016;388:829-40. [PMID: 27560278] doi:10.1016/S0140-6736(16)31277-6

Priori SG, Wilde AA, Horie M, Cho Y, Behr ER, Berul C, et al. HRS/EHRA/APHRS expert consensus statement on the diagnosis and management of patients with inherited primary arrhythmia syndromes: document endorsed by HRS, EHRA, and APHRS in May 2013 and by ACCF, AHA, PACES, and AEPC in June 2013. Heart Rhythm. 2013;10:1932-63. [PMID: 24011539] doi:10.1016/j.hrthm.2013.05.014

Zipes DP, Camm AJ, Borggrefe M, Buxton AE, Chaitman B, Fromer M, et al; American College of Cardiology/American Heart Association Task Force. ACC/AHA/ESC 2006 Guidelines for Management of Patients With Ventricular Arrhythmias and the Prevention of Sudden Cardiac Death: a report of the American College of Cardiology/American Heart Association Task Force and the European Society of Cardiology Committee for Practice Guidelines (writing committee to develop Guidelines for Management of Patients With Ventricular Arrhythmias and the Prevention of Sudden Cardiac Death): developed in collaboration with the European Heart Rhythm Association and the Heart Rhythm Society. Circulation. 2006;114:e385-484. [PMID: 16935995]

Valvular Heart Disease

Desimone DC, Tleyjeh IM, Correa de Sa DD, Anavekar NS, Lahr BD, Sohail MR, et al; Mayo Cardiovascular Infections Study Group. Incidence of infective endocarditis caused by viridans group streptococci before and after publication of the 2007

American Heart Association's endocarditis prevention guidelines. Circulation. 2012;126:60-4. [PMID: 22689929] doi:10.1161/CIRCULATIONAHA.112.095281

Eikelboom JW, Connolly SJ, Brueckmann M, Granger CB, Kappetein AP, Mack MJ, et al; RE-ALIGN Investigators. Dabigatran versus warfarin in patients with mechanical heart valves. N Engl J Med. 2013;369:1206-14. [PMID: 23991661] doi:10.1056/NEJMoa1300615

Holmes DR Jr, Rich JB, Zoghbi WA, Mack MJ. The heart team of cardiovascular care. J Am Coll Cardiol. 2013;61:903-7. [PMID: 23449424] doi:10.1016/j.jacc.2012.08.1034

Li JS, Sexton DJ, Mick N, Nettles R, Fowler VG Jr, Ryan T, et al. Proposed modifications to the Duke criteria for the diagnosis of infective endocarditis. Clin Infect Dis. 2000;30:633-8. [PMID: 10770721]

Mack MJ, Leon MB, Smith CR, Miller DC, Moses JW, Tuzcu EM, et al; PARTNER 1 trial investigators. 5-year outcomes of transcatheter aortic valve replacement or surgical aortic valve replacement for high surgical risk patients with aortic stenosis (PARTNER 1): a randomised controlled trial. Lancet. 2015;385:2477-84. [PMID: 25788234] doi:10.1016/S0140-6736(15)60308-7

Michelena HI, Khanna AD, Mahoney D, Margaryan E, Topilsky Y, Suri RM, et al. Incidence of aortic complications in patients with bicuspid aortic valves. JAMA. 2011;306:1104-12. [PMID: 21917581] doi:10.1001/jama.2011.1286

Nishimura RA, Otto CM, Bonow RO, Carabello BA, Erwin JP 3rd, Fleisher LA, et al. 2017 AHA/ACC focused update of the 2014 AHA/ACC guideline for the management of patients with valvular heart disease: a report of the American College of Cardiology/American Heart Association Task Force on Clinical Practice Guidelines. Circulation. 2017;135:e1159-e1195. [PMID: 28298458] doi:10.1161/CIR.0000000000000503

Nishimura RA, Otto CM, Bonow RO, Carabello BA, Erwin JP 3rd, Guyton RA, et al; American College of Cardiology/American Heart Association Task Force on Practice Guidelines. 2014 AHA/ACC guideline for the management of patients with valvular heart disease: executive summary: a report of the American College of Cardiology/American Heart Association Task Force on Practice Guidelines. J Am Coll Cardiol. 2014;63:2438-88. [PMID: 24603192] doi:10.1016/j.jacc.2014.02.537

Pibarot P, Dumesnil JG. Low-flow, low-gradient aortic stenosis with normal and depressed left ventricular ejection fraction. J Am Coll Cardiol. 2012;60:1845-53. [PMID: 23062546] doi:10.1016/j.jacc.2012.06.051

Suri RM, Vanoverschelde JL, Grigioni F, Schaff HV, Tribouilloy C, Avierinos JF, et al. Association between early surgical intervention vs watchful waiting and outcomes for mitral regurgitation due to flail mitral valve leaflets. JAMA. 2013;310:609-16. [PMID: 23942679] doi:10.1001/jama.2013.8643

Turpie AG, Gent M, Laupacis A, Latour Y, Gunstensen J, Basile F, et al. A comparison of aspirin with placebo in patients treated with warfarin after heart-valve replacement. N Engl J Med. 1993;329:524-9. [PMID: 8336751]

Myocardial Disease

Ammash NM, Seward JB, Bailey KR, Edwards WD, Tajik AJ. Clinical profile and outcome of idiopathic restrictive cardiomyopathy. Circulation. 2000;101:2490-6. [PMID: 10831523]

Butany J, Nair V, Naseemuddin A, Nair GM, Catton C, Yau T. Cardiac tumours: diagnosis and management. Lancet Oncol. 2005;6:219-28. [PMID: 15811617]

Elliott PM, Anastasakis A, Borger MA, Borggrefe M, Cecchi F, Charron P, et al; Authors/Task Force members. 2014 ESC Guidelines on diagnosis and management of hypertrophic cardiomyopathy: the Task Force for the Diagnosis and Management of Hypertrophic Cardiomyopathy of the European Society of Cardiology (ESC). Eur Heart J. 2014;35:2733-79. [PMID: 25173338] doi:10.1093/eurheartj/ehu284

Garcia MJ. Constrictive pericarditis versus restrictive cardiomyopathy? J Am Coll Cardiol. 2016;67:2061-76. [PMID: 27126534] doi:10.1016/j.jacc.2016.01.076

Gersh BJ, Maron BJ, Bonow RO, Dearani JA, Fifer MA, Link MS, et al. 2011 ACCF/AHA guideline for the diagnosis and treatment of hypertrophic cardiomyopathy: executive summary: a report of the American College of Cardiology Foundation/American Heart Association Task Force on Practice Guidelines. J Am Coll Cardiol. 2011;58:2703-38. [PMID: 22075468] doi:10.1016/j.jacc.2011.10.825

Liebregts M, Steggerda RC, Vriesendorp PA, van Velzen H, Schinkel AF, Willems R, et al. Long-term outcome of alcohol septal ablation for obstructive hypertrophic cardiomyopathy in the young and the elderly. JACC Cardiovasc Interv. 2016;9:463-9. [PMID: 26965935] doi:10.1016/j.jcin.2015.11.036

Liebregts M, Vriesendorp PA, Mahmoodi BK, Schinkel AF, Michels M, ten Berg JM. A systematic review and meta-analysis of long-term outcomes after septal reduction therapy in patients with hypertrophic cardiomyopathy. JACC Heart Fail. 2015;3:896-905. [PMID: 26454847] doi:10.1016/j.jchf.2015.06.011

Maron BJ. Hypertrophic cardiomyopathy and other causes of sudden cardiac death in young competitive athletes, with considerations for preparticipation screening and criteria for disqualification. Cardiol Clin. 2007;25: 399-414, vi. [PMID: 17961794]

Mogensen J, Kubo T, Duque M, Uribe W, Shaw A, Murphy R, et al. Idiopathic restrictive cardiomyopathy is part of the clinical expression of cardiac troponin I mutations. J Clin Invest. 2003;111:209-16. [PMID: 12531876]

Seward JB, Casaclang-Verzosa G. Infiltrative cardiovascular diseases: cardiomyopathies that look alike. J Am Coll Cardiol. 2010;55:1769-79. [PMID: 20413025] doi:10.1016/j.jacc.2009.12.040

Pericardial Disease

Adler Y, Charron P, Imazio M, Badano L, Barón-Esquivias G, Bogaert J, et al; European Society of Cardiology (ESC). 2015 ESC guidelines for the diagnosis and management of pericardial diseases: The Task Force for the Diagnosis and Management of Pericardial Diseases of the European Society of Cardiology (ESC)Endorsed by: The European Association for Cardio-Thoracic Surgery (EACTS). Eur Heart J. 2015;36:2921-64. [PMID: 26320112] doi:10.1093/eurheartj/ehv318

Finetti M, Insalaco A, Cantarini L, Meini A, Breda L, Alessio M, et al. Long-term efficacy of interleukin-1 receptor antagonist (anakinra) in corticosteroid-dependent and colchicine-resistant recurrent pericarditis. J Pediatr. 2014;164:1425-31.e1. [PMID: 24630353] doi:10.1016/j.jpeds.2014.01.065

Haley JH, Tajik AJ, Danielson GK, Schaff HV, Mulvagh SL, Oh JK. Transient constrictive pericarditis: causes and natural history. J Am Coll Cardiol. 2004;43:271-5. [PMID: 14736448]

Imazio M, Brucato A, Maestroni S, Cumetti D, Dominelli A, Natale G, et al. Prevalence of C-reactive protein elevation and time course of normalization in acute pericarditis: implications for the diagnosis, therapy, and prognosis of pericarditis. Circulation. 2011;123:1092-7. [PMID: 21357824] doi:10.1161/CIRCULATIONAHA.110.986372

Klein AL, Abbara S, Agler DA, Appleton CP, Asher CR, Hoit B, et al. American Society of Echocardiography clinical recommendations for multimodality cardiovascular imaging of patients with pericardial disease: endorsed by the Society for Cardiovascular Magnetic Resonance and Society of Cardiovascular Computed Tomography. J Am Soc Echocardiogr. 2013;26:965-1012.e15. [PMID: 23998693] doi:10.1016/j.echo.2013.06.023

Lilly LS. Treatment of acute and recurrent idiopathic pericarditis. Circulation. 2013;127:1723-6. [PMID: 23609551] doi:10.1161/CIRCULATIONAHA.111.066365

Welch TD, Ling LH, Espinosa RE, Anavekar NS, Wiste HJ, Lahr BD, et al. Echocardiographic diagnosis of constrictive pericarditis: Mayo Clinic criteria. Circ Cardiovasc Imaging. 2014;7:526-34. [PMID: 24633783] doi:10.1161/CIRCIMAGING.113.001613

Zurick AO, Bolen MA, Kwon DH, Tan CD, Popovic ZB, Rajeswaran J, et al. Pericardial delayed hyperenhancement with CMR imaging in patients with constrictive pericarditis undergoing surgical pericardiectomy: a case series with histopathological correlation. JACC Cardiovasc Imaging. 2011;4:1180-91. [PMID: 22093269] doi:10.1016/j.jcmg.2011.08.011

Adult Congenital Heart Disease

Kent DM, Dahabreh IJ, Ruthazer R, Furlan AJ, Reisman M, Carroll JD, et al. Device closure of patent foramen ovale after stroke: pooled analysis of completed randomized trials. J Am Coll Cardiol. 2016;67:907-17. [PMID: 26916479] doi:10.1016/j.jacc.2015.12.023

Krieger EV, Leary PJ, Opotowsky AR. Pulmonary hypertension in congenital heart disease: beyond eisenmenger syndrome. Cardiol Clin. 2015;33:599-609, ix. [PMID: 26471823] doi:10.1016/j.ccl.2015.07.003

Mas JL, Derumeaux G, Guillon B, Massardier E, Hosseini H, Mechtouff L, et al; CLOSE Investigators. Patent foramen ovale closure or anticoagulation vs. antiplatelets after stroke. N Engl J Med. 2017;377:1011-1021. [PMID: 28902593] doi:10.1056/NEJMoa1705915

Messé SR, Gronseth G, Kent DM, Kizer JR, Homma S, Rosterman L, et al. Practice advisory: recurrent stroke with patent foramen ovale (update of practice parameter): report of the Guideline Development, Dissemination, and Implementation Subcommittee of the American Academy of Neurology. Neurology. 2016;87:815-21. [PMID: 27466464] doi:10.1212/WNL.0000000000002961

Opotowsky AR, Moko LE, Ginns J, Rosenbaum M, Greutmann M, Aboulhosn J, et al. Pheochromocytoma and paraganglioma in cyanotic congenital heart disease. J Clin Endocrinol Metab. 2015;100:1325-34. [PMID: 25581599] doi:10.1210/jc.2014-3863

Regitz-Zagrosek V, Blomstrom Lundqvist C, Borghi C, Cifkova R, Ferreira R, Foidart JM, et al; European Society of Gynecology (ESG). ESC guidelines on the management of cardiovascular diseases during pregnancy: the Task Force on the Management of Cardiovascular Diseases during Pregnancy of the European Society of Cardiology (ESC). Eur Heart J. 2011;32:3147-97. [PMID: 21873418] doi:10.1093/eurheartj/ehr218

Saver JL, Carroll JD, Thaler DE, Smalling RW, MacDonald LA, Marks DS, et al; RESPECT Investigators. Long-term outcomes of patent foramen ovale closure or medical therapy after stroke. N Engl J Med. 2017;377:1022-1032. [PMID: 28902590] doi:10.1056/NEJMoa1610057

Søndergaard L, Kasner SE, Rhodes JF, Andersen G, Iversen HK, Nielsen-Kudsk JE, et al; Gore REDUCE Clinical Study Investigators. Patent foramen ovale closure or antiplatelet therapy for cryptogenic stroke. N Engl J Med. 2017;377:1033-1042. [PMID: 28902580] doi:10.1056/NEJMoa1707404

Valente AM, Cook S, Festa P, Ko HH, Krishnamurthy R, Taylor AM, et al. Multimodality imaging guidelines for patients with repaired tetralogy of Fallot: a report from the American Society of Echocardiography: developed in collaboration with the Society for Cardiovascular Magnetic Resonance and the Society for Pediatric Radiology. J Am Soc Echocardiogr. 2014;27:111-41. [PMID: 24468055] doi:10.1016/j.echo.2013.11.009

Van Hare GF, Ackerman MJ, Evangelista JA, Kovacs RJ, Myerburg RJ, Shafer KM, et al; American Heart Association Electrocardiography and Arrhythmias Committee of Council on Clinical Cardiology, Council on Cardiovascular Disease in Young, Council on Cardiovascular and Stroke Nursing, Council on Functional Genomics and Translational Biology, and American College of Cardiology. Eligibility and disqualification recommendations for competitive athletes with cardiovascular abnormalities: task force 4: congenital heart disease: a scientific statement from the American Heart Association and American College of Cardiology. Circulation. 2015;132:e281-91. [PMID: 26621645] doi:10.1161/CIR.0000000000000240

Warnes CA, Williams RG, Bashore TM, Child JS, Connolly HM, Dearani JA, et al; American College of Cardiology. ACC/AHA 2008 guidelines for the management of adults with congenital heart disease: a report of the American College of Cardiology/American Heart Association Task Force on Practice Guidelines (Writing Committee to Develop Guidelines on the Management of Adults With Congenital Heart Disease). Developed in Collaboration With the American Society of Echocardiography, Heart Rhythm Society, International Society for Adult Congenital Heart Disease, Society for Cardiovascular Angiography and Interventions, and Society of Thoracic Surgeons. J Am Coll Cardiol. 2008;52:e143-263. [PMID: 19038677] doi:10.1016/j.jacc.2008.10.001

Diseases of the Aorta

Amarenco P, Cohen A, Hommel M, Moulin T, Leys D, Bousser M-G; French Study of Aortic Plaques in Stroke Group. Atherosclerotic disease of the aortic arch as a risk factor for recurrent ischemic stroke. N Engl J Med. 1996;334:1216-21. [PMID: 8606716]

Chaikof EL, Brewster DC, Dalman RL, Makaroun MS, Illig KA, Sicard GA, et al. SVS practice guidelines for the care of patients with an abdominal aortic aneurysm: executive summary. J Vasc Surg. 2009;50:880-96. [PMID: 19786241] doi:10.1016/j.jvs.2009.07.001

De Bruin JL, Baas AF, Buth J, Prinssen M, Verhoeven EL, Cuypers PW, et al; DREAM Study Group. Long-term outcome of open or endovascular repair of abdominal aortic aneurysm. N Engl J Med. 2010;362:1881-9. [PMID: 20484396] doi:10.1056/NEJMoa0909499

Erbel R, Aboyans V, Boileau C, Bossone E, Bartolomeo RD, Eggebrecht H, et al; ESC Committee for Practice Guidelines. 2014 ESC guidelines on the diagnosis and treatment of aortic diseases: document covering acute and chronic aortic diseases of the thoracic and abdominal aorta of the adult. The Task Force for the Diagnosis and Treatment of Aortic Diseases of the European Society of Cardiology (ESC). Eur Heart J. 2014;35:2873-926. [PMID: 25173340] doi:10.1093/eurheartj/ehu281

Freeman LA, Young PM, Foley TA, Williamson EE, Bruce CJ, Greason KL. CT and MRI assessment of the aortic root and ascending aorta. AJR Am J Roentgenol. 2013;200:W581-92. [PMID: 23701088] doi:10.2214/AJR.12.9531

Greenhalgh RM, Brown LC, Powell JT, Thompson SG, Epstein D, Sculpher MJ; United Kingdom EVAR Trial Investigators. Endovascular versus open repair of abdominal aortic aneurysm. N Engl J Med. 2010;362:1863-71. [PMID: 20382983] doi:10.1056/NEJMoa0909305

Hiratzka LF, Bakris GL, Beckman JA, Bersin RM, Carr VF, Casey DE Jr, et al; American College of Cardiology Foundation/American Heart Association Task Force on Practice Guidelines. 2010 ACCF/AHA/AATS/ACR/ASA/SCA/ SCAI/SIR/STS/SVM guidelines for the diagnosis and management of patients with thoracic aortic disease. A report of the American College of Cardiology Foundation/American Heart Association Task Force on Practice Guidelines, American Association for Thoracic Surgery, American College of Radiology, American Stroke Association, Society of Cardiovascular Anesthesiologists, Society for Cardiovascular Angiography and Interventions, Society of Interventional Radiology, Society of Thoracic Surgeons, and Society for Vascular Medicine. J Am Coll Cardiol. 2010;55:e27-e129. [PMID: 20359588] doi:10.1016/j.jacc.2010.02.015

Rogers IS, Massaro JM, Truong QA, Mahabadi AA, Kriegel MF, Fox CS, et al. Distribution, determinants, and normal reference values of thoracic and abdominal aortic diameters by computed tomography (from the Framingham Heart Study). Am J Cardiol. 2013;111:1510-6. [PMID: 23497775] doi:10.1016/j.amjcard.2013.01.306

Peripheral Artery Disease

Aboyans V, Criqui MH, Abraham P, Allison MA, Creager MA, Diehm C, et al; American Heart Association Council on Peripheral Vascular Disease. Measurement and interpretation of the ankle-brachial index: a scientific statement from the American Heart Association. Circulation. 2012;126:2890-909. [PMID: 23159553] doi:10.1161/CIR.0b013e318276fbcb

Bonaca MP, Bhatt DL, Storey RF, Steg PG, Cohen M, Kuder J, et al. Ticagrelor for prevention of ischemic events after myocardial infarction in patients with peripheral artery disease. J Am Coll Cardiol. 2016;67:2719-2728. [PMID: 27046162] doi:10.1016/j.jacc.2016.03.524

Creager MA, Kaufman JA, Conte MS. Clinical practice. Acute limb ischemia. N Engl J Med. 2012;366:2198-206. [PMID: 22670905] doi:10.1056/NEJMcp1006054

Gerhard-Herman MD, Gornik HL, Barrett C, Barshes NR, Corriere MA, Drachman DE, et al. 2016 AHA/ACC guideline on the management of patients with lower extremity peripheral artery disease: a report of the American College of Cardiology/American Heart Association Task Force on Clinical Practice Guidelines. Circulation. 2017;135:e726-e779. [PMID: 27840333] doi:10.1161/CIR.0000000000000471

Morrow DA, Braunwald E, Bonaca MP, Ameriso SF, Dalby AJ, Fish MP, et al; TRA 2P-TIMI 50 Steering Committee and Investigators. Vorapaxar in the secondary prevention of atherothrombotic events. N Engl J Med. 2012;366:1404-13. [PMID: 22443427] doi:10.1056/NEJMoa1200933

Patel MR, Conte MS, Cutlip DE, Dib N, Geraghty P, Gray W, et al. Evaluation and treatment of patients with lower extremity peripheral artery disease: consensus definitions from Peripheral Academic Research Consortium (PARC). J Am Coll Cardiol. 2015;65:931-41. [PMID: 25744011] doi:10.1016/j.jacc.2014.12.036

Whelton PK, Carey RM, Aronow WS, Casey DE Jr, Collins KJ, Dennison Himmelfarb C, et al. 2017 ACC/AHA/AAPA/ABC/ACPM/AGS/APhA/ASH/ ASPC/NMA/PCNA guideline for the prevention, detection, evaluation, and management of high blood pressure in adults: A Report of the American College of Cardiology/American Heart Association Task Force on Clinical Practice Guidelines. J Am Coll Cardiol. 2017. [PMID: 29146535] doi:10.1016/j.jacc.2017.11.006

Cardiovascular Disease in Cancer Survivors

Armenian SH, Lacchetti C, Lenihan D. Prevention and monitoring of cardiac dysfunction in survivors of adult cancers: American Society of Clinical Oncology clinical practice guideline summary. J Oncol Pract. 2017;13:270-275. [PMID: 27922796] doi:10.1200/JOP.2016.018770

Groarke JD, Nguyen PL, Nohria A, Ferrari R, Cheng S, Moslehi J. Cardiovascular complications of radiation therapy for thoracic malignancies: the role for non-invasive imaging for detection of cardiovascular disease. Eur Heart J. 2014;35:612-23. [PMID: 23666251] doi:10.1093/eurheartj/eht114

Hall PS, Harshman LC, Srinivas S, Witteles RM. The frequency and severity of cardiovascular toxicity from targeted therapy in advanced renal cell carcinoma patients. JACC Heart Fail. 2013;1:72-8. [PMID: 24621801] doi:10.1016/j.jchf.2012.09.001

Jaworski C, Mariani JA, Wheeler G, Kaye DM. Cardiac complications of thoracic irradiation. J Am Coll Cardiol. 2013;61:2319-28. [PMID: 23583253] doi:10.1016/j.jacc.2013.01.090

Kongbundansuk S, Hundley WG. Noninvasive imaging of cardiovascular injury related to the treatment of cancer. JACC Cardiovasc Imaging. 2014;7:824-38. [PMID: 25124015] doi:10.1016/j.jcmg.2014.06.007

Lipshultz SE, Rifai N, Dalton VM, Levy DE, Silverman LB, Lipsitz SR, et al. The effect of dexrazoxane on myocardial injury in doxorubicin-treated children with acute lymphoblastic leukemia. N Engl J Med. 2004;351:145-53. [PMID: 15247354]

Mehta LS, Watson KE, Barac A, Beckie TM, Bittner V, Cruz-Flores S, et al; American Heart Association Cardiovascular Disease in Women and Special Populations Committee of the Council on Clinical Cardiology; Council on Cardiovascular and Stroke Nursing; and Council on Quality of Care and Outcomes Research. Cardiovascular disease and breast cancer: where these entities intersect: a scientific statement from the American Heart Association. Circulation. 2018 Feb 1. [Epub ahead of print] [PMID: 29437116] doi:10.1161/CIR.0000000000000556

Yeh ET, Bickford CL. Cardiovascular complications of cancer therapy: incidence, pathogenesis, diagnosis, and management. J Am Coll Cardiol. 2009;53:2231-47. [PMID: 19520246] doi:10.1016/j.jacc.2009.02.050

Bibliography

Pregnancy and Cardiovascular Disease

Arany Z, Elkayam U. Peripartum cardiomyopathy. Circulation. 2016;133:1397-409. [PMID: 27045128] doi:10.1161/CIRCULATIONAHA.115.020491

Drenthen W, Boersma E, Balci A, Moons P, Roos-Hesselink JW, Mulder BJ, et al; ZAHARA Investigators. Predictors of pregnancy complications in women with congenital heart disease. Eur Heart J. 2010;31:2124-32. [PMID: 20584777] doi:10.1093/eurheartj/ehq200

McNamara DM, Elkayam U, Alharethi R, Damp J, Hsich E, Ewald G, et al; IPAC Investigators. Clinical outcomes for peripartum cardiomyopathy in North America: results of the IPAC Study (Investigations of Pregnancy-Associated Cardiomyopathy). J Am Coll Cardiol. 2015;66:905-14. [PMID: 26293760] doi:10.1016/j.jacc.2015.06.1309

Nishimura RA, Otto CM, Bonow RO, Carabello BA, Erwin JP 3rd, Guyton RA, et al; American College of Cardiology/American Heart Association Task Force on Practice Guidelines. 2014 AHA/ACC guideline for the management of patients with valvular heart disease: executive summary: a report of the American College of Cardiology/American Heart Association Task Force on Practice Guidelines. J Am Coll Cardiol. 2014;63:2438-88. [PMID: 24603192] doi:10.1016/j.jacc.2014.02.537

Regitz-Zagrosek V, Blomstrom Lundqvist C, Borghi C, Cifkova R, Ferreira R, Foidart JM, et al; European Society of Gynecology (ESG). ESC Guidelines on the management of cardiovascular diseases during pregnancy: the Task Force on the Management of Cardiovascular Diseases during Pregnancy of the European Society of Cardiology (ESC). Eur Heart J. 2011;32:3147-97. [PMID: 21873418] doi:10.1093/eurheartj/ehr218

Tweet MS, Gulati R, Hayes SN. Spontaneous coronary artery dissection. Curr Cardiol Rep. 2016;18:60. [PMID: 27216840] doi:10.1007/s11886-016-0737-6

van Hagen IM, Roos-Hesselink JW, Ruys TP, Merz WM, Goland S, Gabriel H, et al; ROPAC Investigators and the EURObservational Research Programme (EORP) Team*. Pregnancy in women with a mechanical heart valve: data of the European Society of Cardiology Registry of Pregnancy and Cardiac Disease (ROPAC). Circulation. 2015;132:132-42. [PMID: 26100109] doi:10.1161/CIRCULATIONAHA.115.015242

Cardiovascular Medicine Self-Assessment Test

This self-assessment test contains one-best-answer multiple-choice questions. Please read these directions carefully before answering the questions. Answers, critiques, and bibliographies immediately follow these multiple-choice questions. The American College of Physicians (ACP) is accredited by the Accreditation Council for Continuing Medical Education (ACCME) to provide continuing medical education for physicians.

The American College of Physicians designates MKSAP 18 Cardiovascular Medicine for a maximum of 30 *AMA PRA Category 1 Credits*™. Physicians should claim only the credit commensurate with the extent of their participation in the activity.

Successful completion of the CME activity, which includes participation in the evaluation component, enables the participant to earn up to 30 medical knowledge MOC points in the American Board of Internal Medicine's Maintenance of Certification (MOC) program. It is the CME activity provider's responsibility to submit participant completion information to ACCME for the purpose of granting MOC credit.

Earn Instantaneous CME Credits or MOC Points Online

Print subscribers can enter their answers online to earn instantaneous CME credits or MOC points. You can submit your answers using online answer sheets that are provided at mksap.acponline.org, where a record of your MKSAP 18 credits will be available. To earn CME credits or to apply for MOC points, you need to answer all of the questions in a test and earn a score of at least 50% correct (number of correct answers divided by the total number of questions). Please note that if you are applying for MOC points, you must also enter your birth date and ABIM candidate number.

Take either of the following approaches:

- Use the printed answer sheet at the back of this book to record your answers. Go to mksap.acponline.org, access the appropriate online answer sheet, transcribe your answers, and submit your test for instantaneous CME credits or MOC points. There is no additional fee for this service.

- Go to mksap.acponline.org, access the appropriate online answer sheet, directly enter your answers, and submit your test for instantaneous CME credits or MOC points. There is no additional fee for this service.

Earn CME Credits or MOC Points by Mail or Fax

Pay a $20 processing fee per answer sheet and submit the printed answer sheet at the back of this book by mail or fax, as instructed on the answer sheet. Make sure you calculate your score and enter your birth date and ABIM candidate number, and fax the answer sheet to 215-351-2799 or mail the answer sheet to Member and Customer Service, American College of Physicians, 190 N. Independence Mall West, Philadelphia, PA 19106-1572, using the courtesy envelope provided in your MKSAP 18 slipcase. You will need your 10-digit order number and 8-digit ACP ID number, which are printed on your packing slip. Please allow 4 to 6 weeks for your score report to be emailed back to you. Be sure to include your email address for a response.

If you do not have a 10-digit order number and 8-digit ACP ID number, or if you need help creating a username and password to access the MKSAP 18 online answer sheets, go to mksap.acponline.org or email custserv@acponline.org.

CME credits and MOC points are available from the publication date of July 31, 2018, until July 31, 2021. You may submit your answer sheet or enter your answers online at any time during this period.

Directions

*Each of the numbered items is followed by lettered answers. Select the **ONE** lettered answer that is **BEST** in each case.*

Item 1

A 19-year-old man is evaluated in the emergency department for a 2-week history of abdominal pain and exertional dyspnea. He underwent cardiac transplantation 10 months ago for viral myocarditis. Medications are tacrolimus, prednisone, mycophenolate mofetil, valganciclovir, trimethoprim-sulfamethoxazole, valsartan, calcium–vitamin D supplement, and low-dose aspirin.

On physical examination, vital signs are normal. Neck examination reveals occasional jugular cannon *a* waves with no venous distention. Cardiac examination is significant for an S_3. The remainder of the examination is normal.

An electrocardiogram is shown.

Which of the following tests will most likely establish the diagnosis?

(A) Abdominal CT
(B) Coronary angiography
(C) Echocardiography
(D) Endomyocardial biopsy

Item 2

A 69-year-old man is evaluated in the hospital for four episodes of chest pain at rest in the past 24 hours. Medical history is significant for hyperlipidemia, hypertension, tobacco use, and previous transient ischemic attack. Medications are aspirin, hydrochlorothiazide, atorvastatin, and ramipril.

On physical examination, vital signs are normal. The remainder of the examination is unremarkable.

Laboratory studies are notable for normal serum troponin levels.

An electrocardiogram demonstrates 2-mm ST-segment depressions in leads V_4 through V_6.

Metoprolol, nitrates, clopidogrel, and heparin are initiated.

Which of the following is the most appropriate management?

(A) Adenosine nuclear stress testing
(B) Coronary CT angiography
(C) Exercise stress electrocardiography
(D) Urgent angiography

Item 3

A 65-year-old woman is evaluated during a routine examination. She was diagnosed with a cardiac murmur in early adulthood. She is active, healthy, and without symptoms. She takes no medications.

On physical examination, vital signs are normal. A grade 3/6 holosystolic murmur preceded by multiple clicks is present at the apex. Physical findings are otherwise unremarkable.

An echocardiogram demonstrates a left ventricular ejection fraction of 50%. The left ventricle is moderately dilated with an end-systolic dimension of 42 mm. Myxomatous

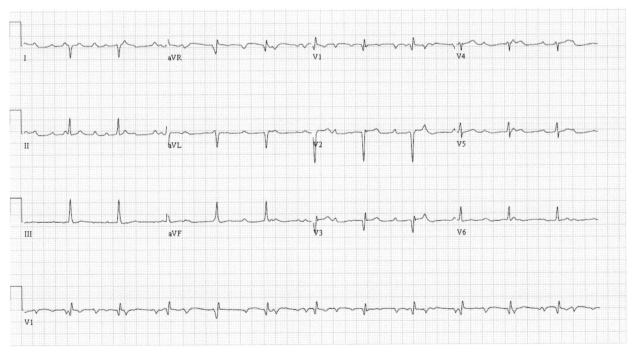

ITEM 1

degeneration of the mitral valve is present with severe regurgitation due to posterior leaflet prolapse.

Which of the following is the most appropriate next step in management?

(A) Serial clinical and echocardiographic evaluations
(B) Surgical mitral valve repair
(C) Surgical mitral valve replacement
(D) Transcatheter mitral valve repair

Item 4

A 60-year-old woman is evaluated for new-onset hypertension. Medical history is significant for metastatic cervical cancer for which she began chemotherapy 2 months ago. She has no history of hypertension. Medications are bevacizumab, cisplatin, paclitaxel, dexamethasone, promethazine, and ranitidine.

On physical examination, temperature is normal, blood pressure is 172/106 mm Hg, pulse rate is 82/min, and respiration rate is 18/min. The remainder of the examination is unremarkable.

Which of the following medications is the most likely cause of this patient's hypertension?

(A) Bevacizumab
(B) Cisplatin
(C) Dexamethasone
(D) Paclitaxel

Item 5

A 52-year-old woman is evaluated in the emergency department for progressive dyspnea. Medical history is notable for aortic stenosis and long-standing hypertension. Family history is unremarkable. Medications are metoprolol and chlorthalidone.

On physical examination, temperature is normal, blood pressure is 190/90 mm Hg in both upper extremities, pulse rate is 80/min and regular, and respiration rate is 22/min. The jugular venous pressure is normal. The apical impulse is displaced and sustained. The S_1 is normal, and the S_2 is soft; an S_4 is noted at the apex. An ejection click is heard at the apex and left sternal border. A systolic ejection murmur is noted along the right sternal border, and a separate systolic murmur is noted under the left clavicle and over the left posterior chest. The femoral pulses are diminished, and the radial artery–to–femoral artery pulse is delayed. No bruits are appreciated in the epigastrium or over the femoral vessels.

A chest radiograph is shown (see top of next column).

In addition to aortic stenosis, which of the following is the most likely diagnosis?

(A) Ascending aortic dissection
(B) Coarctation of the aorta
(C) Essential hypertension
(D) Renovascular hypertension

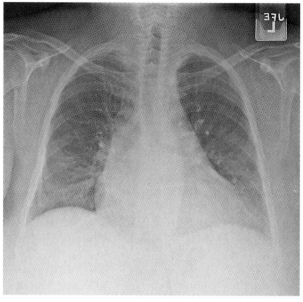

ITEM 5

Item 6

A 64-year-old man is evaluated in the emergency department for acute right lower leg pain that began 2 days ago. The pain is now severe at rest, and he reports coolness of the right foot. He has a 3-year history of intermittent claudication. He underwent right femoral-popliteal bypass graft surgery for life-limiting claudication 1 year ago. Medical history is otherwise significant for hypertension, hyperlipidemia, and type 2 diabetes mellitus. He quit smoking 4 years ago. Medications are low-dose aspirin, ramipril, hydrochlorothiazide, rosuvastatin, and metformin.

On physical examination, vital signs are normal. The right foot is cool and pale, sensation is intact, and muscle strength is normal. The pedal pulses are not palpable in the right leg. Arterial Doppler ultrasound signals are not detectable over the right dorsalis pedis and right posterior tibial arteries.

Intravenous anticoagulation with heparin is initiated.

Which of the following is the most appropriate management?

(A) Arterial duplex ultrasonography
(B) CT angiography
(C) Emergent right leg amputation
(D) Intravenous recombinant tissue plasminogen activator
(E) Urgent invasive angiography

Item 7

A 75-year-old woman is evaluated during a routine visit. Medical history is significant for hypertension and coronary artery disease with placement of a stent in the mid right coronary artery 5 years ago. She is symptom free. Medications are metoprolol succinate, lisinopril, aspirin, and atorvastatin.

On physical examination, temperature is normal, blood pressure is 130/80 mm Hg, pulse rate is 72/min, and respiration rate is 16/min. BMI is 23. The precordial cadence is irregularly irregular. The remainder of the examination is unremarkable.

An electrocardiogram shows atrial fibrillation.

Which of the following is the most appropriate treatment?

(A) Add clopidogrel
(B) Add oral anticoagulation
(C) Discontinue aspirin and begin clopidogrel and oral anticoagulation
(D) Discontinue aspirin and begin oral anticoagulation
(E) No change in therapy

Item 8

A 55-year-old man is evaluated for chest discomfort of several months' duration. He describes the pain as sporadic left-sided chest heaviness that lasts for several minutes. His chest discomfort is generally but not consistently induced by exercise and is often but not always relieved with rest. He has some associated shortness of breath but no other symptoms. He remains active despite the pain and is able to walk without limitations. Medical history is significant for hypertension treated with amlodipine and hydrochlorothiazide.

On physical examination, vital signs and the remainder of the physical examination are normal.

An electrocardiogram is shown.

Which of the following is the most appropriate management?

(A) Coronary angiography
(B) Coronary artery calcium scoring
(C) Exercise stress echocardiography
(D) Exercise stress electrocardiography
(E) Pharmacologic nuclear stress testing

Item 9

A 48-year-old man is hospitalized for a 6-week history of progressive fatigue, dyspnea on exertion, and vague chest "fullness." He has also had pedal edema for the past 2 weeks. He has no history of incarceration or recent travel and is not immunocompromised.

On physical examination, temperature is 37.5 °C (99.5 °F), blood pressure is 132/76 mm Hg with pulsus paradoxus of 16 mm Hg, pulse rate is 100/min, and respiration rate is 16/min. The jugular veins are distended to the angle of the mandible. The lungs are clear to auscultation. No diastolic sound or pericardial friction rub is noted. Hepatomegaly is present. Pitting edema is noted bilaterally at the ankles.

Laboratory studies:

Erythrocyte sedimentation rate	86 mm/h
Leukocyte count	11,000/µL (11×10^9/L) with normal differential
Fourth-generation HIV test	Negative
Antinuclear antibodies	Negative
Interferon-γ release assay	Negative

An electrocardiogram shows sinus tachycardia with a nonspecific ST-T-wave abnormality. A chest radiograph reveals an enlarged cardiac silhouette without pericardial calcification. An echocardiogram shows a moderately sized pericardial effusion. There are diastolic right atrial inversion and a 30% inspiratory reduction in mitral inflow velocity.

Pericardiocentesis reveals an intrapericardial pressure of 16 mm Hg before drainage and 0 to 1 mm Hg after drainage. The right atrial mean pressure and left ventricular end-diastolic pressures before drainage were each 16 mm Hg.

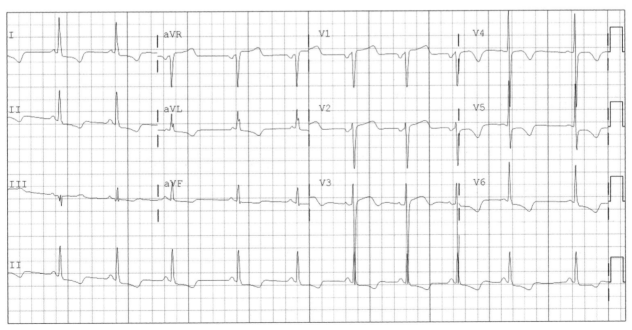

ITEM 8

After pericardiocentesis, there is no change in the intracardiac pressure readings. Pericardial fluid is negative for adenosine deaminase.

Which of the following is the most appropriate management?

(A) Ibuprofen and colchicine

(B) Isoniazid, rifampin, pyrazinamide, and ethambutol

(C) Pericardiectomy

(D) Surgical pericardial window

Item 10

An 80-year-old woman is evaluated for a 6-month history of worsening exertional dyspnea. Two nights ago, she awoke with sudden-onset dyspnea that was relieved with ambulation. She has not had chest pain. Medical history is significant for myocardial infarction 8 years ago. She also has a history of left ventricular dysfunction but has been previously well compensated. Her medications are lisinopril, aspirin, metoprolol, and rosuvastatin.

On physical examination, temperature is normal, blood pressure is 95/60 mm Hg, pulse rate is 56/min, and respiration rate is 18/min. The lungs are clear. The carotid upstroke is low in volume. The apical impulse is laterally displaced and enlarged. S_1 is soft; the aortic component of S_2 is diminished. There is no S_3 or S_4. A grade 2/6 mid-peaking systolic murmur is heard throughout the precordium. The remainder of the examination is normal.

An echocardiogram demonstrates a left ventricular ejection fraction of 32%. The aortic valve is slightly calcified. The stroke volume is markedly decreased (23 mL/m²). The mean aortic gradient is 20 mm Hg (consistent with mild to moderate stenosis), and the aortic valve area is calculated to be 0.7 cm² (consistent with severe stenosis).

Which of the following is the most appropriate next step in management?

(A) Aortic valve replacement

(B) Coronary angiography

(C) Dobutamine echocardiography

(D) Switch lisinopril to valsartan-sacubitril

Item 11

A 75-year-old woman is hospitalized for a 3-week history of progressive exertional dyspnea, increasing peripheral edema, and mental status changes. For the past 4 nights, she has been sleeping in a recliner instead of her bed. She reports no chest pain. She has a 6-year history of ischemic cardiomyopathy, for which she takes low-dose aspirin, furosemide, carvedilol, lisinopril, digoxin, spironolactone, and as-needed metolazone.

On physical examination, the patient is afebrile, blood pressure is 84/52 mm Hg, pulse rate is 118/min, and respiration rate is 28/min. Oxygen saturation is 95% breathing ambient air. She is confused. Jugular venous distention is present. Cardiac examination reveals an S_3. There is ascites on abdominal examination. The extremities are cool, and there is lower extremity edema to the knees.

Laboratory studies:

Alanine aminotransferase	172 U/L
Aspartate aminotransferase	163 U/L
Creatinine	2.9 mg/dL (256.4 µmol/L) (baseline, 1.2 mg/dL [106.1 µmol/L])
Potassium	4.7 mEq/L (4.7 mmol/L)
Sodium	132 mEq/L (132 mmol/L) (baseline, 140 mEq/L [140 mmol/L])
Digoxin	0.3 ng/mL (0.38 nmol/L) (normal range, 0.5-2.0 ng/mL [0.64-2.56 nmol/L])

An electrocardiogram shows no acute changes. An echocardiogram shows a left ventricular ejection fraction of 20%.

Which of the following is the most appropriate initial treatment?

(A) Increase carvedilol

(B) Increase digoxin

(C) Increase lisinopril

(D) Start dobutamine

Item 12

A 78-year-old man is evaluated for palpitations, worsening fatigue, and exercise intolerance. Two months ago, he was diagnosed with atrial flutter and subsequently underwent cardioversion to normal sinus rhythm. Ambulatory electrocardiographic monitoring following cardioversion demonstrated recurrent atrial flutter with an average ventricular rate of 69/min. Medical history is significant for hypertension and coronary artery disease. Medications are warfarin, metoprolol, lisinopril, low-dose aspirin, and atorvastatin.

On physical examination, pulse rate is 73/min and irregular. Other vital signs and findings on physical examination are normal.

Laboratory studies are significant for normal serum thyroid-stimulating hormone and serum N-terminal B-type natriuretic peptide levels.

An electrocardiogram is shown (see top of next page). A stress echocardiogram demonstrates normal wall motion at rest and during stress. The left ventricular ejection fraction is greater than 55%.

Which of the following is the most appropriate treatment?

(A) Amiodarone

(B) Cardiac catheterization

(C) Cardioversion

(D) Catheter ablation

Item 13

An 18-year-old man is evaluated for a murmur detected during a college sports physical examination. He reports no symptoms and has no history of cardiac disease. He takes no medications.

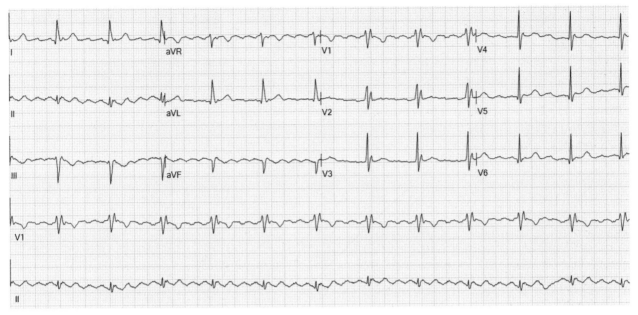

ITEM 12

On physical examination, vital signs are normal. He has a normal central venous pressure, waveform, precordial palpation, and S$_1$. A continuous murmur is heard beneath the left clavicle that envelops the S$_2$. The remainder of the examination is unremarkable.

Which of the following is the most likely cause of this patient's murmur?

(A) Bicuspid aortic valve with aortic regurgitation

(B) Patent ductus arteriosus

(C) Pulmonary regurgitation

(D) Ventricular septal defect

Item 14

A 48-year-old woman is evaluated for exertional substernal chest pain of several weeks' duration. The chest pain consistently subsides with rest. Medical history is significant for episodic migraine. She has no history of hypertension, hyperlipidemia, or other medical problems. She is a nonsmoker. She takes no medications other than naproxen as needed.

On physical examination, vital signs are normal. Oxygen saturation is 98% breathing ambient air. The remainder of the examination is unremarkable.

An electrocardiogram demonstrates baseline 1.5-mm lateral ST-segment depressions. Nuclear stress testing reveals a mild anterior wall perfusion defect, and a subsequent coronary angiogram demonstrates normal coronary arteries.

Which of the following is the most likely diagnosis?

(A) Acute coronary syndrome with spontaneous recanalization

(B) Cardiac syndrome X

(C) Somatic symptom disorder

(D) Takotsubo cardiomyopathy

Item 15

A 56-year-old woman is evaluated for a 6-month history of progressive left calf discomfort. Her symptoms begin as calf tightness after vigorous walking for two blocks, and discomfort causes her to stop walking after four blocks. The symptoms subside after 5 minutes of rest. She reports no rest pain. Medical history is significant for hypertension and hyperlipidemia. She has a 50-pack-year smoking history, but she quit smoking 6 months ago. Medications are low-dose aspirin, amlodipine, cilostazol, high-intensity rosuvastatin, and losartan.

On physical examination, vital signs are normal. Femoral and popliteal pulses are diminished bilaterally. Pedal pulses are not palpable in the left leg. No skin ulceration is noted. The remainder of the examination is unremarkable.

The ankle-brachial index is 0.68 on the left and 0.86 on the right.

Which of the following is the most appropriate management?

(A) Add clopidogrel

(B) Initiate a supervised exercise program

(C) Obtain a magnetic resonance angiogram

(D) Refer for vascular surgery

Item 16

A 69-year-old man is evaluated during a routine examination. He is asymptomatic. Medical history is significant for hypertension. He has a 50-pack-year smoking history but quit smoking 7 years ago. Medications are aspirin, lisinopril, and amlodipine.

On physical examination, vital signs are normal. A bruit is heard over the abdomen, and a pulsatile mass is present in the epigastrium. The remainder of the examination is unremarkable.

A Duplex ultrasound of the abdomen shows an abdominal aortic aneurysm with transverse diameter of 6.2 cm.

Which of the following is the most appropriate next step in management?

(A) CT angiography of the abdominal aorta and iliac vessels
(B) Endovascular repair
(C) Open surgical repair
(D) Switch amlodipine to metoprolol

Item 17

A 52-year-old man is evaluated during a visit to establish care. He is asymptomatic, but he is seeking advice on how to modify his risk for cardiovascular disease. He drinks one glass of wine with dinner most nights, and he quit smoking 12 years ago. Family history is significant for a myocardial infarction in his father at age 61 years. He takes no medications. The patient is Hispanic.

On physical examination, temperature is normal, blood pressure is 128/76 mm Hg, and pulse rate is 74/min. BMI is 28. The remainder of the physical examination is unremarkable.

Laboratory studies:
Total cholesterol   200 mg/dL (5.18 mmol/L)
HDL cholesterol   30 mg/dL (0.78 mmol/L)
LDL cholesterol   130 mg/dL (3.37 mmol/L)
Triglycerides   200 mg/dL (2.26 mmol/L)

Which of the following risk factors most increases this patient's risk for cardiovascular disease?

(A) Alcohol use
(B) Ethnicity
(C) Family history
(D) Hyperlipidemia
(E) Smoking history

Item 18

A 67-year-old man is evaluated during a follow-up visit. Medical history is significant for a 7-year history of heart failure with placement of an implantable cardioverter-defibrillator 6 years ago. He has New York Heart Association functional class II symptoms and is currently stable. Since his last visit 6 months ago, he has had no changes in medications, symptoms, or other medical issues. Medications are valsartan-sacubitril, carvedilol, furosemide, and spironolactone.

On physical examination, the patient is afebrile, blood pressure is 108/74 mm Hg, and pulse rate is 64/min. He has no jugular venous distention or S_3. No edema is noted.

An echocardiogram obtained 1 year ago demonstrated a left ventricular ejection fraction of 25% and left ventricular end-diastolic diameter of 6.7 cm; these findings are unchanged from 2 years ago.

Heart failure education and the need for diet and medication adherence are reinforced.

Which of the following is the most appropriate testing to perform at this visit?

(A) Echocardiography
(B) 24-Hour ambulatory electrocardiographic monitoring
(C) Serum B-type natriuretic peptide level measurement
(D) Serum electrolyte measurement and kidney function studies

Item 19

A 25-year-old woman is evaluated for intermittent palpitations associated with occasional episodes of shortness of breath and lightheadedness. These episodes last from 30 to 90 minutes. Medical history is notable for a similar episode of symptoms during college that required an emergency department visit; supraventricular tachycardia was diagnosed. She takes no medications.

On physical examination, vital signs are normal. Cardiac examination is normal. The remainder of the physical examination is unremarkable.

A 12-lead electrocardiogram is shown (see top of next page). A resting echocardiogram demonstrates normal left ventricular ejection fraction and a structurally normal heart.

Which of the following is the most appropriate next step in management?

(A) Atenolol
(B) Electrophysiology study
(C) Flecainide
(D) Verapamil

Item 20

A 26-year-old woman is evaluated for a preconception assessment. She has Marfan syndrome. She reports no cardiovascular symptoms. Her only medication is long-acting metoprolol.

On physical examination, blood pressure is 110/60 mm Hg, and pulse rate is 60/min and regular. The patient has facial and skeletal features of Marfan syndrome. The estimated central venous pressure is normal. Cardiac examination reveals a normal apical impulse, normal S_1 and S_2, and a grade 2/6 late-peaking systolic murmur and midsystolic click over the apex. The lungs are clear to auscultation. No edema is noted.

Transthoracic echocardiogram demonstrates a dilated proximal ascending aorta with a dimension of 4.6 cm. No aortic regurgitation is appreciated. Bileaflet mitral valve prolapse is noted with mild mitral regurgitation. The left ventricular size and function are normal. There is no recent echocardiogram for comparison.

Which of the following is the most appropriate management?

(A) Advise against pregnancy
(B) Proceed with mitral valve intervention
(C) Repeat echocardiography in 12 months
(D) Switch metoprolol to losartan

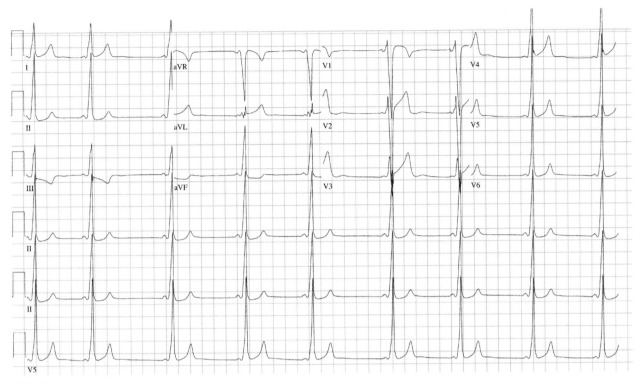

ITEM 19

Item 21

A 62-year-old man is evaluated in the emergency department for a 3-hour history of transient right arm and right leg weakness. His symptoms resolve while in the emergency department. Medical history is otherwise unremarkable, and he takes no medications.

On physical examination, vital signs are normal, and the remainder of the examination is unremarkable.

Laboratory studies are notable for an erythrocyte sedimentation rate of 16 mm/h and LDL cholesterol level of 70 mg/dL (1.81 mmol/L).

A 12-lead electrocardiogram is normal. Carotid duplex ultrasound shows no evidence of hemodynamically significant plaque. CT of the head without contrast demonstrates no evidence of hemorrhage. MRI of the brain reveals a small left internal capsular infarction. A transesophageal echocardiogram is obtained. Representative mid-esophageal four-chamber images at end-systole (*top panel*) and end-diastole (*bottom panel*) are shown.

Which of the following is the most likely diagnosis?

(A) Bacterial endocarditis
(B) Left atrial myxoma
(C) Nonbacterial thrombotic endocarditis
(D) Papillary fibroelastoma

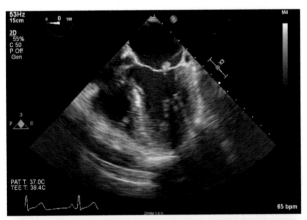

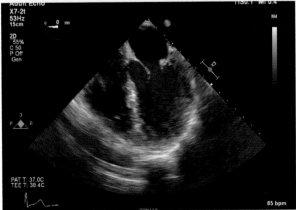

ITEM 21

Item 22

A 47-year-old woman is evaluated for recent fatigue and dyspnea. She underwent an abdominal hysterectomy for recurrent severe menorrhagia 3 weeks ago and has had persistent fatigue and exertional dyspnea since the procedure. She has no other symptoms. Medical history is significant for Eisenmenger syndrome related to a ventricular septal defect. Medications are sildenafil and bosentan.

On physical examination, temperature is normal, blood pressure is 98/60 mm Hg, pulse rate is 80/min and regular, and respiration rate is 20/min. The estimated central venous pressure is elevated with a prominent *a* wave. The apical impulse is normal, and a prominent parasternal impulse is noted at the left sternal border. The S_1 is normal, and the S_2 is loud. Digital clubbing and central cyanosis are noted. The abdominal wound is healing well.

Laboratory testing reveals a hemoglobin level of 10.2 g/dL (102 g/L). The hemoglobin level was 15 g/dL (150 g/L) before hysterectomy. One year ago, the hemoglobin level was 18.5 g/dL (185 g/L).

Which of the following is the most appropriate management?

(A) Erythropoietin
(B) Heart-lung transplantation
(C) Intravenous epoprostenol
(D) Short-course iron therapy

Item 23

A 48-year-old man is evaluated in the emergency department for epigastric discomfort and nausea that began 45 minutes ago. Medical history is significant for hypertension, tobacco use, and hyperlipidemia. His only medication is atorvastatin.

On physical examination, temperature is normal, blood pressure is 110/60 mm Hg, pulse rate is 90/min, and respiration rate is 18/min. Oxygen saturation is 98% breathing ambient air. The remainder of the physical examination is unremarkable.

Laboratory studies are notable for an elevated initial serum troponin I level.

An electrocardiogram shows 3-mm ST-segment elevations in leads II, III, and aVF. A chest radiograph is normal.

The patient is administered aspirin, clopidogrel, and a bolus of heparin. Transport to the nearest hospital capable of percutaneous coronary intervention would take 4 hours.

Which of the following is the most appropriate management?

(A) Fondaparinux and ticagrelor
(B) Full-dose reteplase
(C) Half-dose reteplase with abciximab
(D) Immediate transfer for primary percutaneous coronary intervention
(E) Nitroprusside

Item 24

A 72-year-old man is evaluated for exertional left calf and foot pain. Three weeks ago, the patient developed an ulcer on the medial aspect of the left great toe. His medical history is significant for coronary artery disease, type 2 diabetes

mellitus, hypertension, and hyperlipidemia. Medications are low-dose aspirin, lisinopril, metoprolol, metformin, and atorvastatin.

On physical examination, blood pressure is 155/84 mm; other vital signs are normal. There are no palpable pulses in the left leg. Right femoral, popliteal, and pedal pulses are faint.

Ankle-brachial index testing:

Right systolic brachial pressure	155 mm Hg
Left systolic brachial pressure	145 mm Hg
Left posterior tibialis pressure	255 mm Hg
Left dorsalis pedis pressure	255 mm Hg

Which of the following is the most appropriate diagnostic test to perform next?

(A) Exercise ankle-brachial index
(B) Lower extremity CT angiography
(C) Toe-brachial index
(D) Venous duplex ultrasonography

Item 25

A 33-year-old woman was hospitalized 8 days ago for fever and severe dyspnea. Her current symptoms began 1 month ago with chills, malaise, and low-grade fever. She was diagnosed 5 years ago with a bicuspid aortic valve with regurgitation but had been healthy otherwise. On admission, an echocardiogram demonstrated a 12-mm vegetation involving the aortic valve with severe regurgitation and preserved left ventricular function. Blood cultures grew *Staphylococcus aureus* that was sensitive to oxacillin. After 8 days of intravenous antimicrobial therapy, she has continued to be febrile, and her dyspnea has progressed such that she has symptoms at rest.

On physical examination, temperature is 38.1 °C (100.6 °F), blood pressure is 110/60 mm Hg, pulse rate is 96/min, and respiration rate is 23/min. Lung examination demonstrates bilateral crackles. The estimated central venous pressure is 10 cm H_2O. There is a grade 3/6 diastolic decrescendo murmur along the left sternal border. An S_3 is present.

Repeat blood cultures performed yesterday continue to grow *S. aureus* sensitive to oxacillin. An echocardiogram obtained today shows findings similar to those on the initial study done at admission. A transesophageal echocardiogram confirms the valve findings without evidence of additional complications.

Which of the following is the most appropriate next step in management?

(A) Cardiac catheterization
(B) Cardiac valve surgery
(C) Intra-aortic balloon pump placement
(D) Switch oxacillin to vancomycin

Item 26

A 44-year-old man is evaluated in the office during a routine visit. Medical history is significant for HIV diagnosed at age 25 years, hypertension, and hyperlipidemia. He is a current smoker. Medications are chlorthalidone, tenofovir-emtricitabine, and raltegravir.

On physical examination, the patient is afebrile, and blood pressure is 126/74 mm Hg. Cardiac examination reveals a regular rate and rhythm. S₁ and S₂ are normal; there is an S₄.

Laboratory tests are significant for a fasting plasma glucose level of 98 mg/dL (5.43 mmol/L), a total cholesterol level of 210 mg/dL (5.43 mmol/L), and an HDL cholesterol level of 50 mg/dL (1.29 mmol/L).

An electrocardiogram shows normal sinus rhythm and left ventricular hypertrophy with repolarization abnormalities. A chest radiograph is normal.

To determine his need for statin therapy, his estimated 10-year risk for atherosclerotic cardiovascular disease using the Pooled Cohort Equations will be calculated.

Which of the following risk factors will result in underestimation of the risk for atherosclerotic cardiovascular disease in this patient?

(A) Age
(B) Antihypertensive medication use
(C) Blood pressure
(D) HDL cholesterol level
(E) HIV status

Item 27

A 52-year-old woman is evaluated for a 6-week history of chest pressure. The symptom occurs when she walks up an incline on her daily 2-mile walk and is relieved with rest. She also had chest pressure during a stressful meeting at work last week. She reports no associated symptoms. Medical history is significant for hypertension and hyperlipidemia. Medications are hydrochlorothiazide, lisinopril, and atorvastatin.

On physical examination, vital signs and the remainder of the examination are normal.

An electrocardiogram is normal.

Which of the following is the most appropriate diagnostic test to perform next?

(A) Adenosine single-photon emission CT
(B) Coronary artery calcium scoring
(C) Exercise electrocardiography
(D) Stress echocardiography

Item 28

A 72-year-old man is evaluated in the hospital for heart failure. In the past month, he has developed progressive dyspnea, such that he cannot walk 50 meters without stopping to catch his breath. He has a history of hypertension and ischemic cardiomyopathy. During the hospitalization, a perfusion imaging study demonstrated no ischemia, and an echocardiogram revealed a left ventricular ejection fraction of 20%. Medications are aspirin, ramipril, isosorbide mononitrate, and furosemide.

On physical examination, the patient is afebrile, blood pressure is 120/68 mm Hg, pulse rate is 73/min, and respiration rate is 22/min. The estimated central venous pressure is 9 cm H₂O. A paradoxical split S₂ and an S₃ are present. Lungs are clear to auscultation.

A 12-lead electrocardiogram is shown.

In addition to diuresis, which of the following is the most appropriate treatment before discharge?

(A) Add carvedilol
(B) Add ivabradine
(C) Cardiac resynchronization therapy
(D) Implantable cardioverter-defibrillator placement

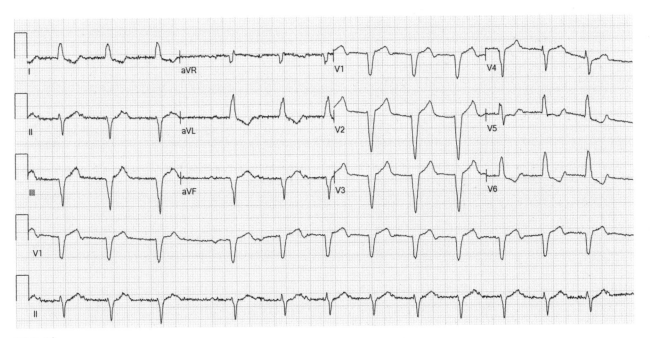

ITEM 28

Item 29

A 64-year-old woman is hospitalized for progressive fatigue, dyspnea, orthopnea, and peripheral edema that have been present for the last 18 months. During this time, she has been hospitalized several times for heart failure with preserved ejection fraction. Her medical history is otherwise notable for hypertension. Her current medications are spironolactone, furosemide, and amlodipine.

On physical examination, temperature is normal, blood pressure is 136/84 mm Hg, pulse rate is 90/min, and respiration rate is 16/min. Jugular venous distention is present. Crackles are noted at the bases of both lungs. A loud S_3 is heard at the apex. A grade 2/6 holosystolic murmur is heard at the left lower sternal border and increases in intensity during inspiration. Abdominal ascites and bilateral pitting edema to the knees are present.

Laboratory studies reveal a serum ferritin level of 180 ng/mL (180 µg/L) and a B-type natriuretic peptide level of 560 pg/mL (560 ng/L). Serum protein electrophoresis and urine protein electrophoresis are unremarkable.

Right heart catheterization demonstrates diastolic equalization of pressures at 18 mm Hg. Simultaneous right and left ventricular hemodynamics demonstrate concordant rise and fall of systolic pressures with respiration. Cardiac magnetic resonance imaging with intravenous gadolinium contrast shows a pericardial thickness of 2 mm without enhancement and marked late gadolinium enhancement of the papillary muscle. Echocardiogram shows symmetric left ventricular wall thickness of 11 mm, normal left ventricular cavity size, a left ventricular ejection fraction of 55%, and severe biatrial dilatation. Right ventricular size and function are normal. Tricuspid regurgitation is noted, and the right ventricular systolic pressure is estimated at 72 mm Hg. There is no pericardial effusion.

Which of the following is the most likely diagnosis?

(A) Constrictive pericarditis
(B) Fabry disease
(C) Hemochromatosis
(D) Primary restrictive cardiomyopathy

Item 30

A 64-year-old woman is evaluated in the emergency department 4 hours after the abrupt onset of sharp, tearing chest and back pain. Medical history is significant for hyperlipidemia. Her only medication is atorvastatin.

On physical examination, temperature is 36.8 °C (98.2 °F), blood pressure is 173/99 mm Hg, and pulse rate is 90/min. Blood pressure measurements in both arms are equal. The remainder of the physical examination is unremarkable.

CT angiography shows a descending thoracic aortic aneurysm with a maximal diameter of 6.8 cm and aortic dissection originating just distal to the left subclavian artery and extending to just below the diaphragm; there is no involvement of the renal arteries.

Which of the following is the most appropriate initial management?

(A) Immediate endovascular stenting
(B) Immediate open surgical repair
(C) Medical therapy
(D) Repeat CT angiography in 12 hours

Item 31

A 58-year-old man is hospitalized for a 1-day history of worsening dyspnea and a 1-month history of increasing weight and peripheral edema. He has a long-standing history of poorly controlled hypertension and stage IV chronic kidney disease. Minoxidil and hydralazine were added to his medical regimen 2 months ago. His other medications are labetalol, a clonidine patch, and furosemide.

On physical examination, he is in distress, with increased work of breathing and diaphoresis. Temperature is normal, blood pressure is 90/60 mm Hg with pulsus paradoxus of 16 mm Hg, pulse rate is 118/min, and respiration rate is 25/min. Oxygen saturation is 90% breathing ambient air. Jugular venous distention is present. Heart sounds are distant, and no pericardial friction rub or murmur is noted. Crackles are noted at the lower quarter of both lung fields. Pitting edema is present to the knees.

Laboratory studies reveal a blood urea nitrogen level of 86 mg/dL (30.7 mmol/L), a serum creatinine level of 5.1 mg/dL (451 µmol/L), and a serum potassium level of 5.0 mEq/L (5.0 mmol/L).

A chest radiograph shows an enlarged cardiac silhouette, prominent pulmonary vasculature, and evidence of pulmonary edema. Echocardiographic findings are compatible with cardiac tamponade.

Which of the following is the most appropriate management?

(A) Hemodialysis
(B) Intravenous nitroglycerin
(C) Pericardiocentesis
(D) Right heart catheterization

Item 32

A 52-year-old woman is evaluated during a follow-up visit. She was discharged from the hospital 3 weeks ago following a small non–ST-elevation myocardial infarction treated with drug-eluting stent placement in the right coronary artery. An echocardiogram obtained during hospitalization showed normal left ventricular function and normal valvular function. Her hospital course was uncomplicated. Since discharge, she has had shortness of breath. Medical history is significant for hyperlipidemia. Medications are aspirin, ticagrelor, lisinopril, metoprolol, and atorvastatin.

On physical examination, vital signs are normal. Oxygen saturation is 99% breathing ambient air. The estimated central venous pressure is normal. Cardiac examination reveals no S_3 or murmurs. The lungs are clear to auscultation.

A chest radiograph is normal. An electrocardiogram is unchanged from those obtained in the hospital.

Which of the following is the most likely cause of this patient's dyspnea?

(A) Heart failure
(B) In-stent restenosis

(C) Stent thrombosis

(D) Ticagrelor-mediated side effect

(E) Ventricular septal rupture

Item 33

A 68-year-old woman is evaluated in the emergency department for acute-onset dyspnea, palpitations, and chest pain. The symptoms began shortly after her dog was attacked by another dog. She is otherwise healthy and takes no medications.

On physical examination, the patient is afebrile, blood pressure is 150/78 mm Hg, and pulse rate is 88/min. Cardiac examination reveals no evidence of increased central venous pressure. There is no heart murmur, but an S_3 is present. The lungs are clear to auscultation.

Laboratory studies are significant for a serum troponin I level of 5.2 ng/mL (5.2 µg/L).

An electrocardiogram demonstrates sinus rhythm and anterior hyperacute T-wave elevations suggestive of an ST-elevation myocardial infarction. Cardiac catheterization shows normal coronary arteries. Systolic (*left panel*) and diastolic (*right panel*) images from left ventriculography are shown.

Which of the following is the most likely diagnosis?

(A) Acute myocarditis

(B) Giant cell myocarditis

(C) Tachycardia-mediated cardiomyopathy

(D) Takotsubo cardiomyopathy

Item 34

A 52-year-old woman is evaluated for recent-onset exertional dyspnea. Medical history is noncontributory, and she takes no medications.

On physical examination, vital signs are normal. The central venous pressure is elevated with a prominent *a* wave. Apical impulse is normal, and a prominent parasternal impulse is noted at the left sternal border. The S_1 is normal; the S_2 is soft. A grade 4/6 late-peaking systolic murmur is heard at the left sternal border and second left intercostal space. An ejection click is not audible.

Echocardiogram demonstrates doming of the pulmonary valve with stenosis, a peak instantaneous systolic gradient of 65 mm Hg, and a mean systolic gradient of 50 mm Hg. Trivial pulmonary regurgitation is present. The right ventricular size and function are normal, but right ventricular hypertrophy is present. The left heart size and function are normal.

Which of the following is the most appropriate management of this patient?

(A) Endocarditis prophylaxis

(B) Exercise stress testing

(C) Pulmonary balloon valvuloplasty

(D) Pulmonary valve replacement

Item 35

A 60-year-old man is evaluated in the hospital for a 2-day history of intermittent chest pain and dyspnea on exertion. Medical history is significant for type 2 diabetes mellitus, hypertension, hyperlipidemia, COPD, and peripheral neuropathy. His ability to exercise is limited by his COPD. Medications are metformin, simvastatin, low-dose aspirin, lisinopril, amlodipine, and an albuterol-ipratropium inhaler.

On physical examination, temperature is normal, blood pressure is 128/78 mm Hg, pulse rate is 80/min, and respiration rate is 16/min. Oxygen saturation is 94% breathing ambient air. Pulmonary examination reveals expiratory wheezing bilaterally. Heart sounds are distant. No edema is present.

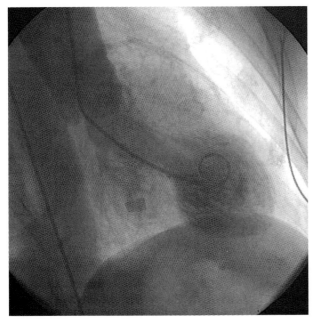
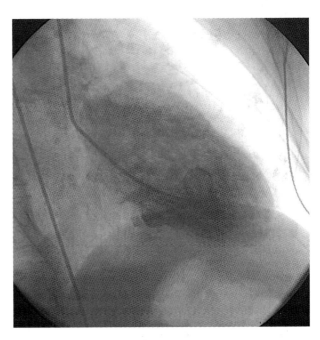

ITEM 33

Serial serum troponin I measurements are negative.

An electrocardiogram demonstrates left ventricular hypertrophy with repolarization abnormalities.

Which of the following is the most appropriate diagnostic test to perform next?

(A) Adenosine single-photon emission CT
(B) Coronary angiography
(C) Coronary CT angiography
(D) Exercise electrocardiography

Item 36

A 35-year-old woman is evaluated for chest discomfort that sometimes occurs at the beginning of exercise but abates completely even though she continues to exercise. She describes the discomfort as sharp in character and notes that it worsens when she breathes in. The pain does not radiate and is not accompanied by other symptoms. She also reports occasionally feeling lightheaded at the end of exercise or as she is "cooling down." She notes that her typical resting heart rate is 49/min. She takes no medications.

On physical examination, pulse rate is 43/min; other vital signs are normal. Oxygen saturation is 99% breathing ambient air. Cardiac examination reveals regular bradycardia. Heart rate varies with respiration. The remainder of the physical examination is normal.

Laboratory studies are significant for normal hemoglobin and serum thyroid-stimulating hormone levels.

A 12-lead electrocardiogram is shown. An echocardiogram demonstrates normal cardiac structure and function.

Which of the following is the most appropriate next step in management?

(A) Chest CT
(B) Coronary angiography
(C) Exercise treadmill stress testing
(D) Pacemaker implantation

Item 37

A 35-year-old woman is evaluated for hypertension. She is at 12 weeks' gestation of her first pregnancy. She reports no symptoms and has no history of hypertension or cardiovascular disease. She has not routinely had her blood pressure checked. Family history is significant for hypertension. Her only medication is a prenatal vitamin.

On physical examination, blood pressure is 166/94 mm Hg in both arms, and pulse rate is 80/min. An S_4 is noted at the apex. There are no murmurs. Pulses are normal throughout. The remainder of the examination is unremarkable.

Serum creatinine level, plasma glucose level, and urinalysis are normal. An ambulatory blood pressure monitor demonstrates an average blood pressure of 162/90 mm Hg.

Which of the following is the most appropriate treatment?

(A) Diet and weight loss alone
(B) Labetalol
(C) Lisinopril
(D) Spironolactone

Item 38

A 55-year-old woman is evaluated during a routine examination. Her medical history is significant for mitral regurgitation. She has no history of cardiovascular symptoms. She is moderately active, plays doubles tennis, and occasionally participates in road cycling. She has no other medical problems and takes no medications.

On physical examination, vital signs are normal. Cardiac auscultation reveals a high-pitched midsystolic click and a grade 3/6 late systolic murmur that is loudest at the apex. Standing results in the click-murmur complex increasing in intensity and moving closer to S_1.

An echocardiogram shows severe mitral regurgitation and myxomatous degeneration of the mitral valve. The left ventricular ejection fraction is 65% with normal chamber size.

After discussion regarding early surgical repair versus surveillance, she chooses to defer surgery.

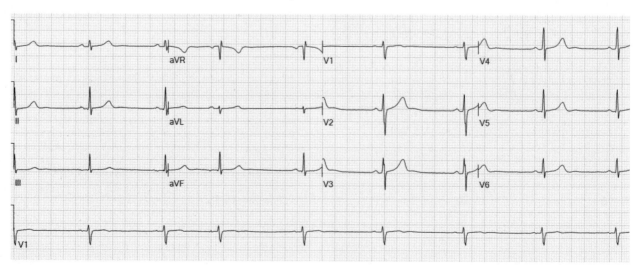

ITEM 36

In the absence of clinical symptoms, which of the following is the most appropriate timing for the next clinical evaluation in this patient?

(A) 3 months
(B) 6 to 12 months
(C) 1 to 2 years
(D) 3 to 5 years

Item 39

A 64-year-old man is evaluated in the office 7 days after discharge from the hospital for non–ST-elevation myocardial infarction. He was treated with percutaneous coronary intervention using a radial artery approach. Right femoral artery access was initially attempted, but the catheter guidewire could not be passed. During the procedure, an abdominal aortogram was obtained (shown). He has not had any symptoms of claudication. Medical history is significant for hyperlipidemia. He is a current smoker with a 40-pack-year history. Medications are low-dose aspirin, ticagrelor, metoprolol, and atorvastatin.

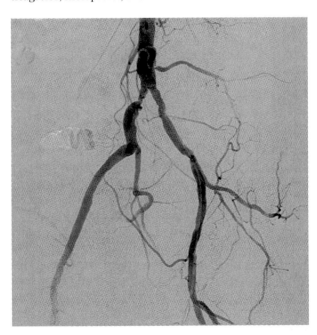

On physical examination, vital signs are stable. The right femoral pulse is faint, and a bruit is heard over the right femoral artery. No foot or toe ulceration is noted.

In addition to aggressive risk factor modification, which of the following is the most appropriate management?

(A) Cilostazol
(B) Cardiac rehabilitation
(C) Endovascular iliac stenting
(D) Vorapaxar

Item 40

An 18-year-old man is evaluated as part of a preparticipation sports examination. He is attending college on a basketball scholarship. He reports no symptoms. Medical history is unremarkable, and he takes no medications.

On physical examination, vital signs are normal. Cardiac examination reveals a brisk carotid upstroke. A grade 3/6 systolic crescendo-decrescendo murmur is heard best along the left sternal border; it decreases with squatting and is more pronounced in the upright position. Lungs are clear to auscultation.

An electrocardiogram shows voltage criteria for left ventricular hypertrophy with abnormal repolarization. An echocardiogram demonstrates asymmetric septal hypertrophy with septal thickness of 18 mm. Systolic anterior motion of the mitral valve is present, and the peak instantaneous left ventricular outflow tract gradient at rest is 30 mm Hg.

Which of the following is the most appropriate management regarding this patient's participation on the basketball team?

(A) Advise the patient that he should not play basketball
(B) Begin β-blocker therapy
(C) Refer for alcohol septal ablation
(D) Refer for implantable cardioverter-defibrillator placement

Item 41

An 80-year-old woman was hospitalized for chest pain and findings of a lateral ST-elevation myocardial infarction. She underwent percutaneous coronary intervention of a marginal branch of the left circumflex artery 16 hours after symptom onset. On hospital day 3, her cardiac examination is normal, but 3 hours later, she develops sudden-onset chest pain and loses consciousness. She is found to have pulseless electrical activity. Heart sounds are significantly diminished.

Which of the following is the most likely diagnosis?

(A) Aortic dissection
(B) In-stent restenosis
(C) Ventricular free wall rupture
(D) Ventricular septal defect

Item 42

A 64-year-old man is hospitalized for persistent low-grade fever, chest discomfort, and lower extremity edema. He underwent triple coronary artery bypass graft surgery 6 weeks ago. His medical history is otherwise notable for hypertension, hyperlipidemia, and previous smoking. His current medications are aspirin, metoprolol succinate, atorvastatin, lisinopril, and furosemide.

On physical examination, temperature is 37.7 °C (99.8 °F), blood pressure is 136/84 mm Hg, pulse rate is 96/min, and respiration rate is 14/min. Jugular venous distention is noted to the angle of the mandible. Decreased breath sounds and dullness to percussion are noted at the left base. No crackles are noted. A pericardial rub is present. There is no gallop. The liver is enlarged. There is bilateral pitting edema to the mid shin.

Laboratory studies:

Erythrocyte sedimentation rate	76 mm/h
Leukocyte count	12,000/µL (12 × 10⁹/L)
Serum creatinine	1.4 mg/dL (123.8 µmol/L)
Troponin (two samples)	Normal
B-type natriuretic peptide	105 pg/mL (105 ng/L)

A 12-lead electrocardiogram demonstrates normal sinus rhythm with nonspecific ST-T-wave abnormalities. A chest radiograph demonstrates bilateral small pleural effusions. An echocardiogram shows no pericardial effusion. A Doppler echocardiogram shows enhanced ventricular interdependence and dilation of the inferior vena cava. Right heart catheterization demonstrates equalization of diastolic pressures in all heart chambers. Gadolinium-enhanced cardiac magnetic resonance imaging demonstrates increased pericardial thickness and evidence of active pericardial inflammation and edema.

Which of the following is the most likely diagnosis?

(A) Heart failure with preserved ejection fraction
(B) Perioperative graft failure with infarction
(C) Restrictive cardiomyopathy
(D) Transient constrictive pericarditis

Item 43

A 72-year-old woman is evaluated during a routine office visit. She has a 3-year history of heart failure with preserved ejection fraction and a long history of hypertension. She has exertional dyspnea with walking around the house, almost nightly paroxysmal nocturnal dyspnea, and peripheral edema. Cardiac catheterization performed 2 years ago revealed normal coronary arteries. Medications are hydrochlorothiazide and diltiazem.

On physical examination, the patient is afebrile, blood pressure is 136/82 mm Hg, pulse rate is 48/min, and respiration rate is 18/min. There is jugular venous distention.

An S₄ is present. Pulmonary examination reveals no wheezes or crackles. Peripheral edema is noted.

Laboratory studies are significant for a serum creatinine level of 1.2 mg/dL (106.1 µmol/L) and a serum sodium level of 139 mEq/L (139 mmol/L).

Which of the following is the most appropriate management?

(A) Add ivabradine
(B) Add valsartan
(C) Discontinue hydrochlorothiazide and diltiazem and start furosemide
(D) Refer for pacemaker placement

Item 44

A 47-year-old man is evaluated for gradually progressive exertional dyspnea and two episodes of self-limited atrial fibrillation during the past 6 months. The atrial fibrillation was attributed to alcohol consumption, and no additional testing was performed. Medical history is otherwise noncontributory. He takes no medications.

On physical examination, vital signs are normal. The estimated central venous pressure is elevated. A parasternal impulse is noted at the left sternal border. Persistent splitting of the S₂ is present. A grade 2/6 systolic murmur is heard at the second left intercostal space, with a separate grade 3/6 holosystolic murmur at the apex. The remainder of the examination is normal.

An electrocardiogram is shown.

Which of the following is the most likely diagnosis?

(A) Coronary sinus atrial septal defect (ASD)
(B) Ostium primum ASD
(C) Ostium secundum ASD
(D) Sinus venosus ASD

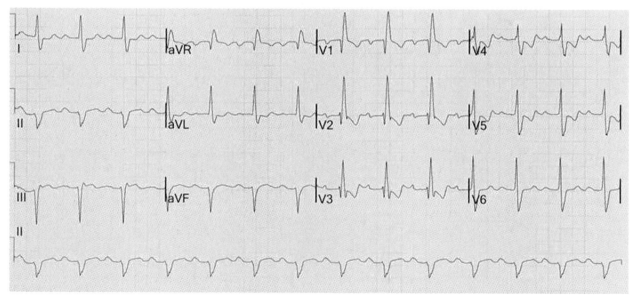

ITEM 44

Item 45

A 59-year-old man is evaluated during a routine examination. He feels well and has no symptoms. Medical history is significant for hypertension. He does not smoke, and he does not have diabetes mellitus. He is active, performing aerobic exercise for 20 to 30 minutes four times per week. Medications are lisinopril and chlorthalidone.

On physical examination, the patient is afebrile, blood pressure is 122/74 mm Hg, and pulse rate is 76/min. Cardiac examination is unremarkable.

Laboratory studies:

Total cholesterol	169 mg/dL (4.38 mmol/L)
HDL cholesterol	36 mg/dL (0.93 mmol/L)
LDL cholesterol	106 mg/dL (2.75 mmol/L)
Triglycerides	135 mg/dL (1.53 mmol/L)

Which of the following is the most appropriate next step in management?

(A) Begin low-intensity statin therapy
(B) Begin moderate-intensity statin therapy
(C) Begin high-intensity statin therapy
(D) Calculate the 10-year atherosclerotic cardiovascular disease risk
(E) Repeat lipid level measurement in 5 years

Item 46

A 66-year-old man has just received an aortic valve replacement with a mechanical prosthesis. He is otherwise healthy and takes no medications.

On physical examination, vital signs are normal. There is a regular rhythm with a normal S$_1$, a mechanical S$_2$, and no murmurs. The remainder of the physical examination is normal.

Which of the following is the most appropriate antithrombotic therapy?

(A) Apixaban
(B) Dabigatran
(C) Warfarin
(D) Warfarin and aspirin
(E) No anticoagulation required

Item 47

A 79-year-old woman is evaluated in the emergency department for palpitations that have occurred intermittently over the past 48 hours. Medical history is significant for hypertension and hyperlipidemia. Medications are low-dose aspirin, atorvastatin, and lisinopril.

On physical examination, temperature is 36.8 °C (98.2 °F), and blood pressure is 110/74 mm Hg. The resting pulse rate is 110/min with intermittent irregularity. The estimated central venous pressure is normal. Cardiac examination reveals tachycardia with a split S$_2$. The lung fields are clear. The extremities are warm and well perfused without edema.

An electrocardiogram is shown.

Which of the following is the most appropriate next step in management?

(A) β-Blocker therapy and anticoagulation
(B) Intravenous adenosine
(C) Intravenous procainamide
(D) Urgent cardioversion

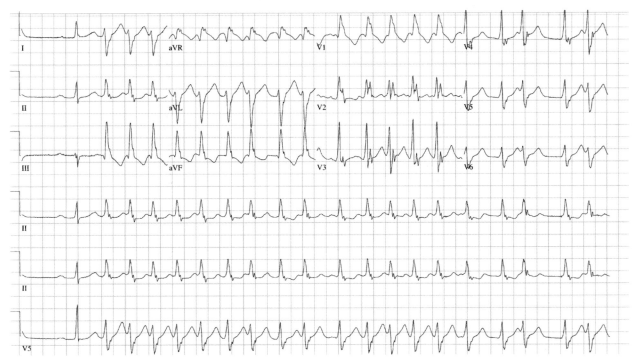

ITEM 47

Item 48

A 60-year-old man is evaluated for a 5-month history of exertional chest discomfort that improves with rest. His symptoms have progressively worsened such that he has reduced his activity to a minimum. Medical history is significant for hypertension and hyperlipidemia. Medications are low-dose aspirin, losartan, hydrochlorothiazide, and atorvastatin.

On physical examination, the patient is afebrile, blood pressure is 122/71 mm Hg, and pulse rate is 74/min. Cardiac examination shows a normal S_1 and S_2. A grade 2/6 crescendo-decrescendo systolic murmur is heard best at the upper sternal border with no radiation. Lung examination is normal.

A stress echocardiogram shows 2-mm ST-segment depression at peak stress, normal left ventricular function at rest, normal valvular function, and anterior hypokinesis at peak stress (normal at rest). A 5.4-cm ascending thoracic aortic aneurysm is noted at the level of the sinuses of Valsalva. Coronary angiogram reveals 80% stenosis of the left main coronary artery bifurcation with no significant disease of the left anterior descending, left circumflex, or right coronary arteries.

Which of the following is the most appropriate next step in the patient's management?

(A) Coronary artery bypass graft surgery
(B) Metoprolol and isosorbide mononitrate
(C) Percutaneous coronary intervention
(D) Simultaneous coronary artery bypass graft surgery and aortic repair

Item 49

A 37-year-old man is evaluated in the emergency department for right-sided weakness. Medical history is significant for heart failure with placement of a left ventricular assist device 2 years ago. Family history is significant for familial cardiomyopathy. Medications are warfarin, aspirin, lisinopril, carvedilol, and furosemide.

On physical examination, temperature is normal, mean arterial pressure measured by Doppler ultrasonography is 106 mm Hg, pulse rate is 98/min, and respiration rate is 16/min. Oxygen saturation is 94% breathing ambient air. There is no jugular venous distention. Neurologic examination demonstrates global aphasia, right arm paralysis, antigravity movement in the right leg, left gaze preference, and decreased blink response to threat from the right side.

CT of the head shows sulcal effacement and loss of gray-white differentiation in the territory of the left middle cerebral artery.

Which of the following is the most likely cause of this patient's stroke?

(A) Carotid artery stenosis
(B) Cryptogenic stroke
(C) Lacunar infarction
(D) Left ventricular assist device–related thrombosis

Item 50

A 48-year-old woman is evaluated during a new-patient visit. She reports no symptoms. She is fairly sedentary but is trying to become more active by joining the local health club. She has noticed that she is "out of shape" but can cycle on a stationary bike with moderate intensity to the end of her 30-minute workout. Medical history is otherwise unremarkable. She takes no medications.

On physical examination, vital signs are normal. The estimated central venous pressure is 6 cm H_2O. The apical impulse is not palpable. Cardiac examination reveals a grade 2/6 midsystolic murmur localized to the left sternal border without radiation. The murmur does not change with respiration or handgrip but does diminish in intensity with standing. The S_2 is physiologically split. There are no clicks. The lungs are clear to auscultation. Peripheral pulses are normal in volume and contour. No edema is present.

Which of the following is the most appropriate management?

(A) Cardiac magnetic resonance imaging
(B) Transesophageal echocardiography
(C) Transthoracic echocardiography
(D) Routine clinical follow-up without imaging

Item 51

An 81-year-old woman is evaluated following drug-eluting stent placement for stable but disabling angina 1 month ago. After stent placement, she was started on aspirin and clopidogrel. She is currently asymptomatic, and she is interested in minimizing the duration of dual antiplatelet therapy because of her age and comorbid illnesses. Medical history is significant for hyperlipidemia, hypertension, stage 3 chronic kidney disease, and previous peptic ulcer disease. Other medications are lisinopril, metoprolol, atorvastatin, and pantoprazole.

On physical examination, vital signs are normal. Oxygen saturation is 98% breathing ambient air. The remainder of the examination is unremarkable.

Which of the following is the most appropriate management of this patient's antiplatelet therapy?

(A) Discontinue clopidogrel now
(B) Discontinue clopidogrel in 5 months
(C) Discontinue clopidogrel in 11 months
(D) Discontinue clopidogrel and aspirin in 11 months
(E) Discontinue clopidogrel in 29 months

Item 52

A 52-year-old woman is evaluated in the hospital for left arm and left leg weakness of 12 hours' duration. She has a 4-month history of progressive dyspnea on exertion, fatigue, low-grade fever, and arthralgia. She takes no medications.

On physical examination, temperature is 38.1 °C (100.5 °F). Other vital signs are normal. On neurologic examination, muscle strength is 4/5 in the left arm and left leg; strength in all other muscle groups is 5/5. Cardiac examination reveals a loud S_1, a soft diastolic rumble heard at the apex, and an early diastolic sound. The remainder of the examination is normal.

Laboratory studies are significant for an erythrocyte sedimentation rate of 87 mm/h; normocytic, normochromic anemia; and a normal leukocyte count.

An electrocardiogram demonstrates normal sinus rhythm. MRI of the brain reveals multiple small infarcts. An echocardiogram is shown. Left ventricular function is normal.

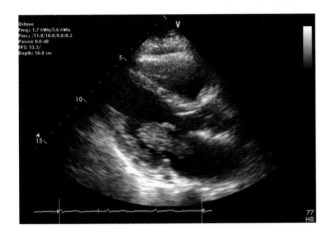

Which of the following is the most appropriate treatment?

(A) Anticoagulation
(B) Chemotherapy and radiotherapy
(C) Empiric broad-spectrum antibiotic therapy
(D) Percutaenous transesophageal echocardiographic–guided biopsy
(E) Surgical excision

Item 53

A 19-year-old man is evaluated for a heart murmur noted on physical examination. He reports no symptoms. Medical history is noncontributory. He takes no medications.

On physical examination, vital signs are normal. The patient is of short stature with hypertelorism, neck webbing, and a low hairline. The central venous pressure is elevated with a prominent *a* wave. Apical impulse is normal, and a prominent impulse is noted at the left upper sternal border. The S_1 is normal; the S_2 is soft. A grade 4/6 late-peaking systolic murmur is heard best at the left sternal border and second left intercostal space. An ejection click is not audible. The remainder of the examination is unremarkable.

Echocardiogram demonstrates a dysplastic pulmonary valve with a peak instantaneous systolic gradient of 65 mm Hg. Pulmonary regurgitation is moderate. The right ventricular size and function are normal, but right ventricular hypertrophy is present. The left heart size and function are normal.

Which of the following is the most likely genetic disorder responsible for this patient's findings?

(A) Down syndrome
(B) Marfan syndrome
(C) Noonan syndrome
(D) Turner syndrome

Item 54

A 51-year-old man is evaluated in the emergency department for an abrupt loss of consciousness while sitting in a restaurant. The event was witnessed, and the patient was noted to shake for several seconds before he regained consciousness. No prodromal symptoms occurred before the episode. After the event, he had no confusion or altered sensorium. Medical history is significant for nonischemic cardiomyopathy. He is slightly limited by shortness of breath during exercise. He has been taking metoprolol succinate and lisinopril for 9 months.

On physical examination, temperature is normal, blood pressure is 134/78 mm Hg, pulse rate is 72/min, and respiration rate is 15/min. Cardiac examination reveals a regular rhythm with intermittent ectopy. The chest is clear to auscultation. The estimated central venous pressure is normal. No edema is present. Carotid massage produces no bradycardia.

Laboratory findings are notable for a negative result on a serum troponin test.

Telemetry in the emergency department demonstrates short runs of nonsustained ventricular tachycardia. A 12-lead electrocardiogram shows premature ventricular contractions. An echocardiogram demonstrates a left ventricular ejection fraction of 25%.

Which of the following is the most appropriate management?

(A) Electroencephalography
(B) Exercise treadmill stress testing
(C) Implantable cardioverter-defibrillator placement
(D) PET of the mediastinum
(E) Tilt-table testing

Item 55

A 45-year-old woman is evaluated for a 12-month history of exertional dyspnea. She experiences shortness of breath during mild exertion, such as house chores and walking on flat surfaces. She describes her symptoms as debilitating, as they have interfered with her activities of daily living. She has not had symptoms at rest, and she has had no palpitations. She takes hydrochlorothiazide for hypertension.

On physical examination, temperature is normal, blood pressure is 112/72 mm Hg, pulse rate is 76/min, and respiration rate is normal. The apical impulse is slightly sustained but not displaced. S_1 is increased. There is an early diastolic sound followed by a soft rumble heard best at the apex. S_2 is normal.

An echocardiogram shows findings consistent with moderate rheumatic mitral stenosis and minimal mitral regurgitation. The mean gradient across the mitral valve is 8 mm Hg, and the mitral valve area is calculated to be 1.8 cm². The mitral valve is pliable. Moderate pulmonary hypertension is present, with an estimated pulmonary artery systolic pressure of 45 mm Hg.

Which of the following is the most appropriate next step in management?

(A) Exercise echocardiography
(B) Medical therapy
(C) Percutaneous balloon mitral valvuloplasty
(D) Surgical mitral valve replacement

Item 56

A 56-year-old man is evaluated in the emergency department for progressive chest pain and dyspnea that began 3 hours ago. Medical history is significant for hypertension treated with lisinopril.

On physical examination, he is confused. Temperature is normal, blood pressure is 86/50 mm Hg, pulse rate is 118/min, and respiration rate is 24/min. Oxygen saturation breathing ambient air is 90%. Cardiac examination reveals an S_3 gallop. Crackles are noted on pulmonary examination. The extremities are cool to the touch.

An electrocardiogram is shown. A chest radiograph reveals pulmonary edema.

Aspirin is initiated in the emergency department.

Which of the following is the most appropriate immediate management?

(A) Admission to the ICU for medical stabilization
(B) Intravenous metoprolol
(C) Percutaneous coronary intervention
(D) Sublingual nitroglycerin
(E) Thrombolytic therapy

Item 57

A 54-year-old man is evaluated during a routine examination. He is asymptomatic, and he exercises regularly without any limitations. Medical history is significant for hypertension and a bicuspid aortic valve with an enlarged aortic root (measuring 5.1 cm 6 months ago). Family history is unremarkable. His only medication is losartan.

On physical examination, blood pressure is 122/74 mm Hg. Cardiac examination reveals a midsystolic ejection click and a grade 2/6 crescendo-decrescendo systolic murmur at the second right intercostal space. The remainder of the examination is unremarkable.

Transthoracic echocardiogram shows normal left ventricular function and a bicuspid aortic valve. The mean gradient across the aortic valve is 20 mm Hg, and the aortic valve area is 1.6 cm². The ascending aorta is 5.1 cm; the descending thoracic aorta is incompletely visualized.

Which of the following is the most appropriate management?

(A) Aortic valve replacement and ascending aortic repair
(B) Ascending aortic repair
(C) Dobutamine stress echocardiography
(D) Repeat echocardiography in 6 months

Item 58

A 36-year-old woman is evaluated in the emergency department for progressive dyspnea. She gave birth 3 weeks ago. The pregnancy and delivery were uncomplicated. She has no history of cardiovascular disease.

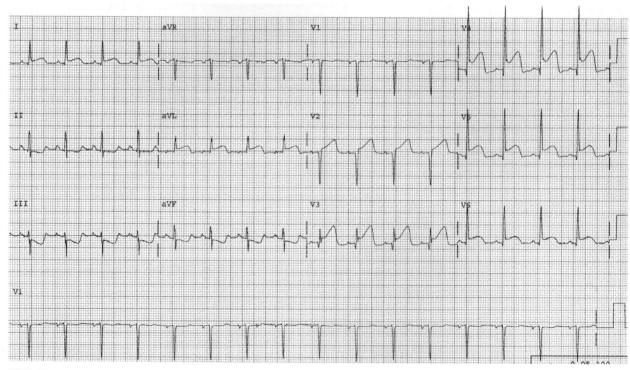

ITEM 56

On physical examination, temperature is normal, blood pressure is 100/72 mm Hg in both arms, pulse rate is 102/min and regular, and respiration rate is 26/min. The estimated central venous pressure is elevated. Cardiac palpation reveals a diffuse apical impulse. The S_1 and S_2 are soft. An S_3 and S_4 are present. A grade 2/6 holosystolic murmur is heard at the apex. Crackles are auscultated bilaterally.

An electrocardiogram demonstrates sinus tachycardia without ST-T-wave changes. Transthoracic echocardiogram reveals ventricular dilatation with global reduction in contractility; the left ventricular ejection fraction is 30%.

Which of the following is the most likely diagnosis?

(A) Acute aortic dissection
(B) Acute pulmonary embolism
(C) Peripartum cardiomyopathy
(D) Takotsubo cardiomyopathy

Item 59

A 48-year-old man is evaluated for a 6-month history of intermittent palpitations with accompanying lightheadedness and near-syncope. The episodes last approximately 5 minutes and occur once or twice per week. He cannot identify any precipitating triggers for his symptoms. Medical history is notable for hypertension. His only medication is chlorthalidone.

On physical examination, vital signs and the remainder of the examination are normal.

An electrocardiogram shows normal sinus rhythm with no evidence of preexcitation.

Which of the following is the most appropriate diagnostic testing option?

(A) Electrophysiology study
(B) External event recorder
(C) 24-Hour ambulatory electrocardiographic monitor
(D) Implantable loop recorder

Item 60

A 70-year-old woman is evaluated in the emergency department for dyspnea. For the past 5 days, she has had progressive shortness of breath associated with a nonproductive cough. Symptoms are greatest with exertion and possibly when lying down. She has had no fever, chest pain, or increase in her chronic lower extremity edema. Her other medical problems are chronic venous insufficiency, COPD, and hypertension. Medications are chlorthalidone, amlodipine, lisinopril, and a tiotropium inhaler.

On physical examination, she is afebrile, blood pressure is 144/88 mm Hg, pulse rate is 90/min, and respiration rate is 22/min. Oxygen saturation is 94% breathing ambient air. BMI is 36. Because her neck is large, it is not possible to estimate central venous pressure. Breath sounds are distant, with occasional end-expiratory wheezing. Heart sounds are distant, and extra sounds or murmurs are not detected. There is 2+ ankle edema with hyperpigmentation localized to the medial aspect of the ankles.

B-type natriuretic peptide level is 128 pg/mL (128 ng/L).

A chest radiograph shows increased radiolucency of the lung, flat diaphragms, and a narrow heart shadow consistent with COPD.

An electrocardiogram shows evidence of left ventricular hypertrophy.

This patient's B-type natriuretic peptide level is most consistent with which of the following causes of dyspnea?

(A) Acute heart failure
(B) Chronic heart failure
(C) Noncardiac disease
(D) Cannot be determined

Item 61

A 77-year-old man is evaluated for a 4-week history of progressive left foot pain that occurs at rest. He also has calf muscle pain that worsens when he ambulates. Medical history is significant for type 2 diabetes mellitus, hypertension, and hyperlipidemia. Medications are low-dose aspirin, metformin, amlodipine, lisinopril, and rosuvastatin.

On physical examination, temperature is 36.8 °C (98.2 °F), blood pressure is 134/74 mm Hg, and pulse rate is 92/min. The left foot is cool. There is a shallow 3.0-cm × 2.5-cm ulceration on the medial aspect of the left first metatarsal. Pedal pulses are diminished on the right and absent on the left. Left foot sensation and muscle strength are intact.

The ankle-brachial index is 0.62 on the right and unobtainable on the left.

Which of the following is the most appropriate next step in management?

(A) Add vorapaxar
(B) Invasive angiography of the left leg
(C) Magnetic resonance angiography
(D) Primary below-knee amputation

Item 62

A 68-year-old woman is evaluated in the emergency department for a 1-hour history of chest pain. Medical history is significant for hypertension and a 20-year history of type 2 diabetes mellitus. Medications are metformin, quinapril, and aspirin.

On physical examination, blood pressure is 95/60 mm Hg, pulse rate is 50/min, and respiration rate is 16/min. The patient is alert and conversant. The precordial cadence is not regular. There is no evidence of pulmonary or peripheral congestion, and the extremities are warm.

Laboratory studies reveal a serum troponin T level of 1.1 ng/mL (1.1 µg/L).

An electrocardiogram is shown (see top of next page).

Which of the following is the most appropriate next step in management of this patient's arrhythmia?

(A) Cardiac catheterization
(B) Echocardiography
(C) Permanent pacemaker implantation
(D) Temporary pacing

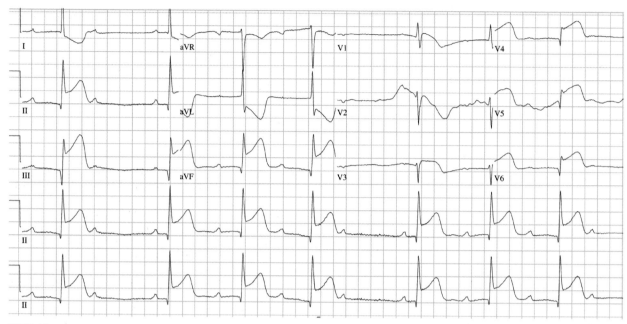

ITEM 62

Item 63

A 73-year-old man is evaluated during a routine examination. He is physically active and participates regularly in charitable running events. He has no cardiac symptoms, and his medical history is unremarkable.

On physical examination, vital signs are normal. The lungs are clear. Jugular venous pulse is normal. Carotid upstrokes are normal. The apical impulse is palpable and not displaced or sustained. There is a grade 3/6 diastolic decrescendo murmur best heard at the left lower sternal border. The remainder of the examination is normal.

A transthoracic echocardiogram shows severe aortic regurgitation. The left ventricular ejection fraction is 65%. The left ventricle is minimally dilated with an end-systolic dimension of 40 mm.

Which of the following is the most appropriate next step in management?

(A) Carvedilol
(B) Lisinopril
(C) Surgical aortic valve replacement
(D) Clinical and echocardiographic follow-up in 6 to 12 months

Item 64

A 65-year-old woman is evaluated in the hospital following primary percutaneous coronary intervention with stent placement in the mid left anterior descending artery. She presented 4 hours ago with findings of an anterior myocardial infarction complicated by heart failure. Medical history is significant for hyperlipidemia, hypertension, type 2 diabetes mellitus, and previous ACE inhibitor–induced cough. Medications are atorvastatin, aspirin, clopidogrel, metformin, and furosemide.

On physical examination, vital signs are normal. Oxygen saturation is 98% on 3 L oxygen by nasal cannula. The estimated central venous pressure is elevated. An S_3 is present. Pulmonary examination reveals bibasilar crackles.

Laboratory studies are notable for normal serum creatinine and serum potassium levels.

A chest radiograph shows pulmonary edema. An echocardiogram demonstrates a left ventricular ejection fraction of 40%.

Which of the following is the most appropriate treatment?

(A) Carvedilol
(B) Diltiazem
(C) Hydralazine–isosorbide dinitrate
(D) Valsartan

Item 65

A 36-year-old man is evaluated for a 3-day history of progressive exertional dyspnea and palpitations. Medical history is notable for hypertrophic cardiomyopathy and mild mitral regurgitation. His only medication is metoprolol succinate.

On physical examination, pulse rate is 116/min and irregularly irregular. Oxygen saturation is 98% breathing ambient air. There is jugular venous distention. A grade 3/6 systolic crescendo-decrescendo murmur is heard along the left sternal border. The remainder of the examination is normal.

An electrocardiogram demonstrates atrial fibrillation with rapid ventricular response. Transesophageal echocardiogram shows asymmetric septal hypertrophy and dynamic left ventricular outflow tract obstruction, with a gradient of 36 mm Hg. There is no evidence of left atrial appendage thrombus.

His CHA_2DS_2-VASc score is 0 points.

In addition to acute anticoagulation with heparin, which of the following is most appropriate for thromboembolic risk reduction in this patient?

(A) Dabigatran

(B) Dose-adjusted warfarin

(C) High-dose aspirin

(D) No further therapy

Item 66

A 78-year-old man is evaluated for exertional dyspnea. He was previously asymptomatic, but 4 months ago he began having shortness of breath during moderate levels of activity. The dyspnea dissipates with rest. He is otherwise healthy and takes no medications.

On physical examination, temperature is normal, supine blood pressure is 132/80 mm Hg, pulse rate is 80/min, and respiration rate is 22/min. The lungs are clear to auscultation. The carotid upstroke is delayed. There is a grade 3/6 late-peaking systolic murmur best heard at the base of the heart with radiation to both carotid arteries. S_1 is normal; the aortic component of S_2 is diminished. The remainder of the examination is unremarkable.

An echocardiogram demonstrates a left ventricular ejection fraction of 65%. There is moderate aortic stenosis, with a mean gradient of 28 mm Hg and an aortic valve area of 1.5 cm².

Which of the following is the most appropriate next step in management?

(A) Cardiac catheterization

(B) Surgical aortic valve replacement

(C) Transcatheter aortic valve replacement

(D) Continued clinical observation

Item 67

A 24-year-old woman undergoes routine evaluation. She has not seen a physician recently but reports no symptoms. She was diagnosed with a ventricular septal defect at age 7 months. Regular evaluation was performed during childhood. Medical history is otherwise noncontributory, and she takes no medications.

On physical examination, vital signs are normal. The jugular venous pressure and apical impulse are normal. No parasternal impulse is noted. The S_1 and S_2 are masked by a loud holosystolic murmur noted at the left lower sternal border. The remainder of the examination is unremarkable.

An electrocardiogram and chest radiograph are normal. A transthoracic echocardiogram demonstrates a membranous ventricular septal defect with a small left-to-right shunt. The left ventricular size and function are normal, with an ejection fraction of 60%. The right heart chambers and valve function are normal. The estimated pulmonary artery pressure is normal.

Which of the following is the most appropriate management?

(A) Cardiac catheterization

(B) Cardiac magnetic resonance imaging

(C) Endocarditis prophylaxis

(D) Follow-up in 3 to 5 years

Item 68

A 35-year-old woman is evaluated in the emergency department for a 3-week history of progressive dyspnea, fatigue, chest "fullness," and bilateral peripheral edema. Her medical history is notable for systemic lupus erythematosus manifested by malar rash, polyarticular arthritis, and previous pleural effusion. Her medications are hydroxychloroquine, ibuprofen, and prednisone.

On physical examination, temperature is 38.1 °C (100.6 °F), blood pressure is 108/68 mm Hg with pulsus paradoxus of 18 mm Hg, pulse rate is 160/min, and respiration rate is 18/min. Oxygen saturation is 97% breathing ambient air. Jugular venous distention to the angle of the mandible is present. Heart sounds are soft. No rubs, murmurs, or diastolic sounds are present. Pitting edema is noted bilaterally to above the ankle.

A chest radiograph and electrocardiogram are shown (see top of next page).

Which of the following is the most likely diagnosis?

(A) Cardiac tamponade

(B) Constrictive pericarditis

(C) Pulmonary embolism

(D) Pulmonary hypertension

Item 69

A 56-year-old man is evaluated for cardiovascular risk assessment. At a recent employee health screening, he was informed that he has elevated cholesterol levels. He feels well and exercises three to four times per week without any symptoms. He does not use tobacco. Medical history is unremarkable. Family history is notable for a myocardial infarction in his father at age 54 years. He takes no medications.

On physical examination, the patient is afebrile, blood pressure is 124/82 mm Hg, and pulse rate is 76/min. BMI is 28. Cardiovascular examination is normal.

Laboratory studies:

Total cholesterol	194 mg/dL (5.02 mmol/L)
HDL cholesterol	38 mg/dL (0.98 mmol/L)
LDL cholesterol	122 mg/dL (3.16 mmol/L)
Triglycerides	170 mg/dL (1.92 mmol/L)

His 10-year risk for atherosclerotic cardiovascular disease using the Pooled Cohort Equations is 7%.

Which of the following is the most reasonable next step in management?

(A) Adenosine cardiac magnetic resonance imaging

(B) Coronary artery calcium scoring

(C) Exercise stress echocardiography

(D) Lipoprotein(a) measurement

(E) Pharmacologic nuclear stress testing

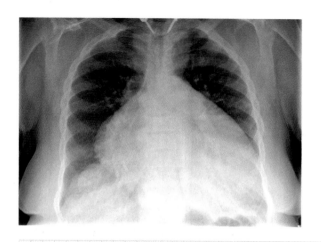

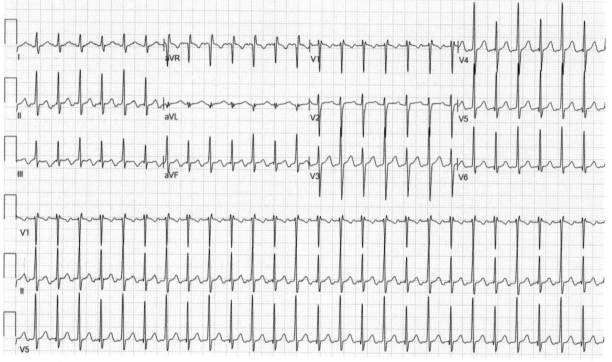

ITEM 68

Item 70

A 69-year-old man is evaluated after a recent hospitalization for heart failure. On hospital admission, he was appropriately treated, and an echocardiogram showed a left ventricular ejection fraction of 30% and left ventricular hypertrophy. He is currently asymptomatic. Medical history is otherwise significant for hypertension and hyperlipidemia. Medications are enalapril, furosemide, low-dose aspirin, and atorvastatin.

On physical examination, vital signs are normal. There is no jugular venous distention. Cardiac examination is normal. No edema is noted.

Which of the following is the most appropriate treatment?

(A) Add bisoprolol
(B) Add diltiazem
(C) Add spironolactone
(D) Discontinue enalapril and add losartan
(E) No additional therapy

Item 71

A 64-year-old man is evaluated following coronary angiography. He initially presented several weeks ago for progressive exertional chest pain and shortness of breath. Nuclear stress testing demonstrated a large anterior stress defect and an ejection fraction of 33%. Coronary angiography was significant for 90% stenosis of the proximal left anterior descending artery, a chronically occluded right coronary artery, and 80% stenosis of the left circumflex artery. He currently has stable dyspnea and chest pressure with moderate activity. Medical history is significant for hyperlipidemia, hypertension, and type 2 diabetes mellitus. He is taking optimal doses of aspirin, lisinopril, carvedilol, amlodipine, atorvastatin, and metformin.

On physical examination, temperature is normal, blood pressure is 125/70 mm Hg, pulse rate is 60/min, and respiration rate is 18/min. The remainder of the physical examination is unremarkable.

Which of the following is the most appropriate next step in management?

(A) Add ticagrelor
(B) Coronary artery bypass graft surgery
(C) Multivessel percutaneous coronary intervention
(D) Percutaneous coronary intervention of the left anterior descending artery
(E) Continue current medical therapy

Item 72

A 42-year-old woman is evaluated for a 3-year history of palpitations and fatigue. She reports no chest pain, dizziness, near-syncope, or syncope. An exercise stress test and echocardiogram were normal when she was evaluated for palpitations 1 year ago. There is no family history of sudden cardiac death or heart failure. Her only medication is metoprolol.

On physical examination, vital signs and the remainder of the examination are unremarkable.

An electrocardiogram is shown. Ambulatory 24-hour electrocardiographic monitoring shows frequent monomorphic premature ventricular contractions (22% of all beats) and frequent ventricular bigeminy. An echocardiogram obtained 1 week ago showed mild to moderate global decreased left ventricular function with a left ventricular ejection fraction of 45%.

Which of the following is the most appropriate management?

(A) Amiodarone
(B) Cardiac catheterization

(C) Cardiopulmonary exercise testing
(D) Catheter ablation of premature ventricular contractions

Item 73

An 86-year-old woman is hospitalized for acute decompensated heart failure. Her medical history is significant for a stroke 4 years ago, hypertension, severe COPD, and stage 3 chronic kidney disease. She underwent diuresis with furosemide overnight and is now resting comfortably. Her outpatient medications are lisinopril, atorvastatin, low-dose aspirin, tiotropium, and as-needed albuterol.

On physical examination, temperature is normal, blood pressure is 95/65 mm Hg, pulse rate is 80/min, and respiration rate is normal. Oxygen saturation is 90% on 2 L of oxygen by nasal cannula. Bilateral crackles are noted in the bottom quarter of the lung fields. The estimated central venous pressure is elevated. S_1 is diminished. A grade 3/6 holosystolic murmur and soft diastolic rumble are present at the apex.

An echocardiogram shows a flail segment involving the posterior leaflet of the mitral valve and severe regurgitation. The left ventricular ejection fraction is 60%.

Cardiac and pulmonary surgical risks are estimated to be high (estimated operative mortality, 10%).

Which of the following is the most appropriate next step in management?

(A) Mitral valve replacement
(B) Surgical mitral valve repair
(C) Transcatheter mitral valve repair
(D) Continue current medical therapy

Item 74

A 62-year-old woman is evaluated for a 2-month history of exertional right leg pain. She has no associated chest pain,

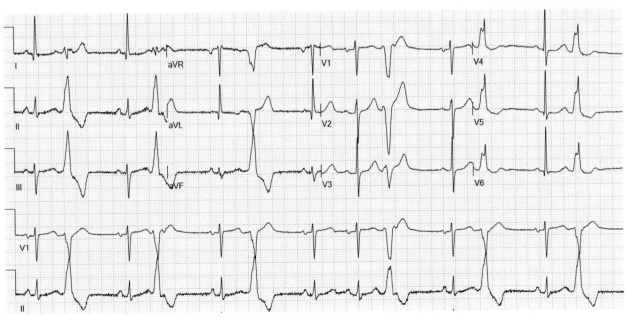

ITEM 72

shortness of breath, or other symptoms. Medical history is significant for hypertension. Medications are lisinopril and chlorthalidone.

On physical examination, vital signs are normal. The right dorsalis pedis and posterior tibialis pulses are faint, and the left dorsalis pedis and posterior tibialis pulses are slightly diminished.

Laboratory studies:

Total cholesterol	180 mg/dL (4.66 mmol/L)
HDL cholesterol	54 mg/dL (1.40 mmol/L)
LDL cholesterol	101 mg/dL (2.62 mmol/L)
Triglycerides	125 mg/dL (1.41 mmol/L)

The right ankle-brachial index is 0.75, and the left is 0.92.

The patient's 10-year risk for atherosclerotic cardiovascular disease is 5.4% based on the American College of Cardiology/American Heart Association Pooled Cohort Equations.

In addition to aspirin and dietary and exercise counseling, which of the following is the most appropriate treatment?

(A) Evolocumab

(B) Ezetimibe

(C) High-intensity atorvastatin

(D) Moderate-intensity pravastatin

(E) No additional therapy

Item 75

A 72-year-old man is evaluated for a 4-month history of progressive exertional dyspnea. He has a 3-year history of ischemic cardiomyopathy, and in the past 6 months, he has had two hospitalizations for heart failure exacerbations. He currently has shortness of breath at rest. Medical history is otherwise significant for renal cell carcinoma treated with surgical resection 4 years ago. Medications are enalapril, bisoprolol, furosemide, atorvastatin, and aspirin.

On physical examination, temperature is normal, blood pressure is 104/80 mm Hg, pulse rate is 98/min, and respiration rate is 18/min. His neck veins are flat. Cardiac examination reveals an S_3. There is no peripheral edema. Extremities are cool.

Laboratory studies show a blood urea nitrogen level of 40 mg/dL (14.3 mmol/L) and a serum sodium level of 134 mEq/L (134 mmol/L). The serum creatinine level is 1.7 mg/dL (150.3 µmol/L), which is increased from 1.4 mg/dL (123.8 µmol/L) 3 months ago.

An electrocardiogram shows a QRS duration of 90 ms. An echocardiogram shows a left ventricular ejection fraction of 15%, left ventricular diastolic diameter of 8.2 cm (normal 3.9-5.3 cm), and moderate mitral regurgitation.

Which of the following is the most appropriate management?

(A) Cardiac resynchronization therapy

(B) Cardiac transplantation

(C) Left ventricular assist device placement

(D) Mitral valve repair

Item 76

A 31-year-old woman undergoes preconception cardiac evaluation. Medical history is significant for tetralogy of Fallot

with a palliative right subclavian artery–to–pulmonary artery (Blalock–Taussig) shunt in infancy and subsequent closure of the shunt and enlargement of the right ventricular outflow tract at 3 years of age. She is asymptomatic.

On physical examination, vital signs are normal. The estimated jugular venous pressure is elevated with a visible *a* wave. The apical impulse is normal; a parasternal impulse is noted at the left sternal border. S_1 is normal, and S_2 is single, with a soft early systolic murmur at the second left intercostal space. A grade 2/6 diastolic decrescendo murmur is noted at the left sternal border that increases with inspiration. The remainder of the examination is normal.

A chest radiograph is shown.

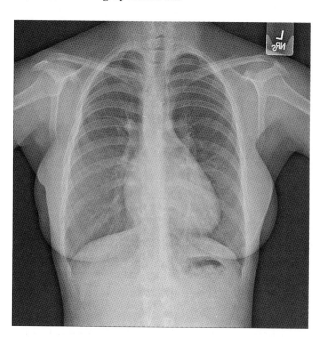

Which of the following is the most likely diagnosis?

(A) Aortic regurgitation

(B) Mitral stenosis

(C) Pulmonary valve regurgitation

(D) Recurrent ventricular septal defect

Item 77

A 68-year-old man is evaluated during a routine examination. He is asymptomatic. Medical history is significant for hypertension and hyperlipidemia. He has a 50-pack-year smoking history but quit smoking at age 45 years. Medications are low-dose aspirin, atorvastatin, and amlodipine.

On physical examination, vital signs are normal.

An abdominal aortic duplex ultrasound shows an abdominal aortic aneurysm with a maximum diameter of 3.5 cm.

Which of the following is the most appropriate management?

(A) Aortic aneurysm repair

(B) CT angiography

(C) Repeat aortic ultrasonography in 24 to 36 months

(D) No further testing

Item 78

A 46-year-old man is evaluated in the hospital for a 6-week history of fatigue and worsening dyspnea. Medical history is significant for a bicuspid aortic valve. He takes no medications.

On physical examination, temperature is 38.1 °C (100.6 °F), blood pressure is 118/58 mm Hg, pulse rate is 92/min, and respiration rate is 18/min. Oxygen saturation is 98% breathing 2 L of oxygen by nasal cannula. Cardiac examination reveals a grade 2/6 diastolic murmur heard best at the left lower sternal border. There are crackles at the lung bases bilaterally. Conjunctival hemorrhage is present in the left eye.

Laboratory studies are notable for a leukocyte count of 15,000/μL (15×10^9/L). Three sets of blood cultures are positive for gram-positive cocci.

An electrocardiogram shows sinus rhythm, a PR interval of 220 ms, and QRS duration of 100 ms.

Which of the following is the most appropriate diagnostic test to perform next?

(A) Cardiac magnetic resonance imaging
(B) Coronary CT angiography
(C) Transesophageal echocardiography
(D) Transthoracic echocardiography

Item 79

A 69-year-old man is evaluated during a follow-up visit. He initially presented with a 3-month history of chest pressure and dyspnea that occurred primarily with exertion. Despite maximal medical therapy, his symptoms have not abated and adversely affect his quality of life. Medical history is significant for type 2 diabetes mellitus, hypertension, and hyperlipidemia. Medications are low-dose aspirin; metformin; long-acting nitroglycerin; and optimal doses of metoprolol, lisinopril, ranolazine, and simvastatin.

On physical examination, blood pressure is 128/73 mm Hg, and pulse rate is 60/min. Cardiac examination reveals a normal S_1 and S_2 without an S_3 or S_4. There is no lower extremity edema.

Coronary angiogram is significant for a normal left main coronary artery and a 90% stenosis in the proximal left anterior descending artery resulting from ulcerated plaque.

Which of the following is the most appropriate management?

(A) β-Carotene
(B) Cardiac rehabilitation

(C) Percutaneous coronary intervention
(D) Ticagrelor

Item 80

A 26-year-old woman seeks preconception counseling. She has a history of mitral stenosis and underwent mitral valve replacement with a tilting-disc mechanical prosthesis 5 years ago. She is asymptomatic. Medications are warfarin, 4 mg/d, and low-dose aspirin.

On physical examination, a normal mechanical S_1 and normal S_2 are appreciated. The remainder of the examination is unremarkable.

Laboratory studies reveal an INR of 3.0 (therapeutic target, 3.0).

An electrocardiogram demonstrates normal sinus rhythm.

In addition to continuing low-dose aspirin, which of the following is the most appropriate anticoagulation regimen for this patient during the first trimester?

(A) Continue INR-adjusted warfarin
(B) Stop warfarin and start apixaban
(C) Stop warfarin and start unfractionated heparin, 5000 units subcutaneously twice daily
(D) Stop warfarin and start weight-based low-molecular-weight heparin

Item 81

A 51-year-old woman is evaluated in the ICU after being admitted 2 days ago for severe community-acquired pneumonia. A chest radiograph demonstrated right lower lobe consolidation, and she was started on moxifloxacin. Today, she developed an arrhythmia that terminated after 20 seconds. An electrocardiogram (ECG) obtained at the time of admission was normal. Medical history is significant for hypertension, hyperlipidemia, and depression. Other medications are venlafaxine, carvedilol, and simvastatin.

On physical examination, temperature is 38.4 °C (101.1 °F), blood pressure is 140/90 mm Hg, pulse rate is 61/min, and respiration rate is 18/min. Diminished breath sounds are located in the right lower posterior thorax. The remainder of the examination is unremarkable.

An ECG at the time of the arrhythmic event is shown. An ECG after the episode reveals a corrected QT interval of 550 ms.

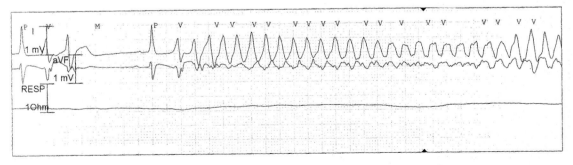

ITEM 81

CONT.

Which of the following medications should be discontinued on the basis of this patient's ECG findings?

(A) Carvedilol
(B) Moxifloxacin
(C) Simvastatin
(D) Venlafaxine

Item 82

A 40-year-old man is evaluated during a routine examination. He has a history of cardiac murmur. He is asymptomatic and active, cycling 12 miles three or four times per week.

On physical examination, vital signs are normal. There is no jugular venous distention. Cardiovascular examination reveals a point of maximal impulse that is displaced laterally and is diffuse. A grade 3/6 early diastolic decrescendo murmur is heard at the left parasternal third intercostal space. Lungs are clear. There are brisk, prominent distal extremity pulses.

A transthoracic echocardiogram demonstrates a bicuspid aortic valve and severe aortic regurgitation. Left ventricular end-systolic dimension is enlarged at 58 mm. Left ventricular ejection fraction is 50%. The proximal ascending aortic diameter is 50 mm (normal, <35 mm).

Which of the following is the most appropriate management?

(A) Aortic valve and root replacement
(B) Clinical and echocardiographic surveillance
(C) Initiation of nifedipine therapy
(D) Treadmill stress echocardiography

Item 83

A 52-year-old man is evaluated before discharge. Medical history is significant for atrial fibrillation and a 7-year history of heart failure with reduced ejection fraction. He was initially hospitalized for a 2-week history of increasing exertional dyspnea, peripheral edema, and a weight gain of 4.1 kg (9 lb). He had not been taking his medications for the past month. He underwent diuresis with a loss of 6.8 kg (15 lb), and he currently feels well. Medications are furosemide, digoxin, warfarin, and low doses of carvedilol and lisinopril.

On physical examination, vital signs are normal. Other than an irregularly irregular rhythm, cardiopulmonary examination is normal. There is no peripheral edema.

Which of the following is the most appropriate management?

(A) Add ivabradine
(B) Add spironolactone
(C) Perform cardioversion
(D) Schedule follow-up within 1 week

Item 84

A 50-year-old man was diagnosed with hypertrophic cardiomyopathy following an episode of syncope. An implantable cardioverter-defibrillator was placed, and metoprolol was initiated. Genetic testing revealed a mutation of the β-myosin heavy-chain gene associated with hypertrophic cardiomyopathy. Medical history is otherwise unremarkable. The patient has a 16-year-old daughter who is asymptomatic.

Which of the following is the most appropriate management of this patient's daughter?

(A) Electrocardiography and echocardiography screening at age 21 years
(B) Electrocardiography and echocardiography screening at age 40 years
(C) Electrocardiography and echocardiography screening if symptoms develop
(D) Genetic counseling and testing

Item 85

A 29-year-old woman is evaluated during a routine office visit. She was recently diagnosed with rheumatoid arthritis, for which she is taking naproxen and methotrexate. She is otherwise well. She does not smoke, drinks one alcoholic beverage daily, and engages in strenuous physical activity 5 days per week for 30 minutes each session. Her mother and father are first-generation Japanese immigrants, both in excellent health.

On physical examination, vital signs are normal. Cardiovascular examination is normal. There is evidence of synovitis involving the second, third, and fourth metacarpophalangeal joints bilaterally.

Her most recent lipid profile showed a total cholesterol level of 128 mg/dL (3.32 mmol/L) and a calculated LDL cholesterol level of 72 mg/dL (1.86 mmol/L).

Which of the following is the most significant risk factor for future cardiovascular disease?

(A) Activity level
(B) Alcohol consumption
(C) Ethnicity
(D) Rheumatoid arthritis

Item 86

A 26-year-old woman is evaluated for palpitations and fatigue of several months' duration. Her symptoms are present at rest and aggravated during light activity, including climbing stairs and walking quickly. She reports no dyspnea, chest pain, orthopnea, lower extremity edema, or syncope. Medical history is otherwise unremarkable, and she takes no medications.

On physical examination, temperature is normal, blood pressure is 110/65 mm Hg, and pulse rate is 115/min. Orthostatic vital signs do not demonstrate any significant changes with posture. Precordial examination reveals mild tachycardia but regular rhythm with no gallops. No thyroid fullness or tremors are noted. The remainder of the examination is normal.

Laboratory studies are significant for a normal complete blood count, serum thyroid-stimulating hormone level, and 24-hour excretion of urine catecholamines.

A 12-lead electrocardiogram is notable for sinus tachycardia with a normal P-wave axis. A 24-hour ambulatory electrocardiographic monitor shows sinus tachycardia throughout the waking hours, with a decline in heart rate to less than 90/min during the night. The average heart rate is 110/min. An echocardiogram reveals a structurally normal heart with normal ventricular function.

Which of the following is the most likely diagnosis?

(A) Generalized anxiety disorder
(B) Inappropriate sinus tachycardia
(C) Somatic symptom disorder
(D) Subclinical hyperthyroidism

Item 87

A 68-year-old man is evaluated for a 2-month history of exertional dyspnea. Medical history is significant for diabetes mellitus, hypertension, and hyperlipidemia. Medications are lisinopril, hydrochlorothiazide, metformin, and atorvastatin.

On physical examination, vital signs are normal. Oxygen saturation is 99% breathing ambient air. Cardiopulmonary examination shows a regular rhythm and a paradoxically split S_2. There is no peripheral edema.

An electrocardiogram is shown.

Which of the following is the most appropriate diagnostic test to perform next?

(A) Adenosine single-photon emission CT
(B) Coronary artery calcium scoring
(C) Exercise single-photon emission CT
(D) Exercise electrocardiography

Item 88

A 27-year-old woman is hospitalized with a 2-month history of progressive exertional dyspnea and edema. She has no history of recent flu-like symptoms, weight change, arthritis, or chest pain.

On physical examination, the patient is afebrile, blood pressure is 118/66 mm Hg, pulse rate is 112/min, and respiration rate is 18/min. Oxygen saturation is 98% breathing ambient air. There is jugular venous distention to the angle of the jaw. Crackles are present at the lung bases. Cardiac examination reveals an S_3. Peripheral edema is noted.

Complete blood count, serum electrolytes, kidney function tests, liver chemistry tests, glucose level, and lipid levels are normal.

An electrocardiogram shows sinus tachycardia with normal intervals and no conduction delay. An echocardiogram demonstrates a left ventricular ejection fraction of 25% and normal left ventricular diastolic diameter.

Which of the following is the most appropriate diagnostic test to perform next?

(A) Acute and convalescent viral titers
(B) Cardiac catheterization
(C) Serum iron and ferritin studies
(D) Thyroid function studies

Item 89

A 66-year-old man is evaluated in the emergency department for chest pain and dyspnea. Three days ago, he experienced the sudden onset of substernal chest pain. His symptoms waxed and waned over a period of 3 hours and then spontaneously subsided. Today, he began experiencing progressive shortness of breath with symptoms occurring at

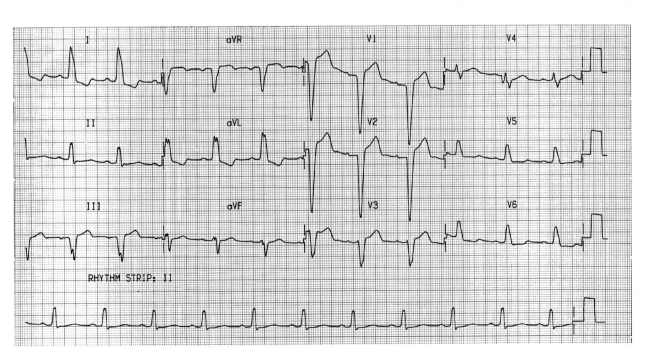

ITEM 87

CONT.

rest. His medical history is significant for hypertension and hyperlipidemia. His medications are hydrochlorothiazide, atenolol, and atorvastatin.

On physical examination, he appears distressed. Temperature is normal, blood pressure is 95/50 mm Hg, pulse rate is 115/min, and respiration rate is 24/min. Oxygen saturation is 90% breathing 4 L of oxygen by nasal cannula. Jugular venous pulse is elevated and visible, with exaggerated x and y descents, and the estimated central venous pressure is 12 cm H_2O. Bilateral crackles are noted. A soft, early systolic murmur with an S_3 is audible in the apical area. An early diastolic rumble is present.

An electrocardiogram demonstrates significant Q waves in the inferolateral leads and elevated ST segments. A chest radiograph confirms the presence of heart failure with cardiomegaly and bilateral pulmonary edema.

Which of the following is the most likely diagnosis?

(A) Aortic stenosis
(B) Cardiac tamponade
(C) Mitral regurgitation
(D) Tricuspid regurgitation

Item 90

A 76-year-old woman is evaluated before discharge. She was diagnosed with a non–ST-elevation myocardial infarction 3 days ago. She declined angiography, and nuclear stress testing revealed a small lateral perfusion defect and normal left ventricular ejection fraction. She has had no further discomfort since admission. Medical history is significant for hyperlipidemia, hypertension, and transient ischemic attack. Medications are low-dose aspirin, ramipril, metoprolol, and atorvastatin.

On physical examination, vital signs and the remainder of the examination are unremarkable.

In addition to low-dose aspirin, which of the following is the optimal antithrombotic regimen for this patient?

(A) Prasugrel
(B) Ticagrelor
(C) Warfarin
(D) No additional antithrombotic therapy

Item 91

A 72-year-old man is evaluated for a 1-year history of bilateral lower extremity edema and abdominal distention. Eight years ago he had esophageal carcinoma treated with radiotherapy. Medical history is otherwise significant for hypertension, type 2 diabetes mellitus, and hypercholesterolemia. Medications are bumetanide, atorvastatin, metformin, and lisinopril.

On physical examination, the patient is afebrile, blood pressure is 170/90 mm Hg, pulse rate is 90/min, and respiration rate is normal. Jugular venous distention is present to the angle of the mandible while seated, with prominent pulsations. Cardiac examination reveals an early diastolic sound at the apex. The liver is palpable

5 cm below the costal margin. The abdomen is distended with ascites. There is bilateral pitting edema to the level of the thighs. Pulmonary examination reveals no crackles.

Laboratory studies are significant for a B-type natriuretic peptide level of 96 pg/mL (96 ng/L).

Chest radiographs are shown. A 12-lead electrocardiogram demonstrates normal sinus rhythm with normal QRS voltage. Echocardiogram demonstrates normal right and left ventricular size and function. Left ventricular wall thickness is normal. Mild tricuspid regurgitation is present. There are respiratory variation in the filling of the right and left ventricles, ventricular septal shift during respiration, and dilation of the inferior vena cava. The estimated right ventricular systolic pressure is 46 mm Hg. There is no pericardial effusion.

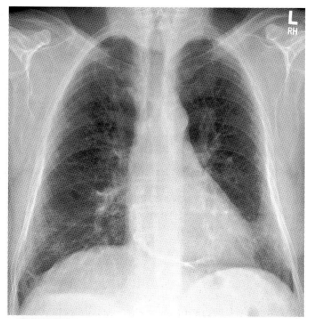

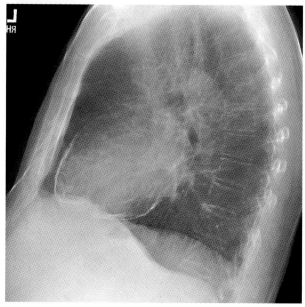

Which of the following is the most likely diagnosis?

(A) Cardiac amyloidosis

(B) Constrictive pericarditis

(C) Heart failure with preserved ejection fraction

(D) Restrictive cardiomyopathy

Item 92

A 35-year-old woman is evaluated for exertional dyspnea of 6 months' duration. She reports no other symptoms. Medical history is unremarkable, and she takes no medications.

On physical examination, vital signs are normal. Oxygen saturation is 96% breathing ambient air. The estimated central venous pressure is elevated. Apical impulse is normal; a parasternal impulse is noted at the left sternal border. A soft systolic murmur is heard at the second left intercostal space, and a diastolic flow rumble is heard at the left sternal border. Fixed splitting of the S_2 is noted throughout the cardiac cycle. The remainder of the physical examination is normal.

An electrocardiogram demonstrates right axis deviation and incomplete right bundle branch block.

Which of the following is the most likely diagnosis?

(A) Atrial septal defect

(B) Bicuspid aortic valve with aortic stenosis

(C) Congenital pulmonary stenosis

(D) Mitral stenosis

Item 93

A 55-year-old woman is evaluated after a recent hospital admission for ischemic stroke. She presented with mild right-sided hemiparesis, but it completely resolved after the second hospital day. An electrocardiogram, transthoracic echocardiogram, and carotid artery ultrasound were normal. A subsequent transesophageal echocardiogram was also normal. She has a 10-year history of hypertension treated with hydrochlorothiazide.

On physical examination, vital signs are normal. Cardiac examination reveals a regular rate and rhythm. Neurologic examination is nonfocal. Hand grip strength, arm flexion, and arm extension are 5/5 on the right and left sides. There is no edema.

A 12-lead electrocardiogram demonstrates normal sinus rhythm.

Which of the following is the most appropriate diagnostic testing option?

(A) Antiphospholipid antibody testing

(B) Cardiac catheterization

(C) 30-Day event-triggered loop recording

(D) 48-Hour ambulatory electrocardiographic monitoring

Item 94

A 72-year-old woman is evaluated in the hospital for a 2-week history of increasing exertional dyspnea and weight gain of 3.3 kg (7.3 lb). Medical history is significant for idiopathic cardiomyopathy with a left ventricular ejection fraction of 25% and hypertension. Medications are lisinopril,

metoprolol succinate, furosemide, spironolactone, and digoxin.

On physical examination, the patient is afebrile, blood pressure is 158/68 mm Hg, pulse rate is 96/min, and respiration rate is 18/min. Oxygen saturation is 98% breathing ambient air. Jugular venous distention is present. Cardiac examination reveals an S_3 and a grade 2/6 apical holosystolic murmur. The lungs have occasional bibasilar crackles. The extremities are warm. Peripheral edema is noted.

Laboratory studies are significant for a serum creatinine level of 1.9 mg/dL (168 μmol/L), a serum potassium level of 4.5 mEq/L (4.5 mmol/L), and a serum sodium level of 139 mEq/L (139 mmol/L).

Which of the following is the most appropriate intravenous treatment?

(A) Dopamine

(B) Furosemide

(C) Milrinone

(D) Nesiritide

Item 95

A 26-year-old man is hospitalized for suspected bacterial endocarditis. He has a long history of injection drug use and has used heroin within the past month. Two weeks ago, he began feeling feverish, and over the past 3 days, he has been increasingly short of breath. He takes no medications.

On physical examination, temperature is 38.7 °C (101.6 °F), blood pressure is 90/50 mm Hg, pulse rate is 95/min, and respiration rate is 16/min. Bilateral lung crackles are present. Jugular venous distention is noted. A grade 2/6 holosystolic murmur is heard at the apex with an S_3. Skin findings are shown.

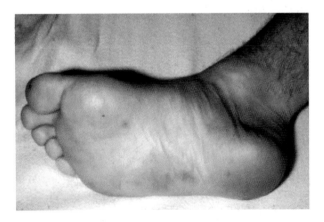

The electrocardiogram is normal. A chest radiograph shows bilateral pulmonary edema and cardiomegaly.

Blood cultures are obtained.

Which of the following is the most appropriate next step in management?

(A) Cardiac CT

(B) Chest MRI

(C) Transesophageal echocardiography

(D) Transthoracic echocardiography

Item 96

A 55-year-old woman is evaluated in the hospital for a single 10-minute episode of chest pain at rest, which occurred 1 hour before presentation. Medical history is significant for hypertension and hyperlipidemia. Medications are hydrochlorothiazide, ramipril, and pravastatin.

On physical examination, vital signs are normal. The remainder of the examination is unremarkable.

Laboratory studies are notable for normal serum troponin levels.

An electrocardiogram demonstrates 1-mm ST-segment depressions in leads V_4 through V_6.

Aspirin and metoprolol are initiated.

Which of the following is the most appropriate management?

(A) Amlodipine

(B) Enoxaparin and eptifibatide

(C) Exercise stress testing

(D) Urgent angiography

Item 97

A 68-year-old man is evaluated for a 4-month history of intermittent left calf pain. He has a history of cigarette smoking but quit 6 months ago. Medical history is otherwise significant for hyperlipidemia. Medications are low-dose aspirin and high-intensity atorvastatin.

On physical examination, vital signs are normal. BMI is 29. Femoral pulses are diminished bilaterally. Popliteal, right dorsalis pedis, and right posterior tibialis pulses are faint. The left dorsalis pedis and posterior tibialis pulses are not palpable. Cardiac examination is normal.

The ankle-brachial index is 0.67 on the left and 0.91 on the right.

He is enrolled in a supervised exercise program. Three months later, the patient calls to report that despite adherence to the exercise program, his symptoms have progressed.

Which of the following is the most appropriate next step to reduce this patient's leg pain?

(A) Add clopidogrel

(B) Discontinue atorvastatin and initiate rosuvastatin

(C) Initiate cilostazol

(D) Refer for invasive angiography

Item 98

A 39-year-old man is evaluated in the emergency department for palpitations and shortness of breath that developed abruptly 45 minutes ago. He has no significant medical history and takes no medications.

On physical examination, blood pressure is 110/48 mm Hg, and pulse rate is 216/min; other vital signs are normal. Cardiac examination reveals a rapid and regular heart rate. The S_1 does not exhibit variable intensity. The rhythm does not change with a Valsalva maneuver.

A 12-lead electrocardiogram obtained in the emergency department is shown.

Which of the following is the most appropriate next step in treatment?

(A) Adenosine

(B) Amiodarone

(C) Ibutilide

(D) Synchronized cardioversion

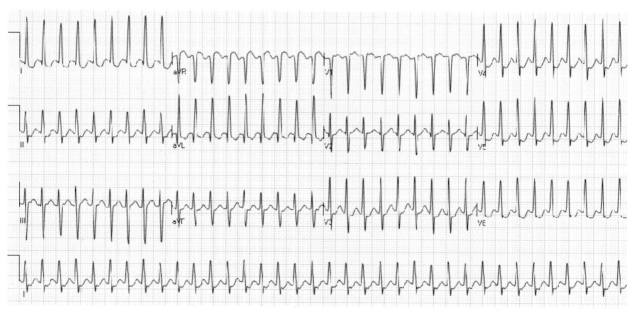

ITEM 98

Item 99

A 62-year-old man is evaluated for a 1-year history of progressive fatigue, dyspnea on exertion, and lower extremity edema. He has been hospitalized twice in the past year for heart failure. Medical history is otherwise unremarkable. His current medications are furosemide, amlodipine, and spironolactone. He is black.

On physical examination, temperature is normal, blood pressure is 106/68 mm Hg, pulse rate is 68/min, and respiration rate is 14/min. Oxygen saturation breathing ambient air is normal. Jugular venous distention is noted. No crackles are present. A grade 2/6 holosystolic murmur is heard at the left lower sternal border and increases with inspiration. There is no S_3 or S_4. The liver is enlarged. Pitting edema is present to the mid shin bilaterally.

An electrocardiogram reveals sinus rhythm, biatrial enlargement, and low voltage of the QRS complexes. Q waves are present in leads V_1 through V_3. Echocardiogram reveals severe concentric left ventricular hypertrophy with wall thickness of 16 mm, moderate biatrial dilatation, normal left ventricular cavity size, a left ventricular ejection fraction of 55%, and no regional wall motion abnormalities. Diastolic dysfunction is noted. Right ventricular size and systolic function are normal, and the right ventricular wall thickness is slightly increased. The estimated right ventricular systolic pressure is 68 mm Hg. Tricuspid regurgitation is present. There is no pericardial effusion.

Which of the following is the most likely diagnosis?

(A) Cardiac amyloidosis
(B) Constrictive pericarditis
(C) Hypertensive heart disease
(D) Hypertrophic cardiomyopathy

Item 100

A 45-year-old man undergoes a pre-employment physical examination. Medical history is notable for aortic coarctation with an end-to-end anastomosis performed at 4 years of age. He reports no symptoms, works full time, and performs regular exercise without limitation. He takes no medications.

On physical examination, vital signs are normal. An ejection click is noted at the left lower sternal border. A grade 2/6 mid-peaking systolic murmur is noted at the second right intercostal space. The femoral pulses are normal, and no radial artery–to–femoral artery pulse delay is present. The remainder of the physical examination is normal.

Which of the following is the most likely cause of this patient's systolic murmur?

(A) Aortic stenosis
(B) Hypertrophic cardiomyopathy
(C) Mitral regurgitation
(D) Recurrent coarctation

Item 101

A 45-year-old man is evaluated during a second follow-up visit after hospitalization for new-onset heart failure with reduced ejection fraction. His ejection fraction at the time of diagnosis 2 months ago was 42%. He reports feeling better, with improving exercise tolerance and no exertional dyspnea. Medications are lisinopril, low-dose carvedilol, and furosemide. He is black.

On physical examination, the patient is afebrile, blood pressure is 120/76 mm Hg, pulse rate is 84/min, and respiration rate is 16/min. The estimated central venous pressure is normal. There is no S_3. Lungs are clear, and there is no peripheral edema.

Which of the following is the most appropriate treatment?

(A) Add digoxin
(B) Add hydralazine and isosorbide dinitrate
(C) Increase carvedilol
(D) Increase furosemide

Item 102

A 65-year-old man was hospitalized 24 hours ago with findings of a large anterior myocardial infarction. He underwent primary percutaneous coronary intervention with stent placement in the proximal left anterior descending artery. He is currently asymptomatic. Medical history is significant for hyperlipidemia and hypertension. Medications are atorvastatin, aspirin, prasugrel, captopril, and metoprolol.

On physical examination, temperature is normal, blood pressure is 110/65 mm Hg, pulse rate is 65/min, and respiration rate is 18/min. Oxygen saturation is 98% breathing ambient air. The remainder of the examination is unremarkable.

An electrocardiogram obtained in the coronary care unit is shown (see top of next page).

Which of the following is the most appropriate treatment?

(A) Atropine
(B) Discontinue metoprolol and observe
(C) Emergent coronary angiography
(D) Emergent pacing

Item 103

A 45-year-old man is evaluated for hypertension. He is otherwise healthy and has not had any symptoms. His father died of an acute myocardial infarction at age 49 years. He takes no medications.

On physical examination, temperature is normal, blood pressure is 172/80 mm Hg, pulse rate is 80/min, and respiration rate is normal. The lungs are clear. Jugular venous pulse is normal. S_1 and S_2 are normal. There is a soft ejection click that precedes a grade 2/6 diastolic decrescendo murmur, which is best heard at the right lower sternal border.

A transthoracic echocardiogram shows a bicuspid aortic valve with mild aortic regurgitation. The left ventricular ejection fraction is 50%. The ascending aorta is enlarged, with a dimension of 42 mm in the mid-portion.

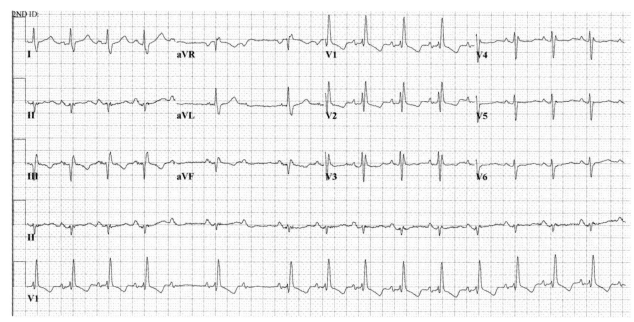

ITEM 102

Which of the following is the most appropriate next step in management?

(A) Annual transthoracic echocardiography
(B) CT angiography of the aorta
(C) Infective endocarditis prophylaxis
(D) Surgical aortic valve replacement

Item 104

A 62-year-old woman is evaluated during a routine examination. She feels well and has no exercise limitations. Medical history is significant for hypertension treated with enalapril. She does not smoke. At her last examination 4 years ago, her blood pressure was 122/76 mm Hg. Laboratory studies at that time revealed a serum total cholesterol level of 184 mg/dL (4.77 mmol/L), serum HDL cholesterol level of 42 mg/dL (1.09 mmol/L), and hemoglobin A_{1c} value of 5.4%. At that time, according to the Pooled Cohort Equations, her 10-year risk for atherosclerotic cardiovascular disease was calculated to be 3.8%. She has gained 5 kg (11 lb) since then.

On physical examination today, blood pressure is 140/90 mm Hg. BMI is 29. The remainder of the physical examination is unremarkable.

Laboratory studies are significant for a serum total cholesterol level of 250 mg/dL (6.47 mmol/L), a serum HDL cholesterol level of 30 mg/dL (0.78 mmol/L), and a hemoglobin A_{1c} value of 6.6%. A subsequent fasting plasma glucose level is 130 mg/dL (7.2 mmol/L).

Which of the following confers the highest risk for atherosclerotic cardiovascular disease in this patient?

(A) Diabetes mellitus
(B) Diastolic blood pressure of 90 mm Hg
(C) HDL cholesterol level of 30 mg/dL (0.78 mmol/L)
(D) Systolic blood pressure of 140 mm Hg
(E) Total cholesterol level of 250 mg/dL (6.47 mmol/L)

Item 105

A 71-year-old man is evaluated for a 10-day history of malaise and fatigue. Two years ago, he underwent dual-chamber pacemaker implantation for third-degree atrioventricular block. He reports discomfort at the site of his pacemaker. He has had no fever, chills, or weight loss. Medical history is otherwise significant for well-controlled hypertension and hyperlipidemia treated with chlorthalidone and atorvastatin.

On physical examination, vital signs are normal. The skin overlying the patient's pacemaker pocket is slightly erythematous and is warm and tender to palpation. The remainder of the physical examination is noncontributory.

A complete blood count and erythrocyte sedimentation rate are ordered.

Which of the following is the most appropriate management?

(A) Blood cultures
(B) Empiric therapy with cephalexin
(C) Pacemaker pocket aspiration
(D) PET/CT scanning

Item 106

A 69-year-old man is evaluated in the emergency department for a 1-week history of progressive exertional dyspnea followed by the development of rest dyspnea. He reports an unchanged nonproductive cough without chest pain. Symptoms were not preceded by a respiratory tract infection. He has been sleeping in a reclining chair at night. Medical history is significant for COPD and ischemic cardiomyopathy with a left ventricular ejection fraction of

20%. He has a 30-year history of cigarette smoking but quit 7 years ago. Current medications are a tiotropium inhaler, lisinopril, carvedilol, furosemide, and low-dose aspirin.

On physical examination, the patient is afebrile, blood pressure is 152/88 mm Hg, pulse rate is 98/min, and respiration rate is 22/min. Oxygen saturation is 95% breathing ambient air. The neck veins cannot be assessed because of large neck size. The heart sounds are distant. Pulmonary examination reveals distant breath sounds and a prolonged expiratory phase but no wheezes. Peripheral edema is noted.

A chest radiograph shows an enlarged cardiac silhouette and no infiltrates. An echocardiogram reveals a left ventricular ejection fraction of 20% and a right ventricular systolic pressure of 40 mm Hg.

Which of the following is the most likely cause of this patient's symptoms?

(A) COPD exacerbation
(B) Heart failure exacerbation
(C) Pneumonia
(D) Pulmonary embolism

Item 107

A 64-year-old man is evaluated in the emergency department for a 1-week history of exertional chest pain and onset of rest pain 3 hours ago. During the evaluation, he develops ventricular fibrillation. The patient undergoes rapid defibrillation. He is currently awake with ongoing chest pain. Medical history is significant for hyperlipidemia, hypertension, type 2 diabetes mellitus, tobacco use, and previous stroke. Medications are aspirin, lisinopril, metoprolol, metformin, and simvastatin.

On physical examination, the patient is alert and oriented. Temperature is normal, blood pressure is 100/60 mm Hg, pulse rate is 110/min, and respiration rate is 24/min. Oxygen saturation is 98% breathing 4 L of oxygen by nasal cannula. Pulmonary examination reveals bibasilar crackles.

An electrocardiogram demonstrates left bundle branch block, a new finding since electrocardiography 8 months ago.

Which of the following is the most appropriate next step in management?

(A) Intravenous amiodarone
(B) Primary percutaneous coronary intervention
(C) Therapeutic hypothermia
(D) Urgent coronary artery bypass graft surgery

Item 108

A 68-year-old man is evaluated for a 4-month history of right arm fatigue and dizziness. Last week, he became dizzy while standing on a 10-foot ladder and cleaning his gutters with his right hand. His symptoms improved after 3 minutes of rest. He reports that right arm activity reproduces his arm fatigue and discomfort, mainly in the forearm. Medical history is significant for hypertension and hyperlipidemia. He has a 60-pack-year smoking history. Medications are lisinopril, amlodipine, and atorvastatin.

On physical examination, temperature is normal, blood pressure is 110/65 mm Hg in the right arm and 145/85 mm Hg

in the left arm, and pulse rate is 72/min. A bruit is heard over the right supraclavicular fossa. Left carotid upstroke is normal. The right radial pulse and right carotid pulse are faint, and the left radial pulse is slightly diminished. Cardiac examination is normal.

Which of the following is the most appropriate diagnostic test to perform next?

(A) Adson maneuver (thoracic outlet maneuver)
(B) Ankle-brachial index
(C) Carotid duplex ultrasonography
(D) CT angiography of the chest and neck

Item 109

A 42-year-old man is evaluated in the emergency department for a 3-hour history of severe chest pain that radiates to the back. The pain is sharp and tearing in character. Medical history is significant for hypertension. Medications are amlodipine and lisinopril.

On physical examination, blood pressure is 128/78 mm Hg in the right arm and 162/99 mm Hg in the left arm, and pulse rate is 110/min. Lungs are clear to auscultation. Other than tachycardia, examination of the heart is normal. Right radial and brachial pulses are diminished.

A chest CT scan is shown.

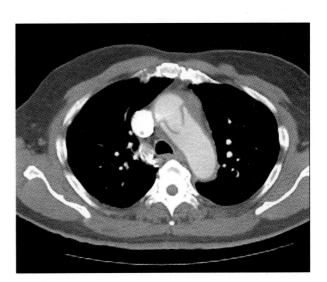

Which of the following is the most appropriate management?

(A) Coronary angiography
(B) Medical therapy alone
(C) Open surgical aortic repair
(D) Thoracic endovascular aortic repair

Item 110

A 48-year-old woman is evaluated during a new-patient visit. She reports no symptoms. She runs 5 miles a day 5 days per week. Medical history is otherwise unremarkable. She takes no medications.

On physical examination, vital signs are normal. The estimated central venous pressure is 6 cm H_2O. Cardiac examination reveals a grade 2/6 holosystolic murmur that is best heard at the apex and radiates toward the axilla. An ejection click is not audible. The lungs are clear to auscultation. No edema is present.

Which of the following is the most appropriate management?

(A) Cardiac magnetic resonance imaging
(B) Transesophageal echocardiography
(C) Transthoracic echocardiography
(D) Routine clinical follow-up without imaging

Item 111

A 62-year-old man is evaluated for a 6-month history of bilateral lower extremity edema. He was started on furosemide 2 months ago, with minimal change in the edema. He has no history of lung disease or recent surgery. His medical history is notable for permanent pacemaker implantation 2 years ago for symptomatic sinus node dysfunction. He takes no medications other than furosemide.

On physical examination, vital signs are normal. The lungs are clear. The estimated central venous pressure is elevated at 10 cm H_2O with a prominent v wave. A mild right ventricular heave is palpable. A grade 3/6 holosystolic murmur is noted at the left lower sternal border. The murmur varies slightly with respiration and is associated with an early diastolic filling sound. S_1 and S_2 are normal. There is no hepatosplenomegaly. Bilateral lower extremity pitting edema is present up to the level of the knees. The remainder of the physical examination is normal.

Which of the following is the most appropriate next step in management?

(A) Cardiac magnetic resonance imaging
(B) Coronary angiography
(C) Right heart catheterization
(D) Transthoracic echocardiography

Item 112

A 64-year-old man is evaluated during a follow-up visit for stable angina. He is currently taking metoprolol and wishes to discontinue this medication owing to side effects. He has normal left ventricular function and no symptoms of heart failure. Medical history is significant for hyperlipidemia, hypertension, and coronary artery disease treated with coronary artery bypass graft surgery. Medications are low-dose aspirin and maximum doses of lisinopril, metoprolol, isosorbide mononitrate, ranolazine, and atorvastatin.

On physical examination, temperature is normal, blood pressure is 120/60 mm Hg, pulse rate is 70/min, and respiration rate is 18/min. Oxygen saturation is 98% breathing ambient air. The remainder of the examination is unremarkable.

The patient is switched to diltiazem.

Which of the following is the most appropriate management of this patient's medication regimen?

(A) Decrease ranolazine
(B) Increase atorvastatin
(C) Switch lisinopril to ramipril
(D) No medication adjustment

Item 113

An 81-year-old man is evaluated before elective hip arthroplasty. Medical history is significant for hypertension and osteoarthritis. He reports no chest pain, palpitations, exertional dyspnea, or other symptoms of cardiovascular disease. His medications are lisinopril and celecoxib.

On physical examination, vital signs are normal. The cardiopulmonary examination is normal. Range of motion of the right hip is limited by pain without overlying erythema or warmth.

Laboratory studies reveal normal kidney function and electrolyte levels.

A 12-lead electrocardiogram is shown. Findings are unchanged from 7 years ago.

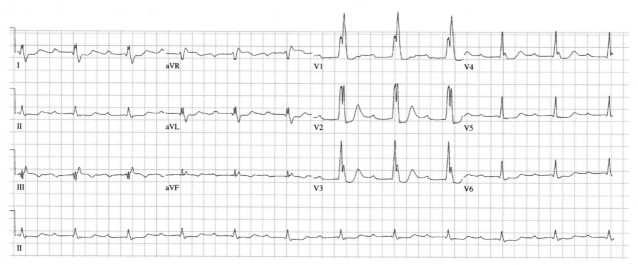

ITEM 113

Which of the following is the most appropriate manage-ment?

(A) Dobutamine echocardiography
(B) Echocardiography
(C) Prophylactic pacemaker insertion
(D) No further testing or intervention

Item 114

A 72-year-old woman is evaluated during a follow-up visit. She has a 3-year history of heart failure with a left ventricular ejection fraction of 25% and New York Heart Association functional class III symptoms. She has an implantable car-dioverter-defibrillator. She reports manageable lighthead-edness with standing. Medications are lisinopril, carvedilol, and spironolactone at maximally tolerated doses.

On physical examination, the patient is afebrile, blood pressure is 98/64 mm Hg, and pulse rate is 68/min. The estimated central venous pressure is 6 cm H_2O. An S_3 is pres-ent. The lungs are clear to auscultation. There is no lower extremity edema.

Which of the following is the most appropriate manage-ment?

(A) Add ivabradine
(B) Add valsartan-sacubitril
(C) Discontinue carvedilol and start ivabradine
(D) Discontinue lisinopril and start valsartan-sacubitril
(E) Continue current medications

Item 115

A 38-year-old woman is evaluated for intermittent palpi-tations. She reports no other symptoms. Medical history is unremarkable, and she takes no medications.

On physical examination, vital signs are normal. The estimated central venous pressure is elevated. Apical impulse is normal, a parasternal impulse is present at the left sternal border, and a soft systolic murmur is heard at the second left intercostal space. Fixed splitting of the S_2 is noted throughout the cardiac cycle. The remainder of the physical examination is normal.

An electrocardiogram demonstrates right-axis deviation and incomplete right bundle branch block. A chest radio-graph shows right heart enlargement. A transthoracic echo-cardiogram demonstrates a 1.5-cm ostium secundum atrial septal defect. The right heart chambers are enlarged and the estimated pulmonary artery systolic pressure is normal.

Which of the following is the best management?

(A) Cardiac magnetic resonance imaging
(B) Device closure of the atrial septal defect
(C) Endocarditis prophylaxis
(D) Measurement of functional aerobic capacity

Item 116

An 88-year-old man is evaluated for chest tightness and dyspnea. His symptoms began 8 months ago and now occur with ambulation. Medical history is significant for type 2 diabetes mellitus, hypertension, chronic kidney disease, and a transient ischemic attack that occurred 4 years ago. Current medications are metformin, atorvastatin, lisinopril, and low-dose aspirin.

On physical examination, temperature is normal, blood pressure is 145/82 mm Hg, pulse rate is 64/min, and respiration rate is normal. The lungs are clear. A grade 3/6 late-peaking systolic murmur is auscultated at the cardiac base with radiation to the carotid arteries. There is no S_3.

Echocardiogram demonstrates severe aortic stenosis with a mean gradient of 62 mm Hg and an aortic valve area of 0.65 cm².

Cardiac surgery assessment estimates the surgical risk to be high (estimated risk for mortality, 10%; estimated risk for major morbidity plus mortality, 38%).

Which of the following is the most appropriate treatment?

(A) Balloon aortic valvuloplasty
(B) Medical therapy
(C) Surgical aortic valve replacement
(D) Transcatheter aortic valve replacement

Item 117

A 66-year-old man is evaluated in the hospital following ST-elevation myocardial infarction treated with primary percutaneous coronary intervention of the left anterior descending artery 4 days ago. His initial presentation was complicated by the presence of heart failure and pulmonary edema. He is asymptomatic and ambulating, and he is nearly ready for discharge. Medical history is significant for hyperlipidemia, type 2 diabetes mellitus, and hypertension. Medications are aspirin, prasugrel, lisinopril, carvedilol, atorvastatin, and basal and prandial insulin.

On physical examination, vital signs are normal. Oxygen saturation is 99% breathing ambient air. The remainder of the examination is unremarkable.

Laboratory studies are significant for a serum creati-nine level of 1.0 mg/dL (88.4 µmol/L) and a serum potassium level of 3.7 mEq/L (3.7 mmol/L).

An echocardiogram shows a left ventricular ejection fraction of 35%.

Which of the following is the most appropriate treatment?

(A) Eplerenone
(B) Isosorbide mononitrate
(C) Valsartan
(D) Warfarin

Item 118

A 63-year-old man is evaluated in the emergency depart-ment for progressive dyspnea. The patient reports increas-ing difficulty breathing while lying flat. He has a history of atrial fibrillation and underwent catheter ablation 1 week ago. Medical history is otherwise significant for hyperten-sion. He has no history of heart failure or left ventricular dysfunction. Medications are warfarin, dronedarone, and lisinopril.

CONT.

On physical examination, temperature is normal, blood pressure is 88/72 mm Hg, pulse rate is 112/min, and respiration rate is 16/min. Pulsus paradoxus of 12 mm Hg is present. Oxygen saturation breathing ambient air is 96%. Cardiac examination reveals elevated estimated central venous pressure. Heart sounds are difficult to auscultate. Lung examination reveals no crackles.

An electrocardiogram demonstrates sinus tachycardia.

Which of the following is most likely responsible for the patient's symptoms?

(A) Atrioesophageal fistula
(B) Cardiac tamponade
(C) Pulmonary vein stenosis
(D) Retroperitoneal bleeding

Item 119

A 43-year-old woman is evaluated during a follow-up visit. Six months ago, she was diagnosed with heart failure and pulmonary sarcoidosis. Cardiac magnetic resonance imaging suggested possible cardiac sarcoidosis. She is feeling better after initiation of therapy, but she still has exertional dyspnea when walking up one flight of stairs. An echocardiogram obtained 1 week ago showed a left ventricular ejection fraction of 30%. Medications are candesartan, carvedilol, and spironolactone. She has also been taking prednisone for cardiac sarcoidosis for the past 6 months.

On physical examination, temperature is normal, blood pressure is 98/60 mm Hg, and pulse rate is 58/min. There is no jugular venous distention. Lungs are clear to auscultation. Cardiac examination is normal. No edema is noted.

An electrocardiogram shows a QRS duration of 158 ms, left bundle branch block, and first-degree atrioventricular block.

Which of the following is the most appropriate management?

(A) Add furosemide
(B) Increase carvedilol
(C) Perform endomyocardial biopsy
(D) Refer for placement of an implantable cardioverter-defibrillator with cardiac resynchronization therapy

Item 120

A 42-year-old man is evaluated in the emergency department for an 8-hour history of acute-onset chest pain. The patient characterizes the pain as sharp and persistent. Medical history is significant for hypertension and hyperlipidemia. Medications are lisinopril and atorvastatin.

On physical examination, temperature is 37.2 °C (99.0 °F), blood pressure is 136/84 mm Hg, and respiration rate is normal. There is no jugular venous distention. The lungs are clear to auscultation. Cardiac examination reveals no rubs, murmurs, or gallops. Peripheral pulses are full and equal.

Laboratory studies reveal an elevated C-reactive protein level and leukocyte count of 9000/µL (9.0×10^9/L). Serum troponin T level is normal on arrival and 1 hour later.

An electrocardiogram is shown. Transthoracic echocardiogram demonstrates normal left ventricular size and function without segmental wall motion abnormalities. There is a small pericardial effusion measuring 4 mm.

Which of the following is the most appropriate management?

(A) Echocardiographic-guided pericardiocentesis
(B) Emergent cardiac catheterization
(C) Exercise treadmill stress testing
(D) High-dose aspirin and colchicine

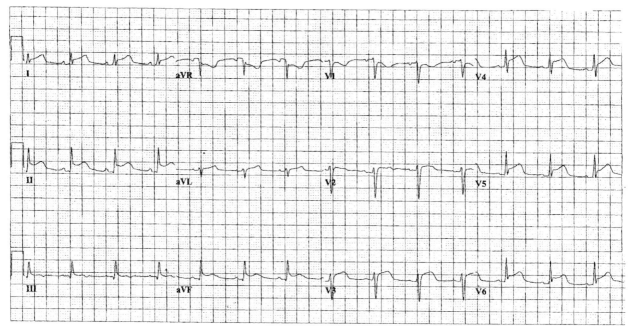

ITEM 120

Answers and Critiques

H **Item 1**   **Answer:**   **D**

Educational Objective: Diagnose acute rejection in a cardiac transplant patient.

Endomyocardial biopsy will most likely establish the diagnosis. For cardiac transplant recipients, the risk for rejection is highest within the first 6 months after transplantation and then within the first year. After that time period, the incidence of rejection is quite low. This post-transplant patient is presenting with signs and symptoms of acute heart failure, including abdominal discomfort, exertional dyspnea, and an S_3. Additionally, the presence of cannon *a* waves suggests complete heart block, and the electrocardiogram is confirmatory, with P waves that march independent of the narrow QRS complex (*arrows*). All of these findings are consistent with acute rejection in a patient within the first year after cardiac transplantation, and the most appropriate test for diagnosis is endomyocardial biopsy. It is important to note that most patients with clinical rejection will not have any symptoms of heart failure; therefore, routine endomyocardial biopsies are performed within the first year after transplantation.

Abdominal CT would not establish the diagnosis. This patient's symptoms are most likely secondary to acute congestion; the patient's complete heart block and other cardiac findings should focus the clinician's attention on the heart. Abdominal CT should be performed only when the abdomen is thought to be the primary cause of the patient's symptoms.

Coronary artery disease is a common long-term complication of cardiac transplantation, and by 5 years after transplantation, vasculopathy is present in almost 50% of patients. Coronary artery disease would be more likely in a patient further removed from transplantation; therefore, coronary angiography would not establish the diagnosis.

Echocardiography will confirm a decreased ejection fraction in this patient but cannot establish the diagnosis of rejection.

> **KEY POINT**
>
> - The risk for cardiac transplant rejection is highest within the first 6 months after transplantation and then within the first year; endomyocardial biopsy should be routinely performed within the first year after cardiac transplantation to diagnose rejection.

Bibliography

Birati EY, Rame JE. Post-heart transplant complications. Crit Care Clin. 2014;30:629-37. [PMID: 24996612] doi:10.1016/j.ccc.2014.03.005

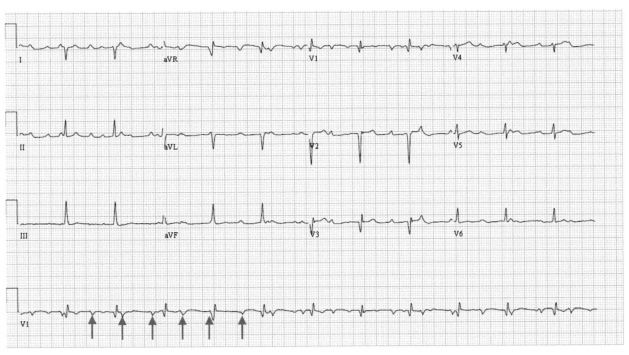

ITEM 1

Item 2   Answer: D

Educational Objective: Treat a patient with a non–ST-elevation acute coronary syndrome with an early invasive strategy.

This patient should undergo urgent angiography. Patients with a non–ST-elevation acute coronary syndrome (NSTE-ACS) should undergo risk stratification before invasive treatment because the link between revascularization and clinical outcomes is less clear in these patients than in patients with ST-elevation myocardial infarction (STEMI). Risk stratification tools, such as the TIMI risk score, can be used to determine which patients with NSTE-ACS should be treated with an invasive strategy versus an ischemia-guided approach. An early invasive strategy benefits patients with high TIMI risk scores (5-7) and intermediate TIMI risk scores (3-4). This patient has a TIMI risk score of 5, as indicated by the presence of three traditional risk factors for coronary artery disease, aspirin use within the last week, age older than 65 years, two or more angina episodes in the past 24 hours, and significant ST-segment deviation on electrocardiogram. His score places him at high risk for death and cardiac ischemic events, and despite the absence of elevated cardiac biomarker levels, urgent coronary angiography is warranted.

Stress testing with adenosine nuclear stress testing or exercise stress electrocardiography could be considered for purposes of risk stratification if this patient declines an early invasive strategy. However, an invasive strategy has been shown to improve the composite clinical endpoint of death, recurrent myocardial infarction, and repeat hospitalization compared with an ischemia-guided approach in patients with NSTE-ACS.

In patients with suspected NSTE-ACS with a normal initial troponin level and inconclusive electrocardiographic findings, further diagnostic studies may be indicated. Coronary CT angiography is appropriate, and rest single-photon emission CT may be appropriate. However, in this patient with a high pretest probability of CAD, coronary CT angiography would only delay critical therapy.

KEY POINT

- Patients with a non–ST-elevation acute coronary syndrome who have a high or intermediate TIMI risk score should be treated with an early invasive strategy.

Bibliography

Amsterdam EA, Wenger NK, Brindis RG, Casey DE Jr, Ganiats TG, Holmes DR Jr, et al; ACC/AHA Task Force Members. 2014 AHA/ACC guideline for the management of patients with non-ST-elevation acute coronary syndromes: executive summary: a report of the American College of Cardiology/American Heart Association Task Force on Practice Guidelines. Circulation. 2014;130:2354-94. [PMID: 25249586] doi:10.1161/CIR.0000000000000133

Item 3   Answer: B

Educational Objective: Treat degenerative mitral regurgitation with surgical mitral valve repair.

The most appropriate next step in management is surgical mitral valve repair. Myxomatous degeneration of the mitral valve is common, affecting 1% to 2% of the general population. In 10% of patients, the valvular lesion can progress, become life threatening, and require surgery. The only definitive therapy for severe mitral regurgitation is mitral valve surgery. Options are mitral valve repair, mitral valve replacement with preservation of part or all of the mitral apparatus, and mitral valve replacement with removal of the mitral apparatus. Mitral valve repair is generally preferred to valve replacement because it is associated with improved survival in retrospective studies. Mitral valve repair is strongly recommended for chronic severe primary mitral regurgitation in (1) symptomatic patients with left ventricular ejection fraction greater than 30%, (2) asymptomatic patients with left ventricular dysfunction (left ventricular ejection fraction of 30%-60% and/or left ventricular end-systolic diameter ≥40 mm), and (3) patients undergoing another cardiac surgical procedure. Additionally, mitral valve repair is reasonable in asymptomatic patients with chronic severe primary mitral regurgitation who have new-onset atrial fibrillation or pulmonary hypertension (pulmonary artery systolic pressure >50 mm Hg). Notably, a left ventricular ejection fraction of 60% or less is used in defining left ventricular systolic dysfunction in mitral regurgitation because aortic emptying into the left atrium contributes to the relatively lower afterload conditions and higher ejection fraction despite impaired left ventricular performance.

Serial evaluations every 6 to 12 months are recommended for patients with severe mitral regurgitation who do not have indications for surgery. This patient meets the criteria for surgery; therefore, serial evaluations would not be appropriate at this time.

Many patients who could benefit from mitral valve repair are denied surgery because of high surgical risk, advanced age, or comorbid conditions. A catheter-based device can improve mitral valve function by delivering a clip percutaneously to approximate the valve leaflet edges and improve leaflet coaptation at the origin of the mitral regurgitation jet. The device is approved for patients with significant symptomatic degenerative mitral regurgitation for whom mitral valve surgery poses a prohibitive risk. This patient is healthy and does not have comorbid conditions that would significantly increase surgical risk; therefore, transcatheter repair is not indicated.

KEY POINT

- Mitral valve repair is strongly recommended for chronic severe primary mitral regurgitation in symptomatic patients with left ventricular ejection fraction greater than 30%, asymptomatic patients with left ventricular dysfunction, and patients undergoing another cardiac surgical procedure.

Bibliography

Foster E. Clinical practice. Mitral regurgitation due to degenerative mitral-valve disease. N Engl J Med. 2010;363:156-65. [PMID: 20647211] doi:10.1056/NEJMcp0906782

Item 4   Answer: A

Educational Objective: Diagnose hypertension related to bevacizumab therapy.

Bevacizumab is the most likely cause of this patient's hypertension. Bevacizumab is a monoclonal antibody that blocks angiogenesis by inhibiting vascular endothelial growth factor (VEGF) A. It is effective in combination with standard chemotherapy for the treatment of metastatic colon and gynecologic cancers. Inhibition of VEGF appears to cause hypertension through several mechanisms, including altered nitric oxide production, increased endothelin-1 production, and alterations in the pressure-natriuresis relationship. As such, bevacizumab-related hypertension is a mechanism-dependent, on-target toxicity, which results directly from inhibition of the VEGF signaling pathway rather than as a nonspecific drug side effect. Bevacizumab-related hypertension affects a high proportion of treated patients, and incidence is dose dependent. Hypertension is most commonly detected at approximately 60 days after therapy initiation and is reversible upon discontinuation of the medication. Because large increases in both diastolic and systolic blood pressures can occur as early as the first week of therapy, all patients taking an angiogenesis inhibitor (such as bevacizumab) should have their blood pressure carefully monitored during therapy, particularly early on. There is no preferred antihypertensive agent for treatment. Interestingly, the development of hypertension may be a marker of a therapeutic response or improved cancer outcome for patients treated with this class of drugs.

Cisplatin has been associated with increased risk for venous thromboembolism, supraventricular tachycardia, myocardial ischemia, and cardiomyopathy, but it has not been associated with hypertension.

Glucocorticoids, such as dexamethasone, may contribute to hypertension through an unclear mechanism. However, the timing and degree of hypertension observed in this patient are typical of a bevacizumab-induced reaction.

The most common cardiotoxicities associated with paclitaxel are bradycardia and heart block. Most of these events are asymptomatic, and routine cardiac monitoring is not advocated. Paclitaxel can uncommonly cause hypertension (1% incidence) but is more likely to cause hypotension (up to 12% incidence). When used in combination with doxorubicin, paclitaxel is associated with cardiomyopathy, which occurs at a higher incidence than with doxorubicin alone.

KEY POINT

- The monoclonal antibody bevacizumab is associated with the development of significant but reversible hypertension.

Bibliography

Robinson ES, Khankin EV, Karumanchi SA, Humphreys BD. Hypertension induced by vascular endothelial growth factor signaling pathway inhibition: mechanisms and potential use as a biomarker. Semin Nephrol. 2010;30:591-601. [PMID: 21146124] doi:10.1016/j.semnephrol.2010.09.007

Item 5   Answer: B

Educational Objective: Diagnose aortic coarctation.

The most likely diagnosis is aortic coarctation. This patient has dyspnea in the setting of aortic stenosis and hypertension, and she has clinical features of upper extremity hypertension and a radial artery–to–femoral artery pulse delay that suggest a mechanical obstruction between the radial and femoral arteries. A systolic murmur heard over the left chest is common in patients with severe aortic coarctation; these murmurs can arise from the obstruction or the collateral blood flow. The patient's chest radiograph demonstrates rib notching (*arrows*) affecting several of the posterior ribs; rib notching results from exaggerated collateral blood flow diverting blood around the area of obstruction. The patient additionally has aortic stenosis associated with a bicuspid aortic valve, which is present in more than 50% of patients with aortic coarctation. Cerebral artery aneurysm also occurs with increased frequency in patients with aortic coarctation.

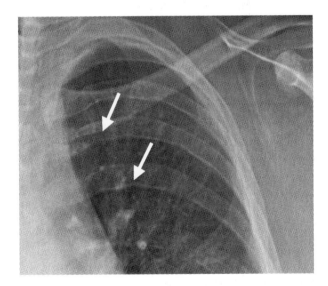

The syndrome of aortic dissection usually presents with sharp or tearing chest and/or back pain. It may be accompanied by syncope, heart failure, or stroke and is rarely asymptomatic. Chest pain with concomitant acute ischemia in a distant arterial bed (stroke, limb ischemia) should prompt consideration of dissection. The chest radiograph does not demonstrate features of aortic dilatation or mediastinal widening characteristic of dissection.

Although the physical examination findings in a patient with severe essential hypertension often include an S_4, blood pressure and pulse differentials between the upper and lower extremities are not expected.

Renovascular hypertension is a common cause of hypertension, occurring primarily in patients with diffuse atherosclerosis. The physical examination in a patient with renovascular hypertension is usually normal, with the exception of hypertension and possible epigastric bruit; blood pressure and pulse differentials between upper and lower extremities are not expected.

KEY POINT

- Aortic coarctation is characterized by clinical features of upper extremity hypertension and a radial artery–to–femoral artery pulse delay as well as radiographic findings of "figure 3 sign" and rib notching.

Bibliography

Tanous D, Benson LN, Horlick EM. Coarctation of the aorta: evaluation and management. Curr Opin Cardiol. 2009;24:509-15. [PMID: 19667980] doi:10.1097/HCO.0b013e328330cc22

Item 6   Answer: E

Educational Objective: Manage a patient with acute limb ischemia.

The most appropriate next step in the management of this patient with acute limb ischemia (ALI) is urgent invasive angiography to determine the extent of disease and to plan treatment. ALI is defined by a sudden or rapid decrease in limb perfusion, often manifested as a new pulse deficit, rest pain, pallor, and/or paralysis. The most common causes of ALI include in situ thrombosis of a lower extremity bypass graft or endovascular stent and thromboembolism. Patients with ALI and a viable extremity are most commonly treated with surgical embolectomy or catheter-directed thrombolysis. This patient is demonstrating several classic signs of ALI, including pulselessness, pallor, and pain, and he is at heightened risk for ALI owing to his history of femoral-popliteal bypass graft surgery. The most appropriate next step is to perform invasive angiography to define the level of occlusion and to determine whether surgical embolectomy or catheter-directed thrombolysis is an option. Delay in treatment may lead to worsening limb perfusion, limb necrosis, or the need for lower extremity amputation.

Noninvasive imaging studies, such as arterial duplex ultrasonography and CT angiography, may be useful to detect the level of stenosis and extent of disease, but these tests will substantially delay the treatment of ALI in this patient.

Emergent lower extremity amputation is necessary in patients with ALI who have a nonviable extremity (gangrene, paralysis); however, this patient exhibits signs of viability (intact sensation and muscle strength) and should not undergo immediate amputation.

In contrast to the treatment of acute ischemic stroke or acute ST-elevation myocardial infarction, systemic thrombolytic therapy (such as with recombinant tissue plasminogen activator) has not been proved beneficial in the treatment of ALI and should not be used in this patient.

KEY POINT

- In patients with acute limb ischemia, invasive angiography should be performed immediately to define the anatomic level of occlusion and plan for revascularization.

Bibliography

Creager MA, Kaufman JA, Conte MS. Clinical practice. Acute limb ischemia. N Engl J Med. 2012;366:2198-206. [PMID: 22670905] doi:10.1056/NEJMcp1006054

Item 7   Answer: D

Educational Objective: Manage antithrombotic therapy in a patient with atrial fibrillation and coronary artery disease.

This patient with coronary artery disease (CAD) and atrial fibrillation should be treated with oral anticoagulation alone. Thromboembolism (stroke or systemic embolism) is the most feared and devastating complication of atrial fibrillation. Patients with atrial fibrillation and a moderate to high risk for stroke (CHA_2DS_2-VASc score ≥ 2) should be treated with oral anticoagulation for stroke prevention. This patient has a CHA_2DS_2-VASc score of 5 (1 point each for female sex, hypertension, and vascular disease; 2 points for age ≥ 75 years) and should receive oral anticoagulation therapy. Dose-adjusted warfarin is an effective low-cost option for stroke prevention in patients with atrial fibrillation. The chief limitations of warfarin are the need for frequent INR monitoring and adjustment as well as the numerous food and drug interactions associated with its use. The FDA has approved several non–vitamin K antagonist oral anticoagulants for the prevention of stroke in patients with nonvalvular atrial fibrillation, including dabigatran, rivaroxaban, edoxaban, and apixaban. These agents are superior, or at least noninferior, to warfarin in the prevention of stroke in patients with nonvalvular atrial fibrillation and do not necessitate routine coagulation monitoring. Warfarin remains the agent of choice in patients with valvular atrial fibrillation.

Antiplatelet therapy with aspirin is typically indicated in patients with CAD; however, aspirin alone or dual antiplatelet therapy (aspirin plus clopidogrel) is insufficient for stroke prevention in patients at high risk, such as this one.

Combination therapy with oral anticoagulation and antiplatelet therapy, such as aspirin or clopidogrel, is associated with significantly increased risk for bleeding and no apparent incremental benefit. This patient already has several risk factors for bleeding, including a low BMI, hypertension, and female sex, and it is important to minimize the risk for bleeding when oral anticoagulation is prescribed. In patients with atrial fibrillation and CAD, it is recommended that antiplatelet therapy be discontinued unless the patient has recent active CAD, defined as acute coronary syndrome or revascularization in the past 12 months. Because this patient has a history of percutaneous coronary intervention performed 5 years ago, there is no indication for concomitant antiplatelet therapy with oral anticoagulation.

KEY POINT

- For most patients with high-risk atrial fibrillation and stable coronary artery disease, oral anticoagulation therapy without an antiplatelet agent is sufficient for prevention of both acute coronary syndromes and thromboembolism.

Bibliography

Steinberg BA, Kim S, Piccini JP, Fonarow GC, Lopes RD, Thomas L, et al; ORBIT-AF Investigators and Patients. Use and associated risks of concomitant aspirin therapy with oral anticoagulation in patients with atrial fibrillation: insights from the Outcomes Registry for Better Informed Treatment of Atrial Fibrillation (ORBIT-AF) Registry. Circulation. 2013;128:721-8.[PMID:23861512]doi:10.1161/CIRCULATIONAHA.113.002927

Item 8   Answer: C

Educational Objective: Evaluate for coronary artery disease in a patient with left ventricular hypertrophy.

This patient should undergo exercise stress echocardiography to evaluate for coronary artery disease (CAD). This patient's symptoms, age, and sex place him at intermediate risk for CAD. His resting electrocardiogram (ECG) demonstrates left ventricular hypertrophy with significant repolarization abnormalities (ST-segment depressions >0.5 mm), findings that limit the ability to interpret the ECG during exercise. Because this patient requires further testing to diagnose obstructive CAD and is able to exercise, he should undergo exercise stress testing with adjunctive imaging, either echocardiography or a nuclear perfusion study. Other uninterpretable ECG findings that should prompt stress testing with imaging include left bundle branch block, ventricular paced complexes, digitalis effect, and preexcitation.

Coronary angiography is an invasive test that carries significant risks. It should be considered in patients who have a high pretest probability for obstructive CAD, including symptomatic patients with abnormal findings on noninvasive testing for CAD or patients with an acute coronary syndrome.

Coronary artery calcium scoring is predominantly used in asymptomatic patients with intermediate risk for CAD to provide additional risk stratification for the purpose of guiding primary prevention.

Exercise stress ECG is inappropriate in this patient with abnormalities on a baseline ECG. Such findings preclude the use of ECG stress testing because they interfere with the ability to accurately interpret changes that may occur with stress.

Exercise stress testing is preferred to pharmacologic stress testing in most clinical scenarios because valuable prognostic information is gained from the patient's exercise capacity. Pharmacologic nuclear stress testing is generally reserved for patients who are unable to exercise.

KEY POINT

- Stress testing with adjunctive imaging should be performed in patients with suspected coronary artery disease who have baseline electrocardiographic (ECG) abnormalities that preclude the use of ECG stress testing, such as ST-segment depressions greater than 0.5 mm, left bundle branch block, ventricular paced complexes, digitalis effect, and preexcitation.

Bibliography

Fihn SD, Gardin JM, Abrams J, et al; American College of Cardiology Foundation.; American Heart Association Task Force on Practice Guidelines.; American College of Physicians; American Association for Thoracic Surgery; Preventive Cardiovascular Nurses Association; Society for Cardiovascular Angiography and Interventions; Society of Thoracic Surgeons. 2012 ACCF/AHA/ACP/AATS/PCNA/SCAI/STS guideline for the diagnosis and management of patients with stable ischemic heart disease: a report of the American College of Cardiology Foundation/American Heart Association Task Force on Practice Guidelines, and the American College of Physicians, American Association for Thoracic Surgery, Preventive Cardiovascular Nurses Association, Society for Cardiovascular Angiography and Interventions, and Society of Thoracic Surgeons. J Am Coll Cardiol. 2012 Dec 18;60(24):e44-e164. [PMID: 23182125]

Item 9   Answer: A

Educational Objective: Treat effusive constrictive pericarditis.

The most appropriate management is ibuprofen and colchicine. This patient has subacute signs of elevated right heart pressure. Pulsus paradoxus is present, and the echocardiogram demonstrates a moderately sized pericardial effusion with evidence of tamponade. The intrapericardial pressure is reduced to normal following drainage, whereas the intracardiac pressures remain elevated and equalized despite drainage, consistent with a diagnosis of effusive constrictive pericarditis. Effusive constrictive pericarditis may occur following idiopathic or infectious pericarditis or radiation therapy. CT or cardiac magnetic resonance imaging may demonstrate thickening of the pericardium, but calcification is usually absent. Fever, leukocytosis, elevated erythrocyte sedimentation rate, and a pericardial friction rub may be present but are not universally so. Similar to acute pericarditis, NSAIDs and colchicine are first-line therapy. Close follow-up is recommended. Pericardiectomy may be required in patients with pericarditis that does not respond to medical therapy.

Isoniazid, rifampin, pyrazinamide, and ethambutol are initial therapy for tuberculous pericarditis; however, this patient does not have risk factors for tuberculosis, and his interferon-γ release assay result is negative. An elevated concentration of adenosine deaminase (>50 U/L) in the pericardial fluid is 100% sensitive for tuberculosis; a negative result rules out tuberculous involvement.

Pericardiectomy is recommended for patients with effusive constrictive pericarditis that does not respond to first-line therapy with NSAIDs and colchicine.

A pericardial subxiphoid window is indicated for patients with recurrent hemodynamically significant pericardial effusion despite medical therapy, as may occur with malignant effusions. This intervention would not provide adequate hemodynamic relief from constriction.

KEY POINT

- Effusive constrictive pericarditis is characterized by findings compatible with constrictive pericarditis and a concomitant effusion; NSAIDs and colchicine are first-line therapy, and close follow-up is recommended.

Bibliography

Syed FF, Ntsekhe M, Mayosi BM, Oh JK. Effusive-constrictive pericarditis. Heart Fail Rev. 2013;18:277-87. [PMID: 22422296] doi:10.1007/s10741-012-9308-0

Item 10   Answer: C

Educational Objective: Differentiate between pseudostenosis and true aortic stenosis.

The most appropriate next step in management is dobutamine echocardiography. This patient has low-flow, low-gradient aortic stenosis. The primary abnormality may be either severe ventricular dysfunction with pseudostenosis or critical aortic stenosis. Severe ventricular dysfunction with diminished cardiac output leads to decreased opening forces on the aortic valve, and the valve area may be calculated to be low even though the valve is not anatomically severe (pseudostenosis). Dobutamine, an inotropic agent, can be used to increase cardiac output and differentiate between these two entities. Dobutamine will cause an increase in the aortic valve area in pseudostenosis, whereas in anatomically severe aortic stenosis, the aortic valve area will not significantly increase.

Aortic valve replacement should be considered for patients with anatomically severe aortic stenosis. This procedure is currently inappropriate for a patient in whom the diagnosis of severe aortic stenosis has not been established.

Coronary angiography is recommended before valve surgery in patients with severe valvular heart disease and a history of coronary artery disease, suspected myocardial ischemia, or left ventricular systolic dysfunction. These patients may require concomitant revascularization at the time of surgery. However, coronary angiography is indicated only in patients for whom valve surgery has been determined to be appropriate.

The 2016 American College of Cardiology/American Heart Association/Heart Failure Society of America heart failure focused update recommends that valsartan-sacubitril be substituted for an ACE inhibitor or an angiotensin receptor blocker in patients with chronic symptomatic heart failure with reduced ejection fraction (New York Heart Association functional class II or III) who have tolerated ACE inhibitor or angiotensin receptor blocker therapy well. In this patient, differentiation of pseudostenosis from true aortic stenosis is most appropriate before initiating an increase in medical therapy.

KEY POINT

- In patients with findings of low-flow, low-gradient aortic stenosis, the primary abnormality may be either severe ventricular dysfunction with pseudostenosis or critical aortic stenosis; dobutamine echocardiography is needed to distinguish between the two entities.

Bibliography

O'Sullivan CJ, Praz F, Stortecky S, Windecker S, Wenaweser P. Assessment of low-flow, low-gradient, severe aortic stenosis: an invasive evaluation is required for decision making. EuroIntervention. 2014;10 Suppl U:U61-8. [PMID: 25256333] doi:10.4244/EIJV10SUA9

Item 11   Answer: D

Educational Objective: Treat cardiogenic shock.

The most appropriate initial treatment of this patient with cardiogenic shock is to start dobutamine. Cardiogenic shock is defined by persistent symptomatic hypotension and end-organ dysfunction. Patients present with acute kidney failure, evidence of liver dysfunction with elevated aminotransferase levels, poor peripheral perfusion with cool extremities, and impaired mental status. Cardiogenic shock secondary to progressive heart failure is generally treated with an inotropic agent, such as dobutamine or milrinone. Patients with peripheral vasoconstriction (increased systemic vascular resistance) often benefit from the addition of a pure vasodilator, such as sodium nitroprusside. In this case, dobutamine would be a better option than milrinone, even in the setting of relative tachycardia, because milrinone is excreted through the kidneys and could build to a toxic level given her current kidney function.

β-Blockers such as carvedilol should be continued during a heart failure hospitalization whenever possible. In a patient with volume overload without signs of low cardiac output, β-blockers can often be continued at the maintenance dose while the patient is undergoing diuresis. However, in a patient with low cardiac output such as this one, β-blockers should be discontinued, owing to their negative inotropic effects, even in the setting of tachycardia.

Digoxin is a weak inotrope that reduces hospitalizations in patients with heart failure. Although this patient's digoxin level is low, the dose should not be increased in the setting of acute kidney failure. Additionally, increasing digoxin would not be expected to adequately improve cardiac output in this patient.

Although afterload reduction is reasonable to decrease myocardial oxygen demand and improve forward flow in patients with acute decompensation, a short-acting intravenous agent, such as nitroprusside or nitroglycerin, would be administered instead of increasing the dosage of an oral ACE inhibitor, such as lisinopril.

KEY POINT

- In patients with cardiogenic shock, inotropes such as dobutamine or milrinone may be considered to improve cardiac function.

Bibliography

Yancy CW, Jessup M, Bozkurt B, Butler J, Casey DE Jr, Drazner MH, et al; American College of Cardiology Foundation. 2013 ACCF/AHA guideline for the management of heart failure: a report of the American College of Cardiology Foundation/American Heart Association Task Force on Practice Guidelines. J Am Coll Cardiol. 2013;62:e147-239. [PMID: 23747642] doi:10.1016/j.jacc.2013.05.019

Item 12   Answer: D

Educational Objective: Treat atrial flutter refractory to medical therapy.

Catheter ablation is the most appropriate treatment for this patient with electrocardiographic evidence of atrial flutter. Atrial flutter is an organized macro-reentrant tachycardia with discrete regular atrial activity on electrocardiogram, usually with a rate of 250/min to 300/min. Typical atrial flutter is characterized electrocardiographically by a sawtooth pattern with inverted flutter waves in leads II, III, and aVF and positive flutter waves in lead V_1. Management of atrial flutter is similar to that for atrial fibrillation and includes catheter ablation, antiarrhythmic drug therapy, and cardioversion. Catheter ablation is the definitive treatment for typical atrial flutter, owing to a very high success rate (>95%) and low complication rate. This patient with typical atrial flutter has symptoms (palpitations, fatigue, and exercise intolerance) despite adequate rate control with metoprolol, and treatment with catheter ablation offers the best balance of benefits and risks.

Antiarrhythmic drug therapy carries a high risk for recurrent atrial flutter and is therefore not the best option for this patient. Additionally, amiodarone is associated with substantial risk for end-organ toxicity, including thyroid dysfunction, neurologic side effects (such as tremor), liver dysfunction, and pulmonary toxicity.

Cardiac catheterization would be appropriate if there were a high pretest probability of obstructive coronary artery disease; however, this patient has normal findings on echocardiogram without evidence of stress-induced wall motion abnormalities.

Cardioversion to restore sinus rhythm could be considered, but this patient is hemodynamically stable and already has experienced a recurrence of atrial flutter after previous cardioversion. Cardioversion may therefore be ineffective for long-term control of the patient's symptoms.

KEY POINT

- Patients with symptomatic atrial flutter despite adequate medical therapy and rate control should undergo catheter ablation.

Bibliography
Page RL, Joglar JA, Caldwell MA, Calkins H, Conti JB, Deal BJ, et al. 2015 ACC/AHA/HRS guideline for the management of adult patients with supraventricular tachycardia: a report of the American College of Cardiology/American Heart Association Task Force on Clinical Practice Guidelines and the Heart Rhythm Society. J Am Coll Cardiol. 2016;67:e27-e115. [PMID: 26409259] doi:10.1016/j.jacc.2015.08.856

Item 13   Answer: B

Educational Objective: Diagnose patent ductus arteriosus.

This patient has a patent ductus arteriosus (PDA). A continuous murmur heard beneath the left clavicle that envelops the S_2 is typical of a PDA; it is often described as a "machinery" murmur. A tiny PDA is generally asymptomatic with an inaudible murmur. Patients with a small PDA may have an audible murmur but no other cardiovascular features. Patients with a moderate-sized PDA may have bounding pulses, a wide pulse pressure, left heart enlargement and dysfunction, and clinical heart failure. A large PDA may present with pulmonary hypertension and shunt reversal (Eisenmenger syndrome) in adults.

Aortic regurgitation due to a bicuspid aortic valve causes a diastolic murmur, most commonly heard along the left sternal border. A brief systolic murmur is also commonly

heard at the second right intercostal space, from increased flow across the bicuspid aortic valve. A systolic ejection click is often heard in patients with bicuspid aortic valve, but a continuous murmur that envelops the S_2 is not expected.

Pulmonary regurgitation occurs most commonly after balloon or surgical intervention for congenital pulmonary stenosis. It is characterized by a diastolic murmur heard along the left sternal border that increases with inspiration; a systolic ejection murmur is also commonly heard from increased flow across the pulmonary valve. Although the pulmonary component of S_2 may be reduced or absent in patients with pulmonary regurgitation, separation between systole and diastole is distinct, and the aortic component should be audible.

A small ventricular septal defect (VSD) presents with a loud holosystolic murmur located at the left sternal border that may obliterate the S_2; a palpable thrill is often present. The pressure gradient between the ventricles determines the murmur quality and duration. A diastolic component of the murmur is not expected. Small VSDs do not cause left heart enlargement or pulmonary hypertension. Progressive pulmonary hypertension results in shortening of the murmur.

KEY POINT

- Patients with a small patent ductus arteriosus may present with a continuous murmur beneath the left clavicle that envelops the S_2 but no other cardiovascular features.

Bibliography
Baumgartner H, Bonhoeffer P, De Groot NM, de Haan F, Deanfield JE, Galie N, et al; Task Force on the Management of Grown-up Congenital Heart Disease of the European Society of Cardiology (ESC). ESC guidelines for the management of grown-up congenital heart disease (new version 2010). Eur Heart J. 2010;31:2915-57. [PMID: 20801927] doi:10.1093/eurheartj/ehq249

Item 14   Answer: B

Educational Objective: Diagnose cardiac syndrome X.

The most likely diagnosis is cardiac syndrome X. This relatively young patient with no traditional risk factors for coronary artery disease has typical angina, abnormal stress testing results, and angiographically normal coronary arteries. Cardiac syndrome X is a frequent cause of chest pain syndromes in women, and patients often present without traditional risk factors for coronary artery disease. The chest pain is often indistinguishable from classic exertional angina, and stress testing results are frequently abnormal. Many hypotheses have been proposed to explain the pathogenesis of cardiac syndrome X, with one of the most accepted centering on microvascular dysfunction as the cause. Although vasodilators should be tried, symptoms can be difficult to treat.

An acute coronary syndrome is unlikely given the lack of risk factors, duration of symptoms, and normal coronary angiogram.

Diagnostic criteria for somatic symptom disorder are as follows: at least one somatic symptom causing distress or interference with daily life; excessive thoughts, behaviors, and feelings related to the somatic symptoms; and persistent somatic symptoms for at least 6 months (does not have to be the same symptom for 6 months). This patient does not fulfill the diagnostic criteria for somatic symptom disorder.

Takotsubo cardiomyopathy, also known as stress cardiomyopathy or apical ballooning syndrome, is a cause of non-exertional chest pain associated with electrocardiographic changes (often ST-segment elevations) and elevated cardiac enzymes. There is often, but not always, an antecedent psychological or physical stressor. The timing and exertional nature of this patient's symptoms are not consistent with the diagnosis of takotsubo cardiomyopathy.

KEY POINT

- Cardiac syndrome X is characterized by angina and stress testing abnormalities in the absence of angiographically significant coronary artery disease.

Bibliography

Löffler AI, Bourque JM. Coronary microvascular dysfunction, microvascular angina, and management. Curr Cardiol Rep. 2016;18:1. [PMID: 26694723] doi:10.1007/s11886-015-0682-9

Item 15   Answer: B

Educational Objective: Treat a patient with intermittent claudication with supervised exercise training.

The most appropriate next step in the management of this patient with established peripheral artery disease (PAD) and symptoms of intermittent claudication is to initiate a supervised exercise program. In addition to medical therapy with cilostazol, supervised exercise training is recommended to improve symptoms and walking distance in patients with intermittent claudication. The recommended program consists of supervised exercise therapy for at least 30 to 45 minutes occurring at least 3 times per week for at least 12 weeks. A meta-analysis of 27 studies demonstrated that supervised exercise training was more effective than home-based exercise training for improvement in walking distance and claudication distance. However, there was no difference in general quality of life or community-based walking at 3 months. Unsupervised exercise programs are defined as walking advice or a structured home-based exercise program.

Antiplatelet therapy with aspirin or clopidogrel is recommended in patients with symptomatic PAD and can be considered in patients with asymptomatic PAD to reduce the risk for myocardial infarction, stroke, or vascular death. Dual antiplatelet therapy is not recommend in patients with PAD in the absence of other indications (drug-eluting stent placement or prosthetic distal lower extremity bypass) because of the increased risk for bleeding and the absence of evidence demonstrating improved clinical outcomes.

Approximately 2% to 4% of patients with stable claudication progress to critical limb ischemia or require surgical revascularization and/or amputation annually. In this patient with stable but progressive intermittent claudication, medical therapy and exercise training are indicated at this time; however, if conservative therapy fails or symptoms become life limiting, anatomic imaging with magnetic resonance angiography or CT angiography and subsequent revascularization (endovascular or surgical) would be appropriate.

KEY POINT

- In patients with intermittent claudication, supervised exercise training is recommended to improve symptoms and walking distance.

Bibliography

Vemulapalli S, Dolor RJ, Hasselblad V, Schmit K, Banks A, Heidenfelder B, et al. Supervised vs unsupervised exercise for intermittent claudication: a systematic review and meta-analysis. Am Heart J. 2015;169:924-937.e3. [PMID: 26027632] doi:10.1016/j.ahj.2015.03.009

Item 16   Answer: A

Educational Objective: Evaluate an abdominal aortic aneurysm with CT angiography before endovascular aneurysm repair.

The most appropriate next step in management of this patient with an abdominal aortic aneurysm (AAA) is CT angiography of the abdominal aorta and iliac vessels to plan for aortic repair. The strongest risk factor for rupture of an AAA is maximal aortic diameter; this measurement is the dominant indication for repair. Aortic repair should be performed in suitable patients with an AAA diameter of 5.5 cm or larger, in patients with rapid expansion in AAA size (>0.5 cm/year), and in patients presenting with symptoms resulting from AAA (abdominal or back pain/tenderness). In patients with an indication for aortic repair, the choice is between open surgical repair and endovascular aneurysm repair (EVAR). Open surgical repair involves abdominal flank incision and opening the aneurysm sac with interposition of a synthetic graft. EVAR is a less invasive method involving intraluminal introduction of a covered stent through the aneurysm sac, with the stent acting as a sleeve. The choice of procedure is driven by several considerations, including the patient's operative risk, expected lifespan, and ability to adhere to the monitoring requirements of EVAR; the location of the AAA; and involvement of the renal and mesenteric arteries. Suprarenal and juxtarenal aneurysms most often necessitate open surgical repair, whereas infrarenal aneurysms may be treated with open surgery or EVAR. In this patient, CT angiography or magnetic resonance angiography should be performed to determine the location and extent of the AAA. Abdominal duplex ultrasonography is insufficient to determine AAA location. In addition, CT measurements exceed ultrasound measurements in 95% of cases.

Although controlling risk factors for cardiovascular disease is essential in patients with AAA, there is little compelling evidence for treating hypertension in these patients with a specific agent, including β-blockers, to prevent aneurysm expansion. Because this patient's blood pressure is well controlled, no change in antihypertensive therapy is indicated. Importantly, an AAA with a diameter of 6.2 cm has a 10% to 20% annual risk for rupture, and definitive surgical therapy is indicated.

KEY POINT

- In patients with an indication for abdominal aortic aneurysm repair, the choice between open surgical repair and endovascular aneurysm repair is driven in part by the location of the aneurysm and involvement of the renal and mesenteric arteries.

Bibliography

Hong H, Yang Y, Liu B, Cai W. Imaging of abdominal aortic aneurysm: the present and the future. Curr Vasc Pharmacol. 2010;8:808-19. [PMID: 20180767]

Item 17   Answer: D

Educational Objective: **Recognize hyperlipidemia as a risk factor for cardiovascular disease.**

This patient's hyperlipidemia most increases his risk for cardiovascular disease (CVD). Most cardiovascular risk can be attributed to modifiable risk factors, and among them, elevated cholesterol levels impart the highest risk for CVD. Reductions in lipid levels can decrease overall risk, and current cholesterol treatment guidelines focus on risk for future cardiovascular events rather than absolute lipid levels. For primary prevention of cardiovascular events, the treatment goal is a reduction in the LDL cholesterol level of at least 50% in high-risk patients and a reduction of 30% to 50% in moderate-risk patients. This patient's 10-year cardiovascular risk based on the American College of Cardiology/American Heart Association Pooled Cohort Equations risk calculator is 7.9%, and statin therapy should be initiated.

Moderate alcohol intake (one to two drinks daily for men, one drink daily for women) has been linked with decreased incidence of CVD; however, heavy alcohol consumption has been shown to increase cardiovascular risk. The deleterious effects of alcohol consumption must be weighed against the potential benefits when patients are counseled about risk modification.

The risk for CVD varies considerably among different ethnic groups. The prevalence of heart disease is lower among persons of Hispanic ethnicity than in most other ethnic groups, and Hispanics tend to have lower rates of traditional modifiable risk factors.

Family history of premature CVD is an independent cardiovascular risk factor but typically adds little precision when included in multivariate risk models. In most studies, premature CVD is defined as CVD in a first-degree male relative younger than 55 years or a first-degree female relative younger than 65 years. A family history of premature CVD doubles the risk for myocardial infarction in men and increases the risk by 70% in women. This patient's father died at age 61 years; therefore, family history is not the most important risk factor for this patient.

Although active smoking remains a strong risk factor for CVD, smoking cessation substantially reduces cardiovascular risk within 2 years, with risk returning to the level of a nonsmoker at approximately 10 years. Smoking status should be addressed at every visit, and cessation counseling should be offered to patients who are actively smoking.

KEY POINT

- Most cardiovascular risk can be attributed to modifiable risk factors; among them, elevated lipid levels impart the highest risk for cardiovascular disease.

Bibliography

Yusuf S, Hawken S, Ounpuu S, Dans T, Avezum A, Lanas F, et al; INTERHEART Study Investigators. Effect of potentially modifiable risk factors associated with myocardial infarction in 52 countries (the INTERHEART study): case-control study. Lancet. 2004;364:937-52. [PMID: 15364185]

Item 18   Answer: D

Educational Objective: **Evaluate a patient with stable chronic heart failure.**

Serum electrolyte measurement and kidney function studies should be performed at this visit. In patients with heart failure, each follow-up visit should include evaluation of current symptoms and functional capacity; assessment of volume status, electrolytes, and kidney function; and review of the patient's medication regimen for adequacy. It is also important to reinforce heart failure education and the need for diet and medication adherence. This patient with stable chronic heart failure is taking appropriate medications, has had no changes in his symptoms or exercise tolerance, and has no evidence of volume overload. Because he is taking a diuretic, an angiotensin receptor blocker, and spironolactone, assessing his electrolyte levels and kidney function is appropriate.

Routine repeat echocardiography is not recommended in a stable patient with heart failure. According to current guidelines, repeat echocardiography should be performed if the patient has had a change in clinical status, received a new medication that might significantly improve ejection fraction (such as a β-blocker), or is being considered for device therapy after medical optimization.

Twenty-four hour ambulatory electrocardiographic monitoring is not indicated to routinely screen for arrhythmias in patients with heart failure in the absence of symptoms or signs worrisome for an arrhythmia.

The B-type natriuretic peptide (BNP) level has prognostic value in patients with heart failure and can be used to determine whether heart failure is progressing. However, determining a prognosis according to an absolute value is difficult, and models that have used BNP levels have different BNP cutpoints and lengths of follow-up. At this time, a BNP level is not routinely obtained in an otherwise stable patient. Other biomarkers of myocardial fibrosis, such as soluble ST2 receptor and galectin-3, have been shown to be predictive of death and hospitalization in small trials, but their role in the management of patients with heart failure is not yet established.

KEY POINT

- In patients with heart failure, each follow-up visit should include evaluation of current symptoms and functional capacity; assessment of volume status, electrolytes, and kidney function; and review of the patient's medication regimen for adequacy.

Bibliography

Yancy CW, Jessup M, Bozkurt B, Butler J, Casey DE Jr, Drazner MH, et al; American College of Cardiology Foundation; American Heart Association Task Force on Practice Guidelines. 2013 ACCF/AHA guideline for the management of heart failure: a report of the American College of Cardiology Foundation/American Heart Association Task Force on Practice Guidelines. J Am Coll Cardiol. 2013 Oct 15;62(16):e147-239. [PMID: 23747642]

Item 19   Answer: B

Educational Objective: Manage Wolff-Parkinson-White syndrome.

The most appropriate next step in management is an electrophysiology study. This young woman with a history of palpitations and paroxysms of dyspnea and lightheadedness likely has atrioventricular reciprocating tachycardia associated with an accessory pathway between the atria and ventricles. Accessory pathway conduction is often observed as preexcitation on electrocardiogram (ECG). Because of early ventricular activation over the accessory pathway, the PR interval is shortened, and the initial part of the QRS complex is slurred (delta wave) because of ventricular depolarization adjacent to the pathway. Wolff-Parkinson-White syndrome is characterized by preexcitation on ECG accompanied by symptoms consistent with tachycardia. Symptoms concerning for arrhythmia in a patient with Wolff-Parkinson-White syndrome should prompt referral to a cardiologist or an electrophysiologist. In these patients, it is also important to obtain an echocardiogram to exclude structural heart disease associated with accessory pathways, including Ebstein anomaly.

In this case, the patient's symptomatic episodes could be caused by supraventricular tachycardia (orthodromic or antidromic reciprocating tachycardia) or preexcited atrial fibrillation. A diagnostic electrophysiology study is indicated to uncover the cause of her palpitations and to determine her risk for sudden cardiac death. The electrophysiology procedure also affords the opportunity to ablate the accessory pathway and potentially cure the arrhythmia. The cure rate of catheter ablation is as high as 95% to 99% in patients with an uncomplicated accessory pathway.

Atenolol and verapamil are atrioventricular nodal blockers and may be unsafe if the patient has anterograde conduction down the accessory pathway during atrial fibrillation. These drugs promote rapid 1:1 conduction from the atria to the ventricles over the accessory pathway during atrial fibrillation, which can lead to very rapid ventricular rates and ventricular fibrillation.

Flecainide is an antiarrhythmic drug that is frequently used to treat paroxysmal atrial fibrillation and other arrhythmias. Flecainide is not indicated in this patient because the

type and mechanism of the arrhythmia are unknown. This patient requires risk stratification, which can be accomplished with an electrophysiology study. Furthermore, the age of the patient should be considered before antiarrhythmic therapy is initiated. Catheter ablation is preferred in young persons to avoid lifelong use of potentially toxic medications. This young woman may also wish to avoid these types of medications if she will be considering pregnancy in the future.

KEY POINT

- Patients suspected of having Wolff-Parkinson-White syndrome should undergo electrophysiology testing for risk stratification for sudden cardiac death.

Bibliography

Delacrétaz E. Clinical practice. Supraventricular tachycardia. N Engl J Med. 2006;354:1039-51. [PMID: 16525141]

Item 20   Answer: A

Educational Objective: Manage a patient with Marfan syndrome who is considering pregnancy.

The most appropriate management is to advise against pregnancy in this patient with Marfan syndrome and a dilated aorta. All women with Marfan syndrome have an increased risk for pregnancy-related aortic dissection and rupture. In women with Marfan syndrome and an ascending aortic diameter of 4.5 cm or greater, aortic repair surgery is recommended before pregnancy to reduce this risk. Some women with Marfan syndrome and an aortic diameter less than 4.5 cm, including those with rapid dilatation of the ascending aorta or a family history of aortic dissection, are at high risk for dissection during pregnancy and are counseled to have surgery before pregnancy. Generally, pregnancy is considered safe if the aortic diameter is smaller than 4.0 cm.

This patient is asymptomatic with normal left ventricular size and function and mild mitral regurgitation; therefore, she does not meet the criteria for mitral valve intervention. Although the mitral valve may warrant intervention at some point, this patient's dilated aorta is the major determinant of pregnancy risk.

Patients with Marfan syndrome who are considering pregnancy should have an aortic dimension smaller than 4.0 to 4.5 cm, with demonstrated stability for 6 months or longer. This patient does not meet these criteria, and repeat imaging demonstrating aortic stability will not provide reassurance about future pregnancy. Owing to the size of the aorta, this patient should be advised to avoid pregnancy and consider elective surgical repair. If she elects not to proceed with pregnancy or surgical repair at this time, repeat aortic root imaging should be performed in 6 months to confirm stability of the aortic dimensions.

Angiotensin receptor blockers, such as losartan, are considered second-line agents to β-blocker therapy for the control of hypertension and slowing aortic root expansion in patients with Marfan syndrome. Furthermore, ACE inhibitors and angiotensin receptor blockers are contraindicated during pregnancy because of fetal toxicity. Fetal exposure to these agents during the first trimester can cause central nervous system and cardiovascular malformations, and exposure during the second trimester can cause developmental malformations of the kidneys and genitourinary system.

KEY POINT

- Women with Marfan syndrome have an increased risk for pregnancy-related aortic dissection and rupture.

Bibliography

Regitz-Zagrosek V, Blomstrom Lundqvist C, Borghi C, Cifkova R, Ferreira R, Foidart JM, et al; European Society of Gynecology (ESG). ESC guidelines on the management of cardiovascular diseases during pregnancy: the Task Force on the Management of Cardiovascular Diseases during Pregnancy of the European Society of Cardiology (ESC). Eur Heart J. 2011;32:3147-97. [PMID: 21873418] doi:10.1093/eurheartj/ehr218

Item 21   Answer: D

Educational Objective: Diagnose a papillary fibroelastoma.

This patient's clinical history, physical examination findings, and echocardiographic features are most consistent with a papillary fibroelastoma (PFE). The echocardiographic images (shown) reveal a PFE (*arrows*) arising from the mitral valve. Most PFEs are small (averaging 12 mm × 9 mm), independently

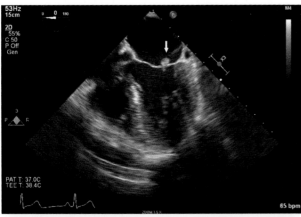

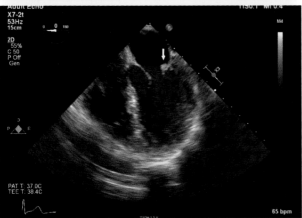

mobile, and attached to the endocardium by a stalk. They are more commonly associated with left-sided valves than right-sided valves or other endocardial surfaces. Patients may present with symptoms of embolism (including stroke or transient ischemic attack), angina, myocardial infarction, and peripheral embolization. PFE may also be discovered incidentally on echocardiogram. Surgery is indicated for symptomatic patients with PFE with acceptable operative risk. The treatment of asymptomatic patients with left heart PFE is controversial, although in one large case series, the risks for stroke and death were higher in patients who did not have surgery.

Bacterial endocarditis is less likely in this patient given the absence of constitutional symptoms, evidence of systemic inflammation, a predisposing valvular lesion, and risk factors for bacteremia (such as dental cleaning or injectable drug use).

Left atrial myxomas may cause cerebral embolic phenomena; however, most myxomas are substantially larger than fibroelastomas and are associated with obstructive symptoms and, in 10% to 15% of patients, an auscultatory "tumor plop." In 75% of cases, myxomas arise within the left atrium attached to the fossa ovalis, not valvular surfaces. Constitutional symptoms, such as fever, anorexia, and weight loss, related to tumor interleukin production may also be present.

Nonbacterial thrombotic endocarditis (NBTE), also known as verrucous, marantic, or Libman-Sacks endocarditis, is likely caused by endothelial injury in the presence of a hypercoagulable state. NBTE occurs on the atrial surface of the mitral valve, the ventricular side of the aortic valve, or both locations. Vegetations are typically small (<1 cm), broad based, and irregularly shaped (wart-like) and are most commonly associated with advanced malignancy or connective tissue disorders. This patient does not have evidence of a predisposing condition for NBTE, and the lesion does not have a wart-like or broad-based appearance.

KEY POINT

- Papillary fibroelastomas are small, independently mobile cardiac tumors that are typically attached to the left-sided valvular endocardium by a stalk; they may be associated with stroke, transient ischemic attack, angina, myocardial infarction, and peripheral embolization.

Bibliography

Val-Bernal JF, Mayorga M, Garijo MF, Val D, Nistal JF. Cardiac papillary fibroelastoma: retrospective clinicopathologic study of 17 tumors with resection at a single institution and literature review. Pathol Res Pract. 2013;209:208-14. [PMID: 23455367] doi:10.1016/j.prp.2013.02.001

Item 22   Answer: D

Educational Objective: Treat iron deficiency anemia in a patient with cyanotic congenital heart disease.

The most appropriate management is initiation of a short course of iron therapy for this patient with Eisenmenger syndrome and symptomatic postoperative anemia. Most patients with cyanosis have compensated erythrocytosis with stable hemoglobin levels. Iron deficiency and resultant microcytosis in these patients is often caused by inappropriate phlebotomy or blood loss. Correction of iron deficiency is associated with increased exercise capacity and improved quality of life. This patient's baseline hemoglobin level was greater than 18 g/dL (180 g/L). She developed preoperative anemia and subsequent perioperative anemia that has persisted and caused dyspnea and fatigue. Oral iron therapy often causes a rapid increase in erythrocyte mass and requires careful monitoring. Administration of ferrous sulfate or ferrous gluconate is recommended with repeat hemoglobin assessment in 7 to 10 days. Once the serum ferritin level or transferrin saturation is within the normal range, iron supplementation may be discontinued. It is important not to exceed the acceptable serum ferritin level. In the absence of dehydration, a hemoglobin level greater than 20 g/dL (200 g/L) and a hematocrit level greater than 65% are associated with hyperviscosity symptoms, such as headache, difficulty concentrating, weakness, and fatigue.

Erythropoietin is used primarily in patients with anemia related to kidney disease. Iron therapy, not erythropoietin, is recommended for patients with cyanotic cardiac disease with iron deficiency anemia. This patient with cyanotic congenital heart disease and relative anemia is likely to have an elevated erythropoietin level; erythropoietin therapy for this patient will be expensive, likely ineffective, and potentially dangerous.

Heart-lung transplantation is an option for end-stage cardiopulmonary disease in patients with Eisenmenger syndrome; however, it is not indicated without a trial of standard medical therapy with iron.

Limited data are available regarding the efficacy of epoprostenol in patients with Eisenmenger syndrome and pulmonary hypertension. Intravenous epoprostenol is typically avoided because of the risk for paradoxical embolism with continuous intravenous therapy in patients with an intracardiac right-to-left shunt. Oral, subcutaneous, and inhaled therapies are preferred. However, this patient's symptoms are likely the result of iron deficiency, and a trial of iron replacement is first-line therapy.

> **KEY POINT**
> - In patients with cyanotic conditions, such as Eisenmenger syndrome, iron deficiency is common, and short-term iron therapy will improve exercise capacity and quality of life.

Bibliography

Tay EL, Peset A, Papaphylactou M, Inuzuka R, Alonso-Gonzalez R, Giannakoulas G, et al. Replacement therapy for iron deficiency improves exercise capacity and quality of life in patients with cyanotic congenital heart disease and/or the Eisenmenger syndrome. Int J Cardiol. 2011;151:307-12. [PMID: 20580108] doi:10.1016/j.ijcard.2010.05.066

Item 23   Answer: B

Educational Objective: Treat ST-elevation myocardial infarction with thrombolytic therapy.

The most appropriate management of this patient with an acute inferior ST-elevation myocardial infarction (STEMI) is to administer full-dose reteplase. All patients who present with STEMI within 12 hours of symptom onset require prompt restoration of flow with primary percutaneous coronary intervention (PCI) or thrombolytic therapy. When a hospital is capable of performing primary PCI or the patient can be transferred from an index hospital to a PCI-capable center quickly (to achieve an expected first medical contact–to–device time of 120 minutes or less), primary PCI is the preferred treatment option. Primary PCI is associated with higher rates of vessel patency and improved overall survival compared with thrombolytic therapy. In this case, transfer time is prohibitively long, and the patient is best treated with immediate thrombolysis with reteplase. After administration of thrombolytic therapy, the patient should be transferred to a PCI-capable center for rescue PCI in case of thrombolytic failure or for nonemergent angiography before discharge.

Evidence supports the efficacy of fondaparinux and ticagrelor as antithrombotic therapies in the setting of STEMI; however, neither agent will likely result in lysis of a clot. These drugs remain adjuvant treatment to a primary thrombolytic strategy.

Half-dose thrombolytic therapy in combination with glycoprotein IIb/IIIa blockade does not offer any additional benefit compared with full-dose thrombolysis in patients with STEMI.

Nitroprusside is a powerful vasodilator and has no role in the management of STEMI. Venodilators, such as nitrates and nitroprusside, must be used with caution in the setting of inferior myocardial infarction because they may result in significant drops in systolic blood pressure, particularly when associated with right ventricular infarction.

> **KEY POINT**
> - Thrombolytic therapy is recommended for patients with ST-elevation myocardial infarction when symptom onset is within 12 hours and primary percutaneous coronary intervention is not available within 120 minutes of first medical contact.

Bibliography

O'Gara PT, Kushner FG, Ascheim DD, Casey DE Jr, Chung MK, de Lemos JA, et al; American College of Cardiology Foundation/American Heart Association Task Force on Practice Guidelines. 2013 ACCF/AHA guideline for the management of ST-elevation myocardial infarction: a report of the American College of Cardiology Foundation/American Heart Association Task Force on Practice Guidelines. Circulation. 2013;127:e362-425. [PMID: 23247304] doi:10.1161/CIR.0b013e3182742cf6

Item 24   Answer: C

Educational Objective: Diagnose peripheral artery disease in a patient with noncompressible arteries.

The most appropriate diagnostic test to perform next in this patient is a toe-brachial index. The diagnostic tool that is most frequently used to identify peripheral artery disease (PAD) is the ankle-brachial index (ABI). To calculate the ABI, the higher ankle pressure in each leg is divided by the higher brachial pressure. An ABI of 0.90 or lower establishes a diagnosis of PAD, whereas an ABI greater than 1.40 indicates the presence of calcified, noncompressible arteries in the lower extremities and is considered uninterpretable. In patients with an ABI greater than 1.40, an appropriate next step is to measure toe pressure or calculate a toe-brachial index (systolic great toe pressure divided by systolic brachial pressure). A great toe systolic pressure below 40 mm Hg or a toe-brachial index below 0.70 is consistent with PAD. Because this patient has a left ABI of 1.65, a toe-brachial index is indicated.

Exercise ABI testing is useful when patients have a borderline ABI (0.91-1.00) or normal ABI (1.00-1.40) and a high likelihood of PAD. The American Heart Association has proposed a postexercise ankle pressure decrease of more than 30 mm Hg or a postexercise ABI decrease of more than 20% as a diagnostic criterion for PAD. Other organizations have proposed a postexercise ABI of less than 0.90 and/or a 30-mm Hg drop in ankle pressure after exercise. This patient's resting ABI value is greater than 1.40; therefore, exercise ABI is not indicated to diagnose PAD.

CT angiography and magnetic resonance angiography are often reserved for planning endovascular or surgical revascularization rather than for diagnosis of PAD.

In patients with venous leg ulcers, venous duplex ultrasonography is indicated to evaluate for chronic venous insufficiency and deep vein thrombosis (acute or chronic). The location of the ulceration and the lack of other findings consistent with venous disease make that diagnosis unlikely, and venous duplex ultrasonography is therefore unnecessary.

KEY POINT

- In patients with an ankle-brachial index greater than 1.40, a toe-brachial index may be used to diagnose peripheral artery disease.

Bibliography

Aboyans V, Criqui MH, Abraham P, Allison MA, Creager MA, Diehm C, et al; American Heart Association Council on Peripheral Vascular Disease. Measurement and interpretation of the ankle-brachial index: a scientific statement from the American Heart Association. Circulation. 2012;126:2890-909. [PMID: 23159553] doi:10.1161/CIR.0b013e318276fbcb

Item 25   Answer: B

Educational Objective: Treat a patient with infective endocarditis and refractory bacteremia with cardiac valve surgery.

The most appropriate next step in management is cardiac valve surgery. This patient has infective endocarditis with refractory bacteremia. For patients such as this one, cardiac surgery is the most appropriate next step when there is evidence of persistent infection lasting longer than 5 to 7 days while the patient is receiving appropriate antimicrobial therapy. Cardiac surgery also is recommended for patients with

infective endocarditis who have the following: symptomatic heart failure; left-sided involvement with *Staphylococcus aureus*, fungal infections, or highly resistant organisms; associated complications, such as heart block, annular or aortic abscess, or destructive penetrating lesions; or prosthetic valve infective endocarditis and relapsing infection.

Cardiac catheterization is not indicated in this patient and may increase the risk for embolization of vegetation or worsen hemodynamic status. Cardiac catheterization before planned cardiac surgery is indicated in patients with risk factors for coronary artery disease, which are not present in this patient.

The most common indications for intervention with an intra-aortic balloon pump are cardiogenic shock unresponsive to other interventions and acute mitral regurgitation. This patient does not have any indication for an intra-aortic balloon pump. Additionally, an intra-aortic balloon pump is contraindicated in the presence of significant aortic regurgitation, as seen in this patient, because it will increase the volume of regurgitant blood flow.

Surgical intervention should not be delayed for observation of the patient's response to another antibiotic once surgical indications have been met. In this patient, switching to another antibiotic without immediate surgical intervention may result in further decompensation of the patient's clinical status and an increased operative risk for intervention at a later time.

KEY POINT

- For patients with infective endocarditis, cardiac surgery is indicated for persistent infection lasting longer than 5 to 7 days while on appropriate antimicrobial therapy; symptomatic heart failure; left-sided involvement with *Staphylococcus aureus*, fungal infections, or highly resistant organisms; complications such as heart block, annular or aortic abscess, or destructive penetrating lesions; and prosthetic valve infective endocarditis and relapsing infection.

Bibliography

Baddour LM, Wilson WR, Bayer AS, Fowler VG Jr, Tleyjeh IM, Rybak MJ, et al; American Heart Association Committee on Rheumatic Fever, Endocarditis, and Kawasaki Disease of the Council on Cardiovascular Disease in the Young, Council on Clinical Cardiology, Council on Cardiovascular Surgery and Anesthesia, and Stroke Council. Infective endocarditis in adults: diagnosis, antimicrobial therapy, and management of complications: a scientific statement for healthcare professionals from the American Heart Association. Circulation. 2015;132:1435-86. [PMID: 26373316] doi:10.1161/CIR.0000000000000296

Item 26   Answer: E

Educational Objective: Recognize the potential for underestimation of cardiovascular risk in patients with HIV infection.

This patient's HIV status will contribute most to the underestimation of his risk for atherosclerotic cardiovascular disease (ASCVD). This young patient has both traditional risk factors (hypertension and smoking) and a nontraditional risk factor (HIV) for ASCVD, which is defined as coronary death or nonfatal myocardial infarction, or fatal or nonfatal stroke. The Pooled Cohort Equations are a risk assessment instrument developed from multiple community-based cohorts; their use as a primary risk assessment tool was recommended in the 2013 American College of Cardiology/American Heart Association (ACC/AHA) Guideline on Assessment of Cardiovascular Risk. The ACC/AHA ASCVD risk calculator based on the Pooled Cohort Equations includes age, sex, race, total and HDL cholesterol levels, systolic blood pressure, blood pressure–lowering medication use, presence of diabetes mellitus, and smoking status. With use of this method of calculating risk, a 10-year risk for ASCVD below 5% is considered low risk, 5% to below 7.5% is classified as intermediate risk, and 7.5% or higher is designated as high risk. This patient's calculated 10-year ASCVD risk is 6.2%.

Large observational studies have demonstrated a 1.5- to 2-fold increase in the risk for ASCVD among patients with HIV infection. The increased risk for ASCVD in HIV-infected patients is likely the result of interactions among the viral infection, host factors, traditional risk factors, and therapies for HIV. Traditional risk models, including the ACC/AHA ASCVD risk calculator based on the Pooled Cohort Equations, underestimate the risk for ASCVD in patients with HIV. Alternative risk models, including one based on the D:A:D (Data Collection on Adverse events of Anti-HIV Drugs) study, have been developed, but they lack validation and have not been widely adopted.

This patient's age, blood pressure, use of antihypertensive medications, and HDL cholesterol level are accounted for in the ACC/AHA ASCVD risk calculator and are not factors responsible for underestimating his ASCVD risk.

KEY POINT

- In patients with HIV infection, there is a 1.5- to 2-fold increased risk for coronary artery disease.

Bibliography
Vachiat A, McCutcheon K, Tsabedze N, Zachariah D, Manga P. HIV and ischemic heart disease. J Am Coll Cardiol. 2017 Jan 3;69(1):73-82. [PMID: 28057253.]

Item 27   Answer: C

Educational Objective: Evaluate for coronary artery disease with exercise electrocardiography.

The most appropriate test to establish a diagnosis of coronary artery disease (CAD) is exercise electrocardiographic (ECG) stress testing. This patient with cardiovascular risk factors (hypertension, hyperlipidemia) is exhibiting typical angina, which has the following characteristics: (1) substernal chest pain or discomfort that (2) is provoked by exertion or emotional stress and (3) is relieved by rest and/or nitroglycerin. Given her age, sex, and symptoms, she has an intermediate pretest probability of CAD (73%) and should undergo stress testing. In patients with a normal baseline ECG and the ability to exercise, exercise ECG is recommended as the initial test

of choice. Exercise ECG can identify flow-limiting lesions indicative of CAD and also further risk stratify this patient. The additional prognostic information available with exercise, including functional capacity and heart rate and blood pressure response, can be used in prediction models, such as the Duke Treadmill Score, which uses several factors (development of symptoms, degree of ST-segment depression, and exercise duration) to provide incremental prognostic information for 5-year mortality risk. Heart rate recovery is another powerful predictor; patients with a heart rate drop of less than 12/min in the first minute after cessation of exercise have a higher mortality rate.

There is no indication for stress testing with additional imaging, such as adenosine single-photon emission CT or stress echocardiography, given this patient's normal baseline ECG findings. If the baseline ECG findings were uninterpretable or the exercise ECG stress test was indeterminate, additional testing with imaging would be warranted.

Coronary artery calcium scoring would identify the presence of CAD, but it would not detect a flow-limiting lesion as the cause of this patient's symptoms. Additionally, the absence of calcification during coronary artery calcium scoring does not exclude the presence of noncalcified plaque.

KEY POINT

- In patients with an intermediate probability of obstructive coronary artery disease, a normal baseline electrocardiogram, and the ability to exercise, exercise electrocardiography is recommended as the initial test of choice.

Bibliography
Mieres JH, Gulati M, Bairey Merz N, Berman DS, Gerber TC, Hayes SN, et al; American Heart Association Cardiac Imaging Committee of the Council on Clinical Cardiology. Role of noninvasive testing in the clinical evaluation of women with suspected ischemic heart disease: a consensus statement from the American Heart Association. Circulation. 2014;130:350-79. [PMID: 25047587] doi:10.1161/CIR.0000000000000061

Item 28   Answer: A

Educational Objective: Treat a patient with heart failure and evidence of conduction delay.

The most appropriate treatment is the addition of carvedilol. This patient with heart failure with reduced ejection fraction has New York Heart Association functional class III symptoms. Guideline-directed medical therapy for heart failure includes treatment with an ACE inhibitor, β-blocker (specifically, metoprolol succinate, carvedilol, or bisoprolol), and an aldosterone antagonist. β-Blockers improve remodeling, increase ejection fraction, and reduce hospitalization and mortality when added to an ACE inhibitor and diuretic therapy. This patient is not taking a β-blocker; therefore, the most important intervention would be initiation of carvedilol to optimize the patient's medical therapy.

In patients with chronic symptomatic heart failure and left ventricular ejection fraction less than or equal to 35% who are in sinus rhythm and taking maximally tolerated doses of a β-blocker, ivabradine reduces heart failure–associated hospitalizations and the combined endpoint of mortality and heart failure hospitalization. Because this patient is not taking a β-blocker, ivabradine is not indicated.

Cardiac resynchronization therapy (CRT) is indicated for primary prevention of sudden cardiac death and to reduce the risk for hospitalization and death in patients with heart failure who have dyssynchrony. Criteria for CRT include an ejection fraction of less than or equal to 35%, New York Heart Association functional class II to IV heart failure symptoms despite guideline-directed medical therapy, sinus rhythm, and left bundle branch block with a QRS complex of 150 ms or greater. This patient fulfills the echocardiographic and electrocardiographic criteria for CRT, and if he continues to have refractory heart failure despite guideline-directed medical therapy for 90 days, he would be a candidate for CRT.

An ICD would protect this patient against sudden cardiac death; however, medical therapy is necessary first to alleviate his heart failure symptoms and improve his functional status. Many patients with new-onset heart failure experience significant improvements in ejection fraction with medical therapy and may not require or benefit from ICD placement.

KEY POINT

- Patients with left ventricular dysfunction due to ischemic cardiomyopathy, left bundle branch block, and heart failure symptoms should receive guideline-directed medical therapy before initiation of device therapy.

Bibliography

Epstein AE, DiMarco JP, Ellenbogen KA, Estes NA 3rd, Freedman RA, Gettes LS, et al; American College of Cardiology Foundation. 2012 ACCF/AHA/HRS focused update incorporated into the ACCF/AHA/HRS 2008 guidelines for device-based therapy of cardiac rhythm abnormalities: a report of the American College of Cardiology Foundation/American Heart Association Task Force on Practice Guidelines and the Heart Rhythm Society. J Am Coll Cardiol. 2013;61:e6-75. [PMID: 23265327] doi:10.1016/j.jacc.2012.11.007

Item 29   Answer: D

Educational Objective: Diagnose primary restrictive cardiomyopathy.

The most likely diagnosis is primary restrictive cardiomyopathy. Patients with constrictive pericarditis and restrictive cardiomyopathy present with similar symptoms and findings on echocardiography, and differentiation is an essential first step in diagnosis. In this patient, several features favor restrictive physiology: the elevated B-type natriuretic peptide level (often <100 pg/mL [100 ng/L] in constrictive pericarditis), the presence of severe pulmonary hypertension, the absence of pericardial thickening on cardiac magnetic resonance imaging, and the presence of delayed enhancement of myocardium consistent with myocardial fibrosis on cardiac magnetic resonance imaging. This patient's simultaneous right and left ventricular hemodynamic recordings demonstrate concordant rise and fall of systolic pressures with respiration. In

constriction, an inverse relationship or discordance is present because of ventricular interdependence: right ventricular systolic pressure rises during inspiration coupled with a simultaneous decrease in left ventricular systolic pressure.

Fabry disease is a lysosomal storage disorder. Clinical manifestations begin in childhood and progress in an orderly fashion, with up to 70% of the following manifestations appearing by age 40 years: neuropathic pain, telangiectasias and angiokeratomas, and proteinuria and chronic kidney disease. The most common cardiac complications are concentric left ventricular hypertrophy, heart failure, coronary artery disease, left-sided valvular dysfunction, and conduction abnormalities. This patient's late onset of cardiac symptoms and lack of other findings make Fabry disease unlikely.

Although wall thickness may be normal in patients with hemochromatosis, the left ventricle is usually dilated, and the serum ferritin level would be greatly elevated in a patient with visceral involvement.

KEY POINT

- Restrictive cardiomyopathy is distinguished from constrictive pericarditis by an elevated B-type natriuretic peptide level and concordant rise and fall of left and right systolic pressures with respiration.

Bibliography

Garcia MJ. Constrictive pericarditis versus restrictive cardiomyopathy? J Am Coll Cardiol. 2016;67:2061-76. [PMID: 27126534] doi:10.1016/j.jacc.2016.01.076

Item 30   Answer: C

Educational Objective: Treat acute descending aortic dissection.

The most appropriate initial step in the management of this patient is initiation of medical therapy. Patients with type B acute aortic dissection without evidence of cardiogenic shock should be initially treated with medical therapy to control heart rate and reduce blood pressure. Intravenous β-blockers are first-line treatment, and sodium nitroprusside can be added if hypertension does not completely respond to β-blocker therapy. Current guidelines recommend reducing systolic blood pressure to 120 mm Hg or less in the first hour in patients with aortic dissection. Pain control is best accomplished with intravenous opioids. In patients with ascending aortic dissection (type A aortic dissection), intramural aortic hematoma, or descending aortic dissection (type B aortic dissection) with complications, immediate repair is warranted. Complications are defined as refractory pain, rapid aneurysmal expansion, rupture, or malperfusion syndrome. This patient has a type B aortic dissection arising just distal to the origin of the left subclavian artery with no evidence of complications. Therefore, medical therapy is the most appropriate treatment.

Endovascular stenting can be used to treat patients with descending aortic aneurysms; however, there is scant evidence to support this as an initial treatment option for

CONT.

aneurysm with dissection. After medical stabilization, thoracic endovascular aortic repair (TEVAR) with stent grafting can be used; typical indications include descending aortic aneurysm diameter greater than 6.0 cm, rapid growth (>0.5 cm/year), or end-organ damage. TEVAR has the advantage over surgical operation of lower morbidity and shorter hospital stay, although there may be complications, including stroke, spinal ischemia, and aortic graft endoleaks. This patient should be treated with stent implantation only after medical stabilization.

Open surgical repair of the descending aorta is not recommended in patients with uncomplicated type B aortic dissection because of high rates of morbidity (such as paraplegia) and mortality. This patient has no signs or symptoms of complications that would prompt immediate surgical repair.

Repeat CT angiography at 12 hours is not indicated unless the patient does not stabilize with medical therapy. Serial imaging (usually magnetic resonance angiography) is typically performed in asymptomatic patients at the time of discharge and then periodically in patients who do not have an indication for aneurysmal repair to screen for extension or recurrence of the dissection, aneurysm formation, and leakage.

KEY POINT

- Patients with uncomplicated type B aortic dissection may be initially treated with medical therapy, including β-blockers, sodium nitroprusside, and opioids.

Bibliography

Mussa FF, Horton JD, Moridzadeh R, Nicholson J, Trimarchi S, Eagle KA. Acute aortic dissection and intramural hematoma: a systematic review. JAMA. 2016;316:754-63. [PMID: 27533160] doi:10.1001/jama.2016.10026

Item 31   Answer: C

Educational Objective: Treat cardiac tamponade.

The most appropriate management is pericardiocentesis. This patient is taking minoxidil and hydralazine, both of which may be associated with the development of a pericardial effusion (PE). Tamponade occurs when intrapericardial pressure exceeds diastolic intracardiac pressures, which leads to compression of cardiac chambers and limits diastolic filling, stroke volume, and cardiac output, with a simultaneous increase in pulmonary capillary wedge pressure that leads to pulmonary edema. Definitive treatment of cardiac tamponade is pericardiocentesis or surgical pericardial drainage. In hemodynamically unstable patients, intravenous normal saline is used to stabilize the patient as a temporizing measure or bridge to definitive therapy. Despite the evidence of fluid overload, intravenous volume loading can help maintain or increase cardiac output. Low systolic blood pressure (<100 mm Hg) is the most readily accessible clinical finding that is predictive of a favorable response to volume loading.

Hemodialysis will decrease right heart filling pressure but not intrapericardial pressure, resulting in further compression of the intracardiac chamber and reduction in cardiac output. Similarly, intravenous loop diuretics or agents that actively dilate capacitance vessels, such as nitroglycerin, should be avoided because they will result in a relative increase in intrapericardial pressure to intracardiac pressure and further impair cardiac output.

Right heart catheterization is not typically performed in the diagnosis of cardiac tamponade. Echocardiography readily detects pericardial effusions and is the primary modality for diagnosing cardiac tamponade. Echocardiographic signs of cardiac tamponade include diastolic collapse of the right atrium and right ventricle, ventricular septal shifting with respiration, and enlargement of the inferior vena cava. An apical four-chamber echocardiographic view demonstrating PE with diastolic inversion (*arrow*) of the right atrium (RA) free wall is shown. With Doppler echocardiography, respiratory variation in mitral inflow can be detected early in the evolution of tamponade. In the pulsed-wave Doppler image, there is a significant and reproducible decrease (>25%) in passive diastolic flow during inspiration, which reflects enhanced ventricular interdependence. Changes in mitral inflow are highly sensitive and may precede changes in cardiac output, blood pressure, and other echocardiographic evidence of tamponade.

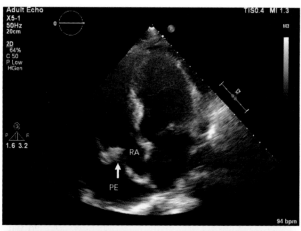

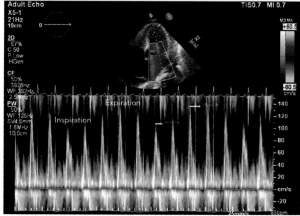

KEY POINT

- Definitive treatment of cardiac tamponade is pericardiocentesis or surgical pericardial drainage.

Bibliography

Adler Y, Charron P, Imazio M, Badano L, Barón-Esquivias G, Bogaert J, et al; European Society of Cardiology (ESC). 2015 ESC guidelines for the diagnosis and management of pericardial diseases: the Task Force for the Diagnosis and Management of Pericardial Diseases of the European Society of Cardiology (ESC) endorsed by: The European Association for Cardio-Thoracic Surgery (EACTS). Eur Heart J. 2015;36:2921-64. [PMID: 26320112] doi:10.1093/eurheartj/ehv318

Item 32   Answer: D

Educational Objective: Diagnose ticagrelor-related dyspnea.

Ticagrelor is the most likely cause of dyspnea in this patient with a normal physical examination, no electrocardiographic changes, and normal findings on imaging studies. Ticagrelor is a $P2Y_{12}$ inhibitor that may be used as a component of dual antiplatelet therapy in select patients with coronary artery disease, including those treated with percutaneous coronary intervention. Dyspnea is a well-recognized side effect of ticagrelor therapy. In clinical trials, 15% to 20% of patients taking ticagrelor experienced dyspnea, although only 5% to 7% required cessation of the drug. In most cases, ticagrelor-mediated dyspnea is self-limited, but it often results in additional testing.

Heart failure can complicate myocardial infarction. In this case, however, the normal findings on physical examination, chest radiograph, and echocardiogram make heart failure an unlikely cause of the patient's symptoms.

In patients with shortness of breath after myocardial infarction, it is important to rule out complications of recent percutaneous coronary intervention, such as in-stent stenosis and stent thrombosis. Patients with in-stent restenosis will exhibit recurrent signs and symptoms of ischemia, including chest pain and dyspnea; however, in-stent restenosis develops months to years after stent implantation, not weeks. In contrast to in-stent restenosis, stent thrombosis is usually a fulminant event, commonly manifesting as acute myocardial infarction or death. The timing and persistent nature of this patient's symptoms, coupled with the unchanged electrocardiographic findings, rule out stent thrombosis as a cause of this patient's symptoms.

Ventricular septal defect (VSD) resulting from rupture of the intraventricular septum is a rare complication of transmural infarction involving the right coronary artery (in which the VSD tends to affect the basal inferior septum) or the left anterior descending artery (in which the VSD is usually located within the apical septum). VSDs typically occur within 3 to 5 days of STEMI presentation. Patients present with worsening heart failure and shock, and a harsh holosystolic murmur may be heard at the left lower sternal border. A small NSTEMI would not result in a VSD, and the laboratory and physical examination findings rule out this diagnosis.

KEY POINT

- Dyspnea is a well-recognized and often self-limited side effect of ticagrelor therapy.

Bibliography

Bonaca MP, Bhatt DL, Cohen M, Steg PG, Storey RF, Jensen EC, et al; PEGASUS-TIMI 54 Steering Committee and Investigators. Long-term use of ticagrelor in patients with prior myocardial infarction. N Engl J Med. 2015;372:1791-800. [PMID: 25773268] doi:10.1056/NEJMoa1500857

Item 33   Answer: D

Educational Objective: Diagnose takotsubo cardiomyopathy.

Takotsubo cardiomyopathy is the most likely diagnosis. This previously healthy patient has symptoms and findings suggestive of an acute coronary syndrome. Cardiac catheterization demonstrates normal coronary arteries and wall motion abnormalities that do not follow one vascular territory, findings that are consistent with takotsubo cardiomyopathy. Takotsubo cardiomyopathy, or stress-induced cardiomyopathy, is a heart failure syndrome that typically occurs in older women and is usually precipitated by a stressful physical or emotional event, such as the death of a loved one, sudden surprise, or other acute stressors. It is associated with electrocardiographic changes suggestive of an acute myocardial infarction or a moderate increase in troponin levels, wall motion changes that extend beyond the territory of a single coronary artery, and normal or near-normal coronary arteries (<50% stenosis). Patients with a drop in ejection fraction should be treated with standard heart failure medications and typically have rapid recovery of left ventricular function.

Acute myocarditis usually presents with heart failure symptoms that develop over a few days to weeks. Occasionally, patients have symptoms for several months before heart failure is discovered. The classic presentation of viral myocarditis includes a viral prodrome with fever, myalgia, and upper respiratory tract symptoms. Patients present with dyspnea, chest pain, and arrhythmias. Electrocardiographic abnormalities are often present, along with evidence of myocardial damage with persistently elevated troponin levels. Acute-onset symptoms following an emotional event and apical ballooning on left ventriculography are not seen in acute myocarditis.

Giant cell myocarditis is an acute, rapidly progressive form of myocarditis associated with ventricular arrhythmias and progressive cardiac dysfunction despite medical therapy. This process usually occurs in persons younger than 40 years. The underlying mechanism is unknown but is thought to be autoimmune in origin. This patient's age and presentation are not compatible with giant cell myocarditis.

Tachycardia-induced cardiomyopathy is related to prolonged tachycardia or frequent premature ventricular contractions. Patients usually have findings related to the tachyarrhythmia (for example, palpitations) and heart failure. This patient's acute presentation is inconsistent with tachycardia-induced cardiomyopathy.

KEY POINT

- Takotsubo cardiomyopathy is a syndrome of reversible ventricular systolic dysfunction that is usually precipitated by an acute emotional or physiologic stressor; the hallmark is wall motion abnormalities that extend beyond a single coronary territory, identified by echocardiography or other imaging studies.

Bibliography

Sharkey SW. A clinical perspective of the takotsubo syndrome. Heart Fail Clin. 2016;12:507-20. [PMID: 27638021] doi:10.1016/j.hfc.2016.06.003

Item 34   Answer: C

Educational Objective: Treat symptomatic severe pulmonary valve stenosis.

Balloon valvuloplasty is the most appropriate management of this patient. The palpable, late-peaking systolic murmur located at the second left intercostal space; absence of an ejection click; and features of right ventricular pressure overload suggest severe pulmonary valve stenosis. The echocardiogram confirms the presence of severe pulmonary valve stenosis with a peak systolic gradient of 65 mm Hg and mean systolic gradient of 50 mm Hg. Balloon valvuloplasty is recommended for symptomatic patients with appropriate valve morphology who have a peak Doppler gradient of greater than 50 mm Hg or a mean gradient greater than 30 mm Hg and favorable valve characteristics for percutaneous intervention.

Patients with pulmonary valve stenosis without a history of endocarditis or pulmonary valve replacement do not require endocarditis prophylaxis.

Exercise stress testing could help determine whether the patient has exercise limitations related to her pulmonary valve stenosis; however, the results would not change the recommendation for intervention.

Surgical pulmonary valve replacement should be considered when the valve is dysplastic or when more than moderate coexisting pulmonary valve regurgitation, a small annulus, severe subvalvar or supravalvar pulmonary valve stenosis, or another cardiac lesion that requires operative intervention is present. It is not the preferred treatment for this patient who has appropriate valve morphology for balloon valvuloplasty.

KEY POINT

- Balloon valvuloplasty is recommended for patients with symptomatic pulmonary valve stenosis who have appropriate valve morphology, a peak Doppler gradient of greater than 50 mm Hg or a mean gradient greater than 30 mm Hg, and valve characteristics favorable for percutaneous intervention.

Bibliography

Warnes CA, Williams RG, Bashore TM, Child JS, Connolly HM, Dearani JA, et al; American College of Cardiology. ACC/AHA 2008 guidelines for the management of adults with congenital heart disease: a report of the American College of Cardiology/American Heart Association Task Force on Practice Guidelines (Writing Committee to Develop Guidelines on the Management of Adults With Congenital Heart Disease). Developed in Collaboration With the American Society of Echocardiography, Heart Rhythm Society, International Society for Adult Congenital Heart Disease, Society for Cardiovascular Angiography and Interventions, and Society of Thoracic Surgeons. J Am Coll Cardiol. 2008;52:e143-263. [PMID: 19038677] doi:10.1016/j.jacc.2008.10.001

Item 35   Answer: C

Educational Objective: Evaluate for coronary artery disease with coronary CT angiography in a patient with COPD.

Coronary CT angiography (CTA) is the most appropriate diagnostic test to perform next. This patient with an intermediate pretest probability of coronary artery disease (CAD) has chest pain without evidence of acute coronary syndrome, and he should undergo risk stratification. Because his baseline electrocardiogram (ECG) has evidence of left ventricular hypertrophy with repolarization abnormalities, which limits the ability to interpret exercise ECG findings, stress testing with adjunctive imaging or anatomic assessment for CAD is indicated. Coronary CTA is a noninvasive anatomic imaging study to evaluate for obstructive CAD. In the PROMISE trial, which compared coronary CTA with functional stress testing among patients with an intermediate pretest probability for CAD, the 2-year composite outcome (death, myocardial infarction, hospitalization for unstable angina, or major procedural complication) was similarly low with both types of diagnostic testing.

Vasodilators, such as regadenoson or adenosine, produce hyperemia and a flow disparity between myocardium supplied by unobstructed vessels and myocardium supplied by the stenotic vessel (in which the distal vasculature is already maximally dilated). In addition to identifying the presence of disease, perfusion imaging can define the location and extent of reduced perfusion and provide additional prognostic information. Single-photon emission CT with the vasodilator adenosine can be performed in patients with underlying reactive airways disease but should be avoided in patients who are actively wheezing, such as this one. The newer selective adenosine A_{2A} receptor agonists are associated with less bronchospasm; however, bronchospasm may still occur as a result of some activation of the A_{2B} and A_3 receptors.

Coronary angiography is an invasive test that carries significant risks. It should be considered in patients who have a high pretest probability for obstructive CAD, including symptomatic patients with abnormal findings on noninvasive testing for CAD or patients with an acute coronary syndrome.

KEY POINT

- Baseline electrocardiogram (ECG) abnormalities that limit the ability to interpret exercise ECG findings are an indication for stress testing with adjunctive imaging or anatomic assessment of coronary arteries.

Bibliography
Douglas PS, Hoffmann U, Patel MR, Mark DB, Al-Khalidi HR, Cavanaugh B, et al; PROMISE Investigators. Outcomes of anatomical versus functional testing for coronary artery disease. N Engl J Med. 2015 Apr 2;372(14):1291-300. [PMID: 25773919]

Item 36   Answer: C
Educational Objective: Evaluate sinus bradycardia.

Exercise treadmill stress testing is the most appropriate next step in management. Sinus bradycardia (sinus rhythm with a heart rate <60/min) may be appropriate in several situations, including in trained athletes or during sleep, when the heart rate may fall as low as 30/min. The most common intrinsic cause of inappropriate or pathologic sinus bradycardia (sinus node dysfunction) is age-related myocardial fibrosis in the vicinity of the sinus node. The most common extrinsic cause of sinus bradycardia is medication use. This young patient has asymptomatic bradycardia and chest pain atypical for cardiac ischemia. However, because of her history of occasional lightheadedness with exercise, this patient should undergo treadmill stress testing to evaluate her heart rate response to exercise (chronotropy) and further exclude symptomatic bradycardia.

Despite the pleuritic component to this patient's chest pain, she has no respiratory distress, has normal oxygen saturation, and can exercise without difficulty. Therefore, CT of the chest to exclude pulmonary embolism is not appropriate.

The utility of any diagnostic test should be interpreted in the context of the pretest likelihood of disease. Patients with a low probability of coronary artery disease, such as younger patients with atypical or nonanginal chest pain, have a higher incidence of false-positive test results and may undergo unnecessary testing without changing patient outcomes. Given this patient's extremely low pretest probability for coronary artery disease, coronary angiography is not indicated. Additionally, if this patient had an intermediate probability of coronary artery disease, noninvasive testing would be performed before angiography.

Pacemakers are indicated in patients with symptomatic bradycardia in the absence of a reversible cause. The decision to implant a pacemaker in this patient should be delayed until after the exercise stress test to ascertain whether she is truly asymptomatic.

KEY POINT
- In patients with sinus bradycardia and equivocal symptoms, exercise stress testing may be used to assess for chronotropic incompetence and determine suitability for pacemaker placement.

Bibliography
Epstein AE, DiMarco JP, Ellenbogen KA, Estes NA 3rd, Freedman RA, Gettes LS, et al; American College of Cardiology Foundation. 2012 ACCF/AHA/HRS focused update incorporated into the ACCF/AHA/HRS 2008 guidelines for device-based therapy of cardiac rhythm abnormalities: a report of the American College of Cardiology Foundation/American Heart Association Task Force on Practice Guidelines and the Heart Rhythm Society. J Am Coll Cardiol. 2013;61:e6-75. [PMID: 23265327] doi:10.1016/j.jacc.2012.11.007

Item 37   Answer: B
Educational Objective: Treat hypertension during pregnancy.

In this pregnant patient, labetalol is the most appropriate treatment to achieve blood pressure control. Hypertension diagnosed before the 20th week of gestation is most consistent with a new diagnosis of chronic hypertension rather than preeclampsia. Pharmacologic treatment of chronic hypertension in pregnancy is recommended to achieve the goal of limiting maternal end-organ damage; there is no evidence that blood pressure control during pregnancy will prevent preeclampsia. The definitive threshold for treatment of chronic hypertension in pregnancy remains controversial. A 2013 guideline published by the American College of Obstetricians and Gynecologists made a strong recommendation for initiation of pharmacologic therapy for pregnant women with persistent chronic hypertension at a systolic blood pressure of 160 mm Hg or higher or a diastolic blood pressure of 105 mm Hg or higher. However, other guidelines, including one from the European Society of Cardiology, continue to recommend initiation of pharmacologic therapy at a systolic blood pressure of 150 mm Hg or higher or a diastolic blood pressure of 95 mm Hg or higher in women without symptoms or evidence of end-organ damage due to hypertension. Although all antihypertensive agents cross the placenta, methyldopa and labetalol appear to be the safest antihypertensive agents in pregnant women.

Diet and weight loss should be used in conjunction with pharmacologic therapy in this patient; however, nonpharmacologic strategies alone are insufficient in a patient with hypertension of this magnitude. Foregoing pharmacologic treatment of chronic hypertension may result in maternal end-organ damage.

ACE inhibitors (such as lisinopril), angiotensin receptor blockers (such as losartan), spironolactone, and direct renin inhibitors (aliskiren) are teratogenic and are therefore contraindicated during pregnancy. During the first trimester, these agents can cause central nervous system and cardiovascular malformations in the fetus. Second-trimester exposure can cause developmental malformations of the kidneys and genitourinary system.

KEY POINT
- Labetalol and methyldopa are the agents of choice in treating pregnant patients with hypertension.

Bibliography
Regitz-Zagrosek V, Blomstrom Lundqvist C, Borghi C, Cifkova R, Ferreira R, Foidart JM, et al; European Society of Gynecology (ESG). ESC guidelines on the management of cardiovascular diseases during pregnancy: the Task Force on the Management of Cardiovascular Diseases during Pregnancy of the European Society of Cardiology (ESC). Eur Heart J. 2011;32:3147-97. [PMID: 21873418] doi:10.1093/eurheartj/ehr218

Answers and Critiques

Item 38   Answer: B

Educational Objective: Manage a patient with severe mitral regurgitation with appropriate surveillance.

In the absence of symptoms, the most appropriate timing for this patient's next clinical evaluation is in 6 to 12 months. Abnormalities in any of the structures of the mitral valve apparatus, including anterior and posterior mitral leaflets, the annulus, the papillary muscles, and the chordae tendineae, can result in mitral regurgitation. Organic, or primary, mitral regurgitation refers to processes involving the leaflets, such as mitral valve prolapse, myxomatous degeneration (the abnormal accumulation of proteoglycans), collagen vascular disease, and infective endocarditis. Processes that affect the support structures, such as coronary artery disease and left ventricular remodeling in the setting of left ventricular dysfunction, result in functional, or secondary, mitral regurgitation. This patient has asymptomatic severe mitral regurgitation resulting from myxomatous degeneration of the mitral valve with preserved left ventricular function. Surgical treatment with repair of the mitral valve is indicated for chronic severe primary mitral regurgitation in (1) symptomatic patients with left ventricular ejection fraction greater than 30%, (2) asymptomatic patients with left ventricular dysfunction (left ventricular ejection fraction of 30%-60% and/or left ventricular end-systolic diameter ≥40 mm), and (3) patients undergoing another cardiac surgical procedure. Mitral valve repair should also be considered in asymptomatic patients with chronic severe primary mitral regurgitation who have new-onset atrial fibrillation or pulmonary hypertension (pulmonary artery systolic pressure >50 mm Hg). Notably, recent studies have suggested a potential mortality benefit of early surgery for patients with asymptomatic severe mitral regurgitation with preserved left ventricular function when the operative risk is low. Therefore, consideration of early surgery, even in the absence of symptoms or an abnormal left ventricle, is appropriate in select candidates and should involve shared decision making with the patient. In this patient who has chosen to defer early surgery, clinical and echocardiographic surveillance is recommended, with follow-up every 6 to 12 months.

KEY POINT

- In patients with asymptomatic severe mitral regurgitation with preserved left ventricular function who do not have an indication for surgery, clinical and echocardiographic surveillance every 6 to 12 months is recommended.

Bibliography

Nishimura RA, Otto CM, Bonow RO, Carabello BA, Erwin JP 3rd, Fleisher LA, et al. 2017 AHA/ACC focused update of the 2014 AHA/ACC guideline for the management of patients with valvular heart disease: a report of the American College of Cardiology/American Heart Association Task Force on Clinical Practice Guidelines. Circulation. 2017;135:e1159-e1195. [PMID: 28298458] doi:10.1161/CIR.0000000000000503

Item 39   Answer: B

Educational Objective: Treat asymptomatic lower extremity peripheral artery disease.

In this patient with asymptomatic peripheral artery disease (PAD) and acute coronary syndrome treated with percutaneous coronary intervention, the most appropriate next step in management is cardiac rehabilitation. Cardiac rehabilitation is indicated in all patients after hospitalization for acute coronary syndrome and percutaneous coronary intervention. In some patients, exercise can provoke symptoms of intermittent claudication; however, the presence of PAD is not a contraindication to cardiac rehabilitation.

Cilostazol, a phosphodiesterase inhibitor with antiplatelet and vasodilatory properties, is not indicated in patients without claudication, such as this one. There is no evidence that cilostazol prevents progression of disease or improves outcomes in asymptomatic patients with PAD.

This patient's iliac artery stenosis could be treated safely and effectively with an endovascular approach; however, endovascular treatment of PAD is not recommended in asymptomatic patients. There is no empiric evidence that endovascular intervention prevents disease progression to intermittent claudication or critical limb ischemia.

Vorapaxar inhibits thrombin-induced and thrombin receptor agonist peptide–induced platelet aggregation. Vorapaxar reversibly inhibits protease-activated receptor-1, although its long half-life makes it effectively irreversible. It does not appear to affect coagulation parameters, nor does it inhibit platelet aggregation due to adenosine diphosphate, collagen, or thromboxane mimetic activities. Vorapaxar has been shown to reduce hospitalizations for acute limb ischemia in patients with symptomatic PAD, an effect that was mostly driven by patients who experienced lower extremity bypass graft thrombosis. When added to standard antiplatelet therapy, vorapaxar was also associated with a significant increase in major bleeding. In this patient with asymptomatic PAD, the benefits of adding vorapaxar to standard therapy are uncertain.

KEY POINT

- Asymptomatic lower extremity peripheral artery disease is managed with aggressive risk factor modification; cilostazol and surgical intervention do not affect progression of disease or prevent acute limb ischemia.

Bibliography

Foley TR, Waldo SW, Armstrong EJ. Medical therapy in peripheral artery disease and critical limb ischemia. Curr Treat Options Cardiovasc Med. 2016;18:42. [PMID: 27181397] doi:10.1007/s11936-016-0464-8

Item 40   Answer: A

Educational Objective: Evaluate the eligibility of a patient with hypertrophic cardiomyopathy for participation in sports.

The most appropriate management is to advise this patient not to play basketball. This asymptomatic patient has findings consistent with hypertrophic cardiomyopathy (HCM). HCM is the single most common cause of sudden death in young athletes, presumably due to ventricular arrhythmia triggered by high-intensity physical activity. The risk for ventricular arrhythmias in competitive athletes with HCM exists in the absence of conventional risk factors for sudden cardiac death. Therefore, the degree and distribution of hypertrophy, the presence and magnitude of left ventricular outflow tract obstruction, and the presence or absence of obstructive symptoms should not influence recommendations regarding athletic participation in patients with phenotypic expression of HCM. According to current recommendations from the American College of Cardiology/American Heart Association, athletes with a probable or unequivocal diagnosis of HCM may participate in competitive sports that are considered static and low intensity (categorized as class Ia sports). Examples of these sports include golf, curling, bowling, and cricket.

In patients with symptoms from HCM (such as dyspnea or syncope/near-syncope), medical therapy and lifestyle modification form the basis of therapy. Nonvasodilating β-blockers titrated to maximum tolerance are first-line treatment for symptomatic patients. However, β-blocker therapy should not be used for the sole purpose of allowing participation in athletics because the ability to effectively prevent sudden cardiac death with this strategy is unknown.

Catheter-based alcohol septal ablation or open surgical septal myectomy should be considered only in patients with HCM who have moderate to severe symptoms of obstruction despite maximal medical therapy or patients with recurrent syncope not related to arrhythmia. These invasive procedures should not be performed for the sole purpose of allowing participation in athletics.

Patients with HCM should be considered for implantable cardioverter-defibrillator therapy if they have any of the following risk factors for sudden cardiac death: (1) massive myocardial hypertrophy (wall thickness ≥30 mm), (2) previous cardiac arrest due to ventricular arrhythmia, (3) blunted blood pressure response or hypotension during exercise, (4) unexplained syncope, (5) nonsustained ventricular tachycardia on ambulatory electrocardiography, and (6) family history of sudden death due to HCM. An implantable cardioverter-defibrillator should not be placed solely for the purpose of allowing a patient to participate in high-intensity sports.

KEY POINT

- Athletes with a probable or unequivocal diagnosis of hypertrophic cardiomyopathy may participate in competitive sports that are considered static and low intensity.

Bibliography

Maron BJ, Udelson JE, Bonow RO, Nishimura RA, Ackerman MJ, Estes NA 3rd, et al. Eligibility and disqualification recommendations for competitive athletes with cardiovascular abnormalities: Task Force 3: hypertrophic cardiomyopathy, arrhythmogenic right ventricular cardiomyopathy and other cardiomyopathies, and myocarditis: a scientific statement from the American Heart Association and American College of Cardiology. J Am Coll Cardiol. 2015;66:2362-71. [PMID: 26542657] doi:10.1016/j.jacc.2015.09.035

Item 41   Answer: C

Educational Objective: Diagnose ventricular free wall rupture as a complication of ST-elevation myocardial infarction.

The most likely diagnosis in this patient with recent ST-elevation myocardial infarction (STEMI) is ventricular free wall rupture. Although the devastating mechanical complications of myocardial infarction have become increasingly rare with the use of reperfusion therapies, clinicians must be able to recognize these complications. The classic presentation of ventricular free wall rupture is sudden-onset chest pain or syncope with rapid progression to pulseless electrical activity, as seen in this patient. Unlike a ventricular septal defect, which results in intracardiac shunting of blood, free wall rupture causes rapid accumulation of blood within the pericardium and consequent tamponade. As a result, mortality rates are extremely high. Free wall rupture is more common in older adults, women, patients with anterior myocardial infarction, those receiving anti-inflammatory agents, and patients with a significant delay in receiving reperfusion therapy (>12 hours).

Although aortic dissection can manifest as sudden death as a result of rupture, aortic dissection is less likely than ventricular free wall rupture to cause pulseless electrical activity 3 days after an anterior myocardial infarction. In patients with a first myocardial infarction without heart failure, pulseless electrical activity is highly predictive of left ventricular free wall rupture.

Patients with in-stent restenosis will exhibit recurrent signs and symptoms of ischemia, including chest pain. Stent restenosis is unlikely in this patient with recent stent placement, as this process occurs over months to years. Additionally, stent restenosis does not present with pulseless electrical activity.

Acquired ventricular septal defect from septal wall rupture may complicate inferior or anterior STEMI. Patients typically present with sudden-onset right-sided heart failure, shock, and a new loud systolic murmur associated with a palpable thrill. The defect develops in the days following the infarction as myocardial necrosis develops, resulting in an often serpiginous defect connecting the left ventricle to the right ventricle. This patient's clinical presentation is inconsistent with postinfarction ventricular septal defect.

KEY POINT

- Ventricular free wall rupture is a rare complication of myocardial infarction that produces sudden-onset chest pain or syncope with rapid progression to pulseless electrical activity.

Bibliography

López-Sendón J, Gurfinkel EP, Lopez de Sa E, Agnelli G, Gore JM, Steg PG, et al; Global Registry of Acute Coronary Events (GRACE) Investigators. Factors related to heart rupture in acute coronary syndromes in the Global Registry of Acute Coronary Events. Eur Heart J. 2010;31:1449-56. [PMID: 20231153] doi:10.1093/eurheartj/ehq061

Item 42   Answer: D

Educational Objective: Diagnose transient constrictive pericarditis.

The most likely diagnosis is transient constrictive pericarditis. This patient has signs of right-sided heart failure accompanied by fever, leukocytosis, an elevated erythrocyte sedimentation rate, and a pericardial friction rub. The echocardiogram demonstrates enhanced ventricular interdependence and equalization of diastolic pressures in all heart chambers. Cardiac magnetic resonance imaging demonstrates pericardial thickening with evidence of active inflammation. These features are consistent with the diagnosis of transient constrictive pericarditis. Transient constrictive pericarditis most often is idiopathic but may follow cardiac surgery. Initial therapy consists of an NSAID plus colchicine.

Patients with chronic constrictive pericarditis are sometimes misdiagnosed as having heart failure with preserved ejection fraction. Although this patient has evidence of right-sided heart failure and has a preserved ejection fraction, Doppler echocardiographic findings of ventricular interdependence and the relative low B-type natriuretic peptide level argue against heart failure with preserved ejection fraction.

Patients with perioperative graft failure with infarction would be more likely to demonstrate pathologic findings of infarction on electrocardiogram, and serum troponin levels may remain elevated.

Although it may be challenging to differentiate restrictive cardiomyopathy from pericardial constriction, the lack of features of heart failure until after coronary artery bypass graft surgery makes the diagnosis of restrictive cardiomyopathy unlikely. Additionally, patients with restrictive cardiomyopathy would not demonstrate evidence of enhanced ventricular interdependence, and the B-type natriuretic peptide level is typically greater than 400 pg/mL (400 ng/L).

KEY POINT

- Some patients with constrictive pericarditis can have reversible or transient pericardial inflammation that responds to anti-inflammatory agents; most cases are idiopathic, whereas others may be associated with recent cardiac surgery.

Bibliography

Gentry J, Klein AL, Jellis CL. Transient constrictive pericarditis: current diagnostic and therapeutic strategies. Curr Cardiol Rep. 2016;18:41. [PMID: 26995404] doi:10.1007/s11886-016-0720-2

Item 43   Answer: C

Educational Objective: Treat heart failure with preserved ejection fraction.

The most appropriate management is to discontinue hydrochlorothiazide and diltiazem and start furosemide. This elderly woman with heart failure with preserved ejection fraction (HFpEF) has signs and symptoms of volume overload in the setting of bradycardia. The cornerstone of treatment for patients with HFpEF is diuretic therapy to maintain euvolemia. Antihypertensive agents should also be used to maintain normal blood pressure in the setting of hypertension. Despite treatment with hydrochlorothiazide, this patient has evidence of volume overload, and she should be switched to furosemide for more efficacious diuresis. This patient is also taking diltiazem, which may be causing her bradycardia, and this agent should be discontinued. If the patient's heart rate fails to improve, she should be referred for pacemaker placement.

Ivabradine is a sinus node modulator that reduces heart failure–associated hospitalizations in select heart failure patients; however, it is indicated as therapy only in patients with a reduced left ventricular ejection fraction and heart rate higher than 70/min while receiving β-blocker therapy.

Although ACE inhibitors, angiotensin receptor blockers (such as valsartan), β-blockers, and aldosterone antagonists have been studied for the treatment of HFpEF, no drugs have been shown to reduce morbidity or mortality in these patients. Most recently, in the TOPCAT trial, there was no difference in the primary combined endpoint of death, aborted cardiac arrest, or heart failure hospitalization with spironolactone compared with placebo; however, spironolactone was associated with a reduction in heart failure hospitalizations. Notably, a retrospective analysis showed that spironolactone reduced the incidence of cardiovascular death and heart failure hospitalization in patients in the Americas compared with those in Eastern Europe, likely because of different patient demographic characteristics across regions.

Pacemaker placement would be indicated only for symptomatic bradycardia in the absence of a reversible cause; the response to diltiazem discontinuation should be assessed before pacemaker placement is considered in this patient.

KEY POINT

- The cornerstone of treatment for patients with heart failure with preserved ejection fraction is diuretic therapy to maintain euvolemia.

Bibliography

Redfield MM. Heart failure with preserved ejection fraction. N Engl J Med. 2016;375:1868-1877. [PMID: 27959663]

Item 44   Answer: B

Educational Objective: Diagnose ostium primum atrial septal defect.

This patient's examination findings and electrocardiogram (ECG) are consistent with a diagnosis of ostium primum atrial septal defect (ASD). The patient has clinical features of ASD, presenting with dyspnea, paroxysmal atrial fibrillation, and features of right heart volume overload with elevation of the central venous pressure and a right ventricular lift. A pulmonary midsystolic flow murmur is caused by increased flow from a large left-to-right shunt. Fixed splitting of the S_2 throughout the cardiac cycle is a characteristic clinical feature of ASD. The apical systolic murmur of mitral regurgitation is related to the mitral valve cleft. This combination of fixed splitting of the S_2, mitral regurgitation murmur, and left-axis deviation on ECG are most consistent with an ostium primum ASD.

Patients with a coronary sinus ASD have features of right heart volume overload but do not have a mitral regurgitation murmur because no mitral valve disease is present. The ECG may be normal or demonstrate first-degree atrioventricular block and incomplete right bundle branch block.

Patients with ostium secundum ASD have right heart volume overload but do not generally have mitral regurgitation. The ECG may demonstrate first-degree atrioventricular block and incomplete right bundle branch block, or it may be normal. This patient's ECG finding of left axis deviation is not seen in patients with ostium secundum ASD.

Patients with sinus venosus ASD have features of right heart volume overload but do not have a mitral regurgitation murmur because no mitral valve disease is present. The ECG may be normal or demonstrate first-degree atrioventricular block, left P-wave axis or abnormal P-wave axis, and incomplete right bundle branch block, but left-axis deviation is not expected.

KEY POINT

- Fixed splitting of the S_2, a mitral regurgitation murmur, and left-axis deviation on electrocardiogram are consistent with an ostium primum atrial septal defect.

Bibliography

Warnes CA, Williams RG, Bashore TM, Child JS, Connolly HM, Dearani JA, et al; American College of Cardiology. ACC/AHA 2008 guidelines for the management of adults with congenital heart disease: a report of the American College of Cardiology/American Heart Association Task Force on Practice Guidelines (Writing Committee to Develop Guidelines on the Management of Adults With Congenital Heart Disease). Developed in Collaboration With the American Society of Echocardiography, Heart Rhythm Society, International Society for Adult Congenital Heart Disease, Society for Cardiovascular Angiography and Interventions, and Society of Thoracic Surgeons. J Am Coll Cardiol. 2008;52:e143-263. [PMID: 19038677] doi:10.1016/j.jacc.2008.10.001

Item 45   Answer: D

Educational Objective: Assess the 10-year risk for atherosclerotic cardiovascular disease with the Pooled Cohort Equations.

The most appropriate next management step is to calculate this patient's 10-year atherosclerotic cardiovascular disease (ASCVD) risk. Results of lipid measurements and patient-specific data (age, race, blood pressure, hypertension treatment, diabetes mellitus, and smoking) allow for the calculation of 10-year ASCVD risk using the Pooled Cohort Equations. In adults aged 40 to 75 years who have at least one ASCVD risk factor (dyslipidemia, diabetes, hypertension, or smoking) and a calculated 10-year ASCVD risk of 10% or greater, the U.S. Preventive Services Task Force (USPSTF) recommends statin therapy for the primary prevention of ASCVD. The USPSTF also recommends that clinicians selectively prescribe statins to adults aged 40 to 75 years without a history of ASCVD who have one or more ASCVD risk factors and a calculated

10-year ASCVD event risk of 7.5% to 10% (grade C recommendation). Because this patient has one ASCVD risk factor (hypertension), it is appropriate that his risk be assessed, and through use of the Pooled Cohort Equations, his 10-year risk for ASCVD is 9.3%. According to the USPSTF recommendation, he should be considered as a potential candidate for statin therapy. The most recent American College of Cardiology/American Heart Association cholesterol treatment guideline recommends that patients without ASCVD or diabetes and a 10-year ASCVD risk of 7.5% or higher receive moderate- or high-intensity statin therapy.

The initiation of statin therapy might be reasonable for this patient but not until his 10-year ASCVD risk is calculated. Such information can be used to determine the need for and intensity of stain therapy.

The optimal interval for assessment of ASCVD risk is undetermined; however, it is reasonable to measure lipid levels every 5 years in adults aged 40 to 75 years. This patient should not wait 5 years to have his ASCVD risk assessed and delay potentially beneficial therapy.

KEY POINT

- Routine screening for lipid disorders and calculation of 10-year atherosclerotic cardiovascular disease risk by using the Pooled Cohort Equations should be performed in adults aged 40 to 75 years.

Bibliography

Bibbins-Domingo K, Grossman DC, Curry SJ, Davidson KW, Epling JW Jr, García FA, et al; US Preventive Services Task Force. Statin use for the primary prevention of cardiovascular disease in adults: US Preventive Services Task Force recommendation statement. JAMA. 2016;316:1997-2007. [PMID: 27838723] doi:10.1001/jama.2016.15450

Item 46   Answer: D

Educational Objective: Manage antithrombotic therapy in a patient with a prosthetic heart valve.

The most appropriate antithrombotic therapy is the combination of warfarin and aspirin. Lifelong oral anticoagulation with warfarin is recommended for all patients with a mechanical prosthesis and those with bioprostheses with other indications for anticoagulation. The target INR is based on prosthesis location, with a target of 2.5 for patients with a mechanical aortic prosthetic valve and 3.0 for patients with a mechanical mitral prosthetic valve and those with a mechanical aortic prosthetic valve and additional risk factors for thromboembolism (atrial fibrillation, left ventricular dysfunction, previous thromboembolism, hypercoagulable condition, or older-generation mechanical aortic valve replacement). The addition of aspirin (75-100 mg/d) is also recommended to reduce the risk for ischemic events. Adding aspirin to warfarin therapy reduces mortality, particularly mortality from vascular causes, and major systemic embolism (1.9% per year versus 8.5% per year). Although there is some increase in bleeding, the risk of the combined treatment was more than offset by the considerable benefit. The need for anticoagulation among patients with bioprosthetic valves is less clear. Oral anticoagulation with warfarin should be considered for at least 3 months and as long as 6 months after implantation of a mitral or aortic bioprosthesis. An INR of 2.5 should be targeted in these patients. Long-term aspirin use is reasonable for all patients with bioprosthetic valves.

Apixaban, a direct factor Xa inhibitor, has not been studied for the prevention of valve thrombosis and thrombo-embolic events in patients with a mechanical valve prosthesis; therefore, it would be inappropriate to initiate apixaban in this patient.

Direct thrombin inhibitors, such as dabigatran, are contraindicated in patients with mechanical valves, owing to the excessive thrombotic complications observed in clinical trials with these agents.

Foregoing anticoagulation would be inappropriate for this patient because lifelong warfarin is indicated in all patients with a mechanical valve prosthesis to decrease the incidence of thromboembolism and the associated morbidity, such as ischemic stroke, cerebrovascular accident, and peripheral systemic embolism.

KEY POINT

- In patients with a mechanical prosthetic valve, low-dose aspirin is recommended in addition to warfarin therapy to reduce the risk for ischemic events.

Bibliography

Turpie AG, Gent M, Laupacis A, Latour Y, Gunstensen J, Basile F, et al. A comparison of aspirin with placebo in patients treated with warfarin after heart-valve replacement. N Engl J Med. 1993;329:524-9. [PMID: 8336751]

Item 47   Answer: A

Educational Objective: **Treat wide-complex tachycardia due to atrial fibrillation with aberrant conduction.**

The most appropriate next step in management is initiation of β-blocker therapy and anticoagulation. This older patient has paroxysmal atrial fibrillation with aberrant conduction, resulting in wide-complex tachycardia. The electrocardiogram (ECG) demonstrates a normal sinus beat followed by an irregularly irregular rhythm, and the QRS morphology (rSR pattern in lead V_1, deep terminal S waves in leads I and V_6) on ECG is consistent with typical right bundle branch block. The physical examination is also notable for a widely split S_2, which is typically heard during right bundle branch block. Atrioventricular nodal blocking agents, such as β-blockers, should be used to control this patient's heart rate and improve her symptoms. This patient is also at moderate to high risk for stroke given her CHA_2DS_2-VASc score of 4 (1 point each for hypertension and female sex; 2 points for age >75 years). Therefore, initiation of oral anticoagulation is also appropriate.

Adenosine is used in the acute treatment of arrhythmias to interrupt atrioventricular conduction and terminate supraventricular tachycardia; however, this patient's arrhythmia is not dependent on the atrioventricular node. Therefore, adenosine would not be of benefit.

Intravenous procainamide would be an appropriate option if the patient had preexcited atrial fibrillation due to an accessory pathway. The presence of an accessory pathway may be indicated on a resting ECG by the presence of two characteristics: a short PR interval when in sinus rhythm (see first beat on the ECG) and a delta wave (a sloping upstroke initiating the QRS complex, which may be wide due to sequential rather than parallel depolarization of the ventricles). This pattern on ECG is referred to as preexcitation, and when present with symptomatic tachycardia, it is called the Wolff-Parkinson-White syndrome. This patient's ECG is most consistent with aberrant conduction in the setting of atrial fibrillation, not preexcited atrial fibrillation.

Urgent cardioversion is unnecessary because the patient is hemodynamically stable and appears to have nonsustained atrial fibrillation on the basis of the intermittent nature of her symptoms. If the patient had a sustained arrhythmia accompanied by hemodynamic instability, emergent cardioversion would be indicated, regardless of the specific cause of the arrhythmia (that is, supraventricular versus ventricular).

KEY POINT

- Atrial fibrillation with aberrant conduction results in an irregularly irregular rhythm and a wide-complex tachycardia with a QRS morphology (rSR pattern in lead V_1, deep terminal S waves in leads I and V_6) on electrocardiogram typical of right bundle branch block.

Bibliography

Link MS. Clinical practice. Evaluation and initial treatment of supraventricular tachycardia. N Engl J Med. 2012;367:1438-48. [PMID: 23050527] doi:10.1056/NEJMcp1111259

Item 48   Answer: D

Educational Objective: **Manage a patient with a thoracic aortic aneurysm and concomitant coronary artery disease.**

The most appropriate management of this patient is simultaneous coronary artery bypass graft (CABG) surgery and aortic repair. On the basis of his angiographic findings (80% stenosis of the left main coronary artery bifurcation), he should undergo revascularization with CABG surgery. In patients with an ascending aorta or aortic root greater than 4.5 cm in diameter who require CABG surgery or surgery to repair valve pathology, aortic repair should be performed at the time of cardiac surgery. Anatomic imaging, such as CT angiography or magnetic resonance angiography, is recommended to plan for open aortic repair before the surgical procedure.

Patients with left main coronary artery disease have traditionally been treated with CABG surgery; however, because this patient has concomitant thoracic aortic aneurysmal disease, CABG surgery without aortic repair is not the best management option.

Patients with established coronary artery disease benefit from optimal medical therapy, including β-blockers and long-acting nitrates. However, given this patient's thoracic aortic aneurysm and severe coronary artery disease, optimal medical therapy in the absence of revascularization and aortic repair is inappropriate.

Percutaneous coronary intervention is not encouraged for patients with complex disease of the left main coronary artery, especially in the presence of a thoracic aortic aneurysm.

KEY POINT

- In patients with a thoracic aortic aneurysm greater than 4.5 cm in diameter who require coronary artery bypass graft surgery or surgery to repair valve pathology, aortic repair should be performed at the time of cardiac surgery.

Bibliography
Hiratzka LF, Bakris GL, Beckman JA, Bersin RM, Carr VF, Casey DE Jr, et al; American College of Cardiology Foundation/American Heart Association Task Force on Practice Guidelines. 2010 ACCF/AHA/AATS/ACR/ASA/ SCA/SCAI/SIR/STS/SVM guidelines for the diagnosis and management of patients with thoracic aortic disease: a report of the American College of Cardiology Foundation/American Heart Association Task Force on Practice Guidelines, American Association for Thoracic Surgery, American College of Radiology, American Stroke Association, Society of Cardiovascular Anesthesiologists, Society for Cardiovascular Angiography and Interventions, Society of Interventional Radiology, Society of Thoracic Surgeons, and Society for Vascular Medicine. Circulation. 2010;121:e266-369. [PMID: 20233780] doi:10.1161/CIR. 0b013e3181d4739e

Item 49   Answer: D

Educational Objective: Diagnose left ventricular assist device–related thrombosis as the cause of stroke.

The most likely cause of stroke in this patient with a left ventricular assist device (LVAD) is LVAD-related thrombosis. Stroke is one of the most common complications after placement of an LVAD. Studies have shown that the incidence of hemorrhagic and embolic strokes approaches 20% at 1 year after LVAD insertion. Other complications of LVAD placement include gastrointestinal bleeding, usually secondary to arteriovenous malformations; pump malfunction; and thrombus formation in the pump that can lead to emboli, hemolysis, or pump stoppage.

Stroke due to large artery atherosclerosis, such as carotid artery stenosis, commonly occurs after local thrombus formation in the area of plaque rupture with subsequent distal embolization. Of the common causes of stroke, extracranial internal carotid artery atherosclerosis has the highest risk for recurrent stroke in the first 2 weeks. Advanced atherosclerotic disease is a much less likely cause of stroke in this 37-year-old man with cardiomyopathy than is thromboembolism related to LVAD placement.

A sizeable proportion of patients will have a cerebral infarction with no definitive cause identified on cardiac or vascular diagnostic testing, termed cryptogenic stroke. However, this diagnosis is not appropriate until a complete evaluation reveals no cause of the stroke, which is not the case for this patient.

Small subcortical infarcts (lacunes) commonly have a diameter of less than 1.5 cm and arise from occlusion of small perforating arteries emanating from the large intracranial vessels. This stroke subtype typically presents with only motor or sensory findings on examination; cortical hemispheric symptoms, such as visual field cuts, aphasia, or hemispatial neglect, are lacking. Lacunar infarction is not compatible with the patient's clinical presentation.

KEY POINT

- The incidence of hemorrhagic and embolic strokes approaches 20% at 1 year after insertion of a left ventricular assist device.

Bibliography
Robertson J, Long B, Koyfman A. The emergency management of ventricular assist devices. Am J Emerg Med. 2016;34:1294-301. [PMID: 27162114] doi:10.1016/j.ajem.2016.04.033

Item 50   Answer: D

Educational Objective: Diagnose a benign heart murmur.

The most appropriate management is routine clinical follow-up without imaging. Cardiac murmurs result from increased blood flow across a normal orifice (such as with anemia, thyrotoxicosis, pregnancy, or atrial septal defect), turbulent flow through a narrowed orifice (such as with aortic stenosis or mitral stenosis), or regurgitant flow through an incompetent valve (such as with aortic regurgitation or mitral regurgitation). Timing in the cardiac cycle, chest wall location, radiation, intensity, configuration, duration, and pitch all assist in the differential diagnosis.

Not all systolic murmurs are pathologic. Asymptomatic patients with short, soft systolic murmurs (grade <3) well localized to the left sternal border and associated with normal heart sounds do not usually require further investigation. Benign murmurs typically decrease in intensity with standing. The presence of any diastolic or continuous murmur, cardiac symptoms (chest pain, dyspnea, syncope), or abnormalities on examination (clicks, abnormal S_2, abnormal pulses) requires evaluation by echocardiography.

Various interventions may alter the intensity of murmurs. The murmur of hypertrophic cardiomyopathy may increase with standing or Valsalva maneuver; both maneuvers decrease venous return, which decreases left ventricular chamber size and increases the degree of obstruction. The click and murmur of mitral valve prolapse may move earlier in systole and increase in intensity as left ventricular volume decreases (standing or Valsalva maneuver). Aortic outflow murmurs increase in intensity in the beat following a premature ventricular contraction due to increased left ventricular volume. Murmurs of mitral regurgitation, ventricular septal defect, and aortic regurgitation increase with handgrip because of increased cardiac output and peripheral resistance. Right-sided heart murmurs may increase during inspiration due to increased venous return.

Characteristics of the S_2 may assist in determining the diagnosis or the severity of a valvular lesion. A fixed split of S_2 (present during inspiration and expiration instead of only inspiration) results from a delay in right ventricular emptying and is strongly associated with atrial septal defect. A paradoxical split of S_2 (present during expiration) indicates a delay in left ventricular emptying, such as with severe aortic stenosis. Presence of a physiologic split (present during inspiration) is helpful for excluding severe aortic stenosis.

Because this patient likely has a benign systolic heart murmur and is asymptomatic, imaging with echocardiography or cardiac magnetic resonance imaging is not necessary.

KEY POINT

• Short, soft systolic murmurs (grade <3) that are well localized to the left sternal border and are not associated with symptoms often do not require further investigation.

Bibliography
Etchells E, Bell C, Robb K. Does this patient have an abnormal systolic murmur? JAMA. 1997;277:564-71. [PMID: 9032164]

Item 51   Answer: B

Educational Objective: Manage dual antiplatelet therapy in a patient with stable angina treated with drug-eluting stent placement.

This patient should receive dual antiplatelet therapy (DAPT) for 5 additional months, after which clopidogrel can be discontinued. In patients who undergo percutaneous coronary intervention (PCI), DAPT with aspirin plus a $P2Y_{12}$ inhibitor is indicated to prevent stent thrombosis and future cardiovascular events. However, recently, there has been considerable movement regarding the optimal duration of DAPT following drug-eluting stent placement. It is important to find the correct balance between blocking platelet activity during the process of reendothelialization of the stent and exposure to the attendant bleeding risk. Current guidelines suggest that the minimum duration for DAPT following drug-eluting stent placement for patients without an acute coronary syndrome is at least 6 months, with the option to continue therapy for a longer duration in those with a high risk for thrombosis-related complications and a favorable bleeding profile. Ultimately, the decision may be individualized at the patient level, such as with this patient, who is at relatively high bleeding risk given her age and comorbid conditions.

In patients who undergo PCI with bare metal stent placement, DAPT may be discontinued after 1 month; however, this patient with a drug-eluting stent requires longer therapy.

Patients with acute coronary syndrome treated with PCI (bare metal or drug-eluting stent placement) should be optimally treated with DAPT for at least 12 months.

Aspirin should be continued indefinitely in patients with coronary artery disease, unless contraindicated. No data support discontinuing both antiplatelet agents following PCI.

A study of DAPT comparing 12 months of therapy with 30 months of therapy suggested a benefit to the longer duration in some patients. Extending DAPT for a longer duration should be individualized on the basis of predicted risk for additional cardiovascular events and risk for bleeding.

KEY POINT

• Dual antiplatelet therapy is recommended for at least 6 months after drug-eluting stent placement for treatment of stable angina.

Bibliography
Levine GN, Bates ER, Bittl JA, Brindis RG, Fihn SD, Fleisher LA, et al. 2016 ACC/AHA guideline focused update on duration of dual antiplatelet therapy in patients with coronary artery disease: a report of the American College of Cardiology/American Heart Association Task Force on Clinical Practice Guidelines. J Thorac Cardiovasc Surg. 2016;152:1243-1275. [PMID: 27751237] doi:10.1016/j.jtcvs.2016.07.044

Item 52   Answer: E   H

Educational Objective: Treat an atrial myxoma.

The most appropriate treatment is surgical excision. This patient's history, physical examination findings, and echocardiographic features are all most consistent with a left atrial myxoma. The parasternal long-axis echocardiographic view (shown) demonstrates a large atrial myxoma (AM) prolapsing across the mitral valve from the left atrium (LA) to the left ventricle (LV) during diastole. Myxomas are connective tissue tumors with cells encompassed within mucopolysaccharide stroma. Most are attached to the left atrial wall in proximity to the fossa ovalis. Patients with an atrial myxoma most often present with symptoms related to obstruction or embolization, or constitutional symptoms related to production of tumor-based interleukin 6, such as fatigue, low-grade fever, and arthralgia. Dyspnea may be related to mitral valvular obstruction, which causes a diastolic rumble resembling mitral stenosis and an early diastolic sound ("tumor plop")

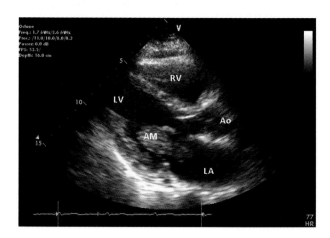

H
CONT.

heard in 10% to 15% of patients. Treatment for an atrial myxoma is urgent surgical excision.

Systemic anticoagulation would be appropriate in patients with a thrombus. Right atrial masses in patients with indwelling cardiac catheters are more likely to represent thrombus. PET and contrast-enhanced MRI/CT may be useful in evaluating metabolic activity and vascularity to differentiate a tumor from a thrombus. This patient has no risk factors for intracardiac thrombus, such as cardiac catheter, atrial fibrillation, or poor left ventricular function, making it an unlikely diagnosis.

Chemotherapy and radiotherapy are used to treat primary cardiac lymphoma. Suspicion for cardiac lymphoma would be higher if this patient were immunocompromised and had presented with a right atrial mass rather than an intra-atrial mass.

Empiric antibiotic therapy would be appropriate for suspected infective endocarditis. Although this patient has a low-grade fever, embolic phenomena, and constitutional symptoms, she has no risk factors for infective endocarditis and no leukocytosis. Additionally, attachment of the tumor to the fossa ovalis, not a valvular surface, makes infective endocarditis unlikely.

Percutaneous biopsy with echocardiographic guidance is sometimes useful in establishing the diagnosis of right-sided masses. However, percutaneous biopsy would not eliminate the need for surgical excision in this patient with embolic events.

KEY POINT

- Patients with an atrial myxoma may present with constitutional symptoms, embolic phenomena from tumor fragmentation, or symptoms referable to intra-cardiac obstruction (dyspnea, syncope); treatment is surgical excision.

Bibliography

Basso C, Rizzo S, Valente M, Thiene G. Cardiac masses and tumours. Heart. 2016 Aug 1;102(15):1230-45. [PMID: 27277840]

Item 53   Answer: C

Educational Objective: Diagnose Noonan syndrome associated with cardiovascular disease.

This patient has features of Noonan syndrome, which is an autosomal dominant disorder commonly associated with congenital cardiac lesions, including pulmonary stenosis; the valve is usually dysplastic. Noonan syndrome should be considered in all patients with pulmonary stenosis, particularly those with short stature, variable intellectual impairment, unique facial features, neck webbing, hypertelorism, and other cardiac abnormalities, including hypertrophic cardiomyopathy, atrial septal defect, and ventricular septal defect. This patient has severe pulmonary stenosis demonstrated by the physical examination findings of a palpable, late-peaking systolic murmur located at the second left intercostal space; absence of an ejection click; and features of right ventricular

pressure overload. An ejection click may be audible in patients with pulmonary stenosis, but as severity progresses, the click disappears owing to loss of valve pliability. The echocardiogram in this patient confirms severe pulmonary stenosis with a peak systolic gradient of 65 mm Hg.

Down syndrome is a genetic disorder caused by the presence of a full or partial extra copy of chromosome 21. Characteristic features include small stature, unique facial features, and intellectual delays. Congenital cardiovascular disease occurs in more than 40% of affected persons, most commonly as a form of atrioventricular septal defect, including ostium primum atrial septal defect, inlet ventricular septal defect, or complete atrioventricular septal defect. Pulmonary stenosis is not typically seen unless associated with tetralogy of Fallot, which is also common in persons with Down syndrome.

Marfan syndrome is a genetic disorder caused by a mutation on chromosome 15. Findings typically include ocular, cardiovascular, skeletal, and systemic features that include tall stature with overgrowth of the long bones. The most common cardiovascular feature is aortic sinus dilatation with a propensity to dissection.

Turner syndrome is a genetic disorder that affects girls and women and is characterized by complete or partial absence of one of the X chromosomes. Affected persons often demonstrate short stature, webbed neck, low-set ears, low hairline, and primary infertility. Cardiac defects occur in about 45% of affected patients; the most common lesions include bicuspid aortic valve, aortic coarctation, and aortic aneurysm. Although pulmonary stenosis can occur in Turner syndrome, this man could not have Turner syndrome.

KEY POINT

- Noonan syndrome is commonly associated with congenital cardiac lesions, including pulmonary stenosis.

Bibliography

Bhambhani V, Muenke M. Noonan syndrome. Am Fam Physician. 2014;89:37-43. [PMID: 24444506]

Item 54   Answer: C

Educational Objective: Prevent sudden cardiac death in a patient with nonischemic cardiomyopathy.

Implantable cardioverter-defibrillator (ICD) placement is the most appropriate management of this patient with nonischemic cardiomyopathy and syncope that is concerning for an arrhythmic cause. He has several high-risk features for ventricular arrhythmia (New York Heart Association functional class II symptoms, ventricular ectopy, and syncope). ICD therapy is indicated to prevent sudden cardiac death.

Electroencephalography is indicated if seizure is suspected as the cause of syncope. However, this patient's presentation was not consistent with a diagnosis of seizure.

Exercise treadmill stress testing is a valuable test when exercise-induced arrhythmias are suspected. This patient's

CONT.

symptoms are not associated with exertion; therefore, exercise treadmill stress testing is unnecessary.

PET can be useful in the evaluation of nonischemic cardiomyopathy when cardiac sarcoidosis is suspected. However, this information would not be helpful in guiding the decision to insert an ICD in this patient at high risk for sudden cardiac death.

Tilt-table testing should be reserved for patients with recurrent syncope without known heart disease or those with heart disease in whom a cardiac cause of the syncope has been excluded. Because cardiac arrhythmias are the most likely cause of this patient's syncope, tilt-table testing is not appropriate.

KEY POINT

- Implantable cardioverter-defibrillator (ICD) therapy is indicated in patients with nonischemic cardiomyopathy who have a left ventricular ejection fraction less than or equal to 35% and who have New York Heart Association functional class II or III symptoms; ICD implantation is also reasonable for patients with nonischemic cardiomyopathy and unexplained syncope and significant left ventricular dysfunction.

Bibliography

Epstein AE, DiMarco JP, Ellenbogen KA, Estes NA 3rd, Freedman RA, Gettes LS, et al; American College of Cardiology Foundation; American Heart Association Task Force on Practice Guidelines; Heart Rhythm Society. 2012 ACCF/AHA/HRS focused update incorporated into the ACCF/AHA/HRS 2008 guidelines for device-based therapy of cardiac rhythm abnormalities: a report of the American College of Cardiology Foundation/American Heart Association Task Force on Practice Guidelines and the Heart Rhythm Society. Circulation. 2013 Jan 22;127(3):e283-352. [PMID: 23255456]

Item 55   Answer: A

Educational Objective: Evaluate symptomatic mitral stenosis with exercise echocardiography.

The most appropriate next step in management is exercise echocardiography. This patient has symptoms typical of severe mitral stenosis (progressive exertional dyspnea) but echocardiographic findings consistent with only moderate mitral stenosis. Symptoms of mitral stenosis can be indolent, with patients remaining asymptomatic for years and then presenting with a gradual decrease in activity. Other symptoms include dyspnea, orthopnea, fatigue, and, less commonly, hemoptysis or systemic embolization. Symptoms typically are not present until the mitral valve area is less than 1.5 cm², although tachycardia may precipitate symptoms at larger valve areas. In patients with a discrepancy between the clinical findings (debilitating symptoms) and the echocardiographic findings (moderate stenosis), additional testing is necessary to ensure that the patient's symptoms can be attributed to mitral stenosis. In this case, exercise echocardiography, using either pharmacologic or physical stressors, should be pursued to assess the response of the mitral gradient and pulmonary pressures. For patients with mitral stenosis, the valve gradient is heavily flow dependent and may become severely

elevated only with exercise. Exercise and the accompanying increases in heart rate augment cardiac output and transvalvular flow and shorten the diastolic filling time in the left ventricle. These conditions can unmask mitral stenosis that does not appear to be functionally severe at rest. With an increase in left atrial pressures during exercise, significant pulmonary hypertension also may become evident.

Medical therapy for mitral stenosis consists of diuretics or long-acting nitrates, which may help alleviate symptoms such as dyspnea. In addition, β-blockers or nondihydropyridine calcium channel blockers can lower heart rate and improve left ventricular diastolic filling time. Medical therapy would be appropriate if the mitral stenosis were not hemodynamically significant or if she were not a surgical candidate.

After hemodynamically significant mitral stenosis is confirmed, percutaneous or surgical therapy can be considered. However, these interventions are not appropriate before confirmation with exercise echocardiography.

KEY POINT

- In patients with mitral stenosis who have a discrepancy between the clinical findings and the echocardiographic findings, exercise echocardiography should be pursued to assess the response of the mitral gradient and pulmonary pressures.

Bibliography

Aviles RJ, Nishimura RA, Pellikka PA, Andreen KM, Holmes DR Jr. Utility of stress Doppler echocardiography in patients undergoing percutaneous mitral balloon valvotomy. J Am Soc Echocardiogr. 2001;14:676-81. [PMID: 11447412]

Item 56   Answer: C

Educational Objective: Treat ST-elevation myocardial infarction complicated by cardiogenic shock.

Immediate percutaneous coronary intervention (PCI) is indicated in this patient with ST-elevation myocardial infarction (STEMI) complicated by cardiogenic shock. Cardiogenic shock is defined by persistent symptomatic hypotension and end-organ dysfunction. Patients have acute kidney failure, evidence of liver dysfunction with elevated aminotransferase levels, poor peripheral perfusion with cool extremities, and decreased mental status. Cardiogenic shock typically occurs as a consequence of a large anterior myocardial infarction, resulting in severely reduced left ventricular systolic function; it carries a mortality rate between 50% and 80%. Despite their instability, patients with cardiogenic shock (particularly those younger than 75 years of age) have a higher rate of survival if they undergo emergent revascularization with primary PCI in the catheterization laboratory.

Medical stabilization with intravenous vasoactive medications and, in severe cases, device-based hemodynamic support without prompt revascularization has been shown to be inferior to revascularization in the setting of shock and is not appropriate.

In the treatment of STEMI, β-blockers are recommended at the time of initial presentation, except in patients with evidence of hypotension, cardiogenic shock, pulmonary congestion, advanced atrioventricular block, or other contraindications to β-blocker therapy. Intravenous metoprolol is the most widely used β-blocker for STEMI treatment. In this case, β-blockade should be withheld and introduced following reperfusion therapy.

Intravenous nitroglycerin can be used to treat patients with STEMI and hypertension or heart failure but should be avoided in the setting of systolic blood pressure less than 90 mm Hg, significant bradycardia or tachycardia, right ventricular infarction, or use of a phosphodiesterase inhibitor (such as sildenafil) in the past 24 to 48 hours.

Because the rates of achieving vessel patency are higher and more reliable with primary PCI than with thrombolysis, primary PCI is the preferred method of treating STEMI. Thrombolytic therapy would be indicated in this patient with STEMI if transfer to a PCI-capable center would result in a first medical contact–to–device time of more than 120 minutes.

KEY POINT

- Patients with ST-elevation myocardial infarction complicated by cardiogenic shock should undergo emergent revascularization with primary percutaneous coronary intervention.

Bibliography

O'Gara PT, Kushner FG, Ascheim DD, Casey DE Jr, Chung MK, de Lemos JA, et al; American College of Cardiology Foundation/American Heart Association Task Force on Practice Guidelines. 2013 ACCF/AHA guideline for the management of ST-elevation myocardial infarction: a report of the American College of Cardiology Foundation/American Heart Association Task Force on Practice Guidelines. Circulation. 2013;127:e362-425. [PMID: 23247304] doi:10.1161/CIR.0b013e3182742cf6

Item 57   Answer: D

Educational Objective: Manage a patient with a bicuspid aortic valve and enlarged aortic root with surveillance echocardiography.

The most appropriate management of this patient with an ascending thoracic aortic aneurysm and a bicuspid aortic valve is repeat echocardiography in 6 months. Patients with a bicuspid aortic valve are prone to enlargement of the ascending aorta, and patients with both a bicuspid aortic valve and enlarged aortic dimensions are at higher risk for aortic dissection. Surveillance echocardiography should be performed in these patients to monitor aortic growth. Patients with a bicuspid aortic valve and a thoracic aortic aneurysm should undergo annual imaging if the aortic diameter has been stable and smaller than 4.5 cm. If the aortic diameter is 4.5 cm or larger or the rate of enlargement exceeds 0.5 cm/year, imaging should be performed every 6 months.

Operative aortic valve repair or replacement is indicated in asymptomatic patients with a bicuspid aortic valve and a thoracic aortic aneurysm diameter of 5.5 cm or larger,

according to American College of Cardiology/American Heart Association guidelines. However, surgical intervention can be beneficial in those patients with a bicuspid aortic valve, thoracic aortic aneurysm diameter of 5.0 cm or larger, and an additional risk factor for dissection/rupture (such as family history of aortic dissection or aortic growth rate ≥0.5 cm/year). In this asymptomatic patient with an ascending aortic diameter of 5.1 cm without additional risk factors, it is premature to repair or replace the aorta.

Some patients with reduced left ventricular (LV) function and calcific aortic stenosis have severe aortic stenosis based on valve area but a gradient that is less than 30 mm Hg. Whether symptoms in this "low-flow/low-gradient" aortic stenosis are caused primarily by aortic valve disease with resultant LV dysfunction or the effective valve area is reduced owing to poor leaflet excursion can be best determined with dobutamine stress echocardiography. In this patient, there is no indication to perform dobutamine stress echocardiography, as he has normal LV function.

KEY POINT

- Patients with a bicuspid aortic valve and a thoracic aortic aneurysm should undergo echocardiography every 6 months if the aortic diameter is larger than 4.5 cm or the rate of enlargement exceeds 0.5 cm/year.

Bibliography

Hiratzka LF, Creager MA, Isselbacher EM, Svensson LG, Nishimura RA, Bonow RO, et al. Surgery for aortic dilatation in patients with bicuspid aortic valves: a statement of clarification from the American College of Cardiology/American Heart Association Task Force on Clinical Practice Guidelines. J Am Coll Cardiol. 2016;67:724-31. [PMID: 26658475] doi:10.1016/j.jacc.2015.11.006

Item 58   Answer: C

Educational Objective: Diagnose peripartum cardiomyopathy.

The most likely diagnosis in this woman who is 3 weeks postpartum is peripartum cardiomyopathy. Peripartum cardiomyopathy is left ventricular systolic dysfunction with onset toward the end of pregnancy or in the months following delivery in the absence of another identifiable cause. Although patients may be asymptomatic, they often present with features of heart failure. Women with peripartum cardiomyopathy should be promptly treated with medical therapy, which may include β-blockers, digoxin, hydralazine, nitrates, or diuretics. ACE inhibitors, angiotensin receptor blockers, and aldosterone antagonists are teratogenic and should be avoided until after delivery.

Acute aortic dissection classically presents with sudden onset of chest or back pain that has a tearing or ripping quality. Dyspnea is less common. Physical examination findings include a blood pressure or pulse differential between the upper extremities. A diastolic murmur of aortic regurgitation may be heard at the cardiac base if the aortic valve is involved. Echocardiography demonstrates an enlarged ascending aorta; the dissection flap may also be visible. Ventricular function is usually normal unless the aortic dissection has involved the coronary arteries, although regional abnormalities may be detected. This patient's clinical findings do not support a diagnosis of acute aortic dissection.

Pulmonary embolism can occur postpartum, particularly when prolonged bed rest is required during or following pregnancy. Patients with pulmonary embolism frequently present with dyspnea; however, this patient's presentation suggests heart failure, given the elevated venous pressure, pulmonary congestion, and global reduction in ejection fraction.

Takotsubo cardiomyopathy, also known as stress cardiomyopathy, is characterized by transient regional cardiac dysfunction, usually involving the apical and mid-portion of the left ventricle. It is usually precipitated by a stressful physical or emotional event. Postpartum cases of takotsubo cardiomyopathy have been reported, especially after cesarean delivery. Patients with takotsubo cardiomyopathy present with features that mimic an acute coronary syndrome: chest pain, ischemic electrocardiographic changes, and elevated cardiac biomarker levels. This patient's clinical picture is inconsistent with takotsubo cardiomyopathy.

KEY POINT

- Peripartum cardiomyopathy is left ventricular systolic dysfunction with onset toward the end of pregnancy or in the months following delivery in the absence of another identifiable cause; patients often present with features of heart failure.

Bibliography

Arany Z, Elkayam U. Peripartum cardiomyopathy. Circulation. 2016;133:1397–409. [PMID: 27045128] doi:10.1161/CIRCULATION AHA.115.020491

Item 59   Answer: B

Educational Objective: Evaluate a patient for an arrhythmia.

An event recorder is the most appropriate diagnostic testing option for this patient. Because he has symptomatic palpitations associated with lightheadedness and near-syncope, evaluation to identify the type and source of any present arrhythmias is important to his care. The intermittent and fleeting nature of arrhythmias can make diagnosis difficult. Diagnostic studies are selected on the basis of the presence and frequency of the patient's symptoms and the duration and timing of the recording. The diagnostic study best suited to capture this patient's symptomatic episodes is an external event recorder. The basic event monitor involves the patient activating or "triggering" the event monitor at the time of symptoms, capturing the rhythm. Some models capture the rhythm only at the time the event recorder is activated or held to the chest, or when electrodes are applied. Other models can capture the rhythm before and after the patient activates the recorder. The newest models are real-time continuous

monitoring systems that automatically record and transmit heart rhythm data from the ambulatory patient to a monitoring station; data can also be sent at the time of patient activation. Patients are encouraged to keep a diary of when symptoms occur so that they may be correlated with arrhythmias shown on the electrocardiographic (ECG) tracing.

An electrophysiology study may be appropriate if this patient's arrhythmia cannot be diagnosed on the basis of less invasive techniques. It may also be helpful therapeutically if the rhythm is amenable to ablation.

Ambulatory ECG monitors are helpful in identifying arrhythmias in patients with daily symptoms. They can also be used to monitor for arrhythmias that may be asymptomatic, such as atrial fibrillation. This patient's symptoms occur once or twice per week; therefore, a 24-hour ambulatory ECG monitor may not capture the arrhythmia.

In patients with very infrequent or rare episodes (>30 days between episodes), an implantable loop recorder may be appropriate; however, these devices should not be used for initial evaluation, given the cost and risks, although minimal, associated with implantation. Implantable loop recorders can remain in place for years to evaluate for infrequent arrhythmias.

KEY POINT

- In patients with infrequent episodes of palpitations, presyncope, or syncope, an event recorder may be used to correlate symptoms with an arrhythmia.

Bibliography

Ruwald MH, Zareba W. ECG monitoring in syncope. Prog Cardiovasc Dis. 2013;56:203–10. [PMID: 24215752] doi:10.1016/j.pcad.2013.08.007

Item 60   Answer: D

Educational Objective: Interpret B-type natriuretic peptide level in an obese patient with dyspnea.

The cause of this patient's dyspnea is indeterminate on the basis of the B-type natriuretic peptide (BNP) level of 128 pg/mL (128 ng/L). In the Breathing Not Properly study of patients who presented to the emergency department with dyspnea, patients with heart failure had a mean BNP level greater than 600 pg/mL (600 ng/L), whereas those with noncardiac causes of dyspnea had levels of approximately 50 pg/mL (50 ng/L). Patients with a history of left ventricular dysfunction but not an acute exacerbation had a BNP level of approximately 200 pg/mL (200 ng/L). In a pooled analysis of 10 studies, BNP values less than 100 pg/mL (100 ng/L) excluded heart failure (90% sensitivity) and greater than 400 pg/mL (400 ng/L) supported the diagnosis of heart failure (74% specificity). BNP levels increase with age and worsening kidney function and are reduced in patients with an elevated BMI. BNP values less than 55 pg/mL (55 ng/L) are likely to rule out heart failure in patients with BMI greater than 35 (sensitivity 90%). In these patients, BNP levels greater than or equal to 170 pg/mL (170 ng/L) are 70% specific for the diagnosis of acute heart failure. This patient's BNP level is not helpful in ruling in or ruling out cardiac disease as the cause of her dyspnea, and further evaluation is required.

KEY POINT

- Common factors other than ventricular wall stress that influence B-type natriuretic peptide (BNP) levels include kidney failure, older age, and female sex, all of which increase BNP levels; obesity reduces BNP levels.

Bibliography

Daniels LB, Clopton P, Bhalla V, Krishnaswamy P, Nowak RM, McCord J, et al. How obesity affects the cut-points for B-type natriuretic peptide in the diagnosis of acute heart failure. Results from the Breathing Not Properly Multinational Study. Am Heart J. 2006;151:999-1005. [PMID: 16644321]

Item 61   Answer: B

Educational Objective: Treat critical limb ischemia.

The most appropriate next step in the management of this patient with critical limb ischemia is to perform invasive angiography of the affected limb with the intent to revascularize. Critical limb ischemia is a severe form of peripheral artery disease (PAD) characterized by ischemic rest pain and ulceration. Clinical findings in a patient with critical limb ischemia include an ankle-brachial index less than 0.40, a flat waveform on pulse volume recording, and low or absent pedal flow on duplex ultrasonography. In patients who undergo successful limb revascularization, the 1-year risk for major amputation is significantly lower than that in patients who do not undergo revascularization.

Vorapaxar inhibits thrombin-induced and thrombin receptor agonist peptide–induced platelet aggregation. In the TRA 2P–TIMI 50 trial, vorapaxar reduced hospitalizations for acute limb ischemia, mainly among patients who had previously undergone revascularization. The role of vorapaxar in patients with PAD is yet to be established.

Owing to the high morbidity and mortality associated with critical limb ischemia, immediate invasive angiography with endovascular revascularization, without additional noninvasive imaging, is often the most effective strategy to preserve tissue viability. Imaging studies such as magnetic resonance angiography would result in treatment time delays in this patient with critical limb ischemia and a viable limb. He should be referred directly for angiography and revascularization.

In patients with critical limb ischemia and a viable limb, angiography and revascularization is always preferred to primary major amputation of the lower extremity. Patients older than 65 years who undergo major amputation have a 1-year mortality rate of nearly 50% and a 3-year mortality rate higher than 70%.

KEY POINT

- In patients with critical limb ischemia, immediate invasive angiography with endovascular revascularization is often the most effective strategy to preserve tissue viability.

Bibliography

Gerhard-Herman MD, Gornik HL, Barrett C, Barshes NR, Corriere MA, Drachman DE, et al. 2016 AHA/ACC guideline on the management of patients with lower extremity peripheral artery disease: executive summary: a report of the American College of Cardiology/American Heart Association Task Force on Clinical Practice Guidelines. J Am Coll Cardiol. 2017;69:1465-1508. [PMID: 27851991] doi:10.1016/j.jacc.2016.11.008

Item 62   Answer: A

Educational Objective: Manage atrioventricular block in the setting of an acute coronary syndrome.

This patient has Mobitz type 1 second-degree atrioventricular (AV) block and evidence of an acute coronary syndrome, and she should undergo cardiac catheterization for emergent revascularization. This patient's chest pain, ST-segment elevation, and elevated troponin T level all indicate acute myocardial infarction. Additionally, the electrocardiogram demonstrates second-degree AV block, which is characterized by nonconducted P waves. The progressive prolongation of the PR interval before loss of AV conduction is consistent with Mobitz type 1 (Wenckebach block). There are many causes of AV block, including fibrosis and sclerosis of the conduction system, ischemic heart disease, and medication use (β-blockers, calcium channel blockers, digoxin). Reversible causes of AV block should always be identified and treated first. In this patient, cardiac catheterization and revascularization are indicated not only to treat the acute coronary obstruction but also to potentially correct the conduction deficit.

Transthoracic echocardiography should be performed in patients with myocardial infarction to evaluate left ventricular function and assess for potential structural complications; however, obtaining an echocardiogram is not the priority in this patient and does not help manage the arrhythmia. The most appropriate next step is cardiac catheterization.

Permanent or temporary pacemaker placement is not required in this case because the patient does not have symptomatic or hemodynamically unstable bradycardia or advanced AV block (Mobitz type 2 second-degree or third-degree AV block). If symptomatic or advanced conduction block persists after revascularization, permanent pacemaker implantation would be recommended.

KEY POINT

- Patients with atrioventricular block and evidence of acute coronary syndrome should undergo cardiac catheterization for diagnosis and possible revascularization.

Bibliography

Epstein AE, DiMarco JP, Ellenbogen KA, Estes NA 3rd, Freedman RA, Gettes LS, et al; American College of Cardiology Foundation. 2012 ACCF/AHA/HRS focused update incorporated into the ACCF/AHA/HRS 2008 guidelines for device-based therapy of cardiac rhythm abnormalities: a report of the American College of Cardiology Foundation/American Heart Association Task Force on Practice Guidelines and the Heart Rhythm Society. J Am Coll Cardiol. 2013;61:e6-75. [PMID: 23265327] doi:10.1016/j.jacc.2012.11.007

Item 63 Answer: D

Educational Objective: Manage aortic regurgitation that does not meet criteria for surgical valve replacement.

The most appropriate next step in management is clinical and echocardiographic follow-up in 6 to 12 months. This asymptomatic patient with severe aortic regurgitation does not currently meet the criteria for surgical aortic valve replacement. For patients with severe aortic regurgitation, surgical aortic valve replacement is recommended in the presence of symptoms attributable to regurgitation, left ventricular ejection fraction less than 50%, or another indication for cardiac surgery. In addition, surgical aortic valve replacement can be beneficial in asymptomatic patients with significant left ventricular dilatation (end-systolic dimension >50 mm or indexed end-systolic dimension >25 mm/m^2). In the absence of these findings, clinical evaluation and surveillance echocardiography every 6 to 12 months is recommended.

The clinical impact of β-blockers, such as carvedilol, in patients with chronic aortic regurgitation is uncertain. Carvedilol is useful in patients with severe aortic regurgitation and heart failure when combined with other standard therapies, such as diuretics, ACE inhibitors, and aldosterone antagonists; however, this patient has no indication for β-blocker therapy.

ACE inhibitors or angiotensin receptor blockers may be used in patients with chronic severe aortic regurgitation and concomitant hypertension, although these agents, as well as dihydropyridine calcium channel blockers, have not been shown to delay the need for surgery in asymptomatic patients without hypertension. Consequently, they are not indicated in this patient in the absence of hypertension.

KEY POINT

- For patients with severe aortic regurgitation, indications for surgery are the presence of attributable symptoms, left ventricular ejection fraction less than 50%, or significant left ventricular dilatation; in the absence of these findings, surveillance echocardiography every 6 to 12 months is recommended.

Bibliography

Nishimura RA, Otto CM, Bonow RO, Carabello BA, Erwin JP 3rd, Guyton RA, et al; American College of Cardiology/American Heart Association Task Force on Practice Guidelines. 2014 AHA/ACC guideline for the management of patients with valvular heart disease: a report of the American College of Cardiology/American Heart Association Task Force on Practice Guidelines. J Am Coll Cardiol. 2014;63:e57-185. [PMID: 24603191] doi:10.1016/j.jacc.2014.02.536

Item 64 Answer: D

Educational Objective: Treat a patient with ST-elevation myocardial infarction and heart failure with renin-angiotensin system inhibition.

The most appropriate treatment of this patient with anterior ST-elevation myocardial infarction (STEMI) complicated by heart failure is valsartan. This patient is at significant risk for short-term and long-term morbidity, and early institution of guideline-directed medical therapy (within 24 hours of presentation) is crucial to improve survival and keep the patient free of symptoms. Although ACE inhibitors are indicated in most patients with STEMI and particularly in patients with impaired left ventricular function and heart failure, angiotensin receptor blockers (such as valsartan) are a suitable alternative and offer similar morbidity and mortality benefits. Additionally, angiotensin receptor blockers are associated with a significantly lower incidence of cough and angioedema than ACE inhibitors. Because this patient has a history of ACE inhibitor–induced cough, valsartan is the most appropriate choice.

In patients with STEMI, β-blockers (such as carvedilol) decrease myocardial oxygen demand, reduce the incidence of ventricular arrhythmias, and improve long-term survival. Whenever possible, β-blockers should be introduced within the first 24 hours of STEMI presentation. The COMMIT/CCS-2 trial demonstrated that early β-blocker initiation was associated with lower risk for reinfarction and lethal ventricular arrhythmias, but it also increased risk for cardiogenic shock. In this case, the patient has evidence of pulmonary edema, and early institution of β-blockade may worsen heart failure and increase the risk for cardiogenic shock. A β-blocker should be initiated once the patient is stabilized.

Like β-blockers, calcium channel blockers (such as diltiazem) are negative inotropic and chronotropic agents. However, unlike β-blockers, calcium channel blockers are generally avoided in the context of STEMI and are contraindicated with left ventricular dysfunction.

Hydralazine–isosorbide dinitrate can be used as a vasodilator, particularly as an add-on therapy in the setting of chronic heart failure, although it has been shown to be inferior to ACE inhibitors in a head-to-head study. Hydralazine–isosorbide dinitrate would not be the preferred agent in this setting, unless the patient had a significantly elevated serum creatinine level or a history of ACE inhibitor–induced angioedema.

KEY POINT

- In patients with ST-elevation myocardial infarction, an ACE inhibitor should be initiated within 24 hours of presentation; an angiotensin receptor blocker may be used if the patient is intolerant of ACE inhibitors.

Bibliography

O'Gara PT, Kushner FG, Ascheim DD, Casey DE Jr, Chung MK, de Lemos JA, et al; American College of Cardiology Foundation/American Heart Association Task Force on Practice Guidelines. 2013 ACCF/AHA guideline for the management of ST-elevation myocardial infarction: a report of the American College of Cardiology Foundation/American Heart Association Task Force on Practice Guidelines. Circulation. 2013;127:e362-425. [PMID: 23247304] doi:10.1161/CIR.0b013e3182742cf6

Item 65 Answer: B

Educational Objective: Treat atrial fibrillation in a patient with hypertrophic cardiomyopathy.

The most appropriate treatment to reduce the risk for thromboembolic events in this patient is dose-adjusted warfarin.

In patients with hypertrophic cardiomyopathy (HCM), atrial fibrillation occurs in 20% to 25% of cases, and dyspnea often develops related to reduced left ventricular diastolic filling and increased left ventricular outflow tract obstruction. Restoration and maintenance of sinus rhythm are important in reducing symptoms. There is also a high incidence of stroke in patients with HCM who have atrial fibrillation, regardless of the type of atrial fibrillation (paroxysmal, persistent, or permanent), and anticoagulation to reduce thromboembolic risk must be considered. In this patient, acute anticoagulation with heparin or low-molecular-weight heparin would be appropriate before cardioversion, followed by administration of dose-adjusted warfarin to achieve an INR of 2 to 3. Two observational studies of patients with atrial fibrillation in the setting of HCM have shown reduced incidence of stroke with this strategy compared with antiplatelet therapy or no treatment.

The use of non–vitamin K antagonist oral anticoagulants, such as dabigatran, for thromboembolic risk reduction in patients with HCM has not been adequately studied, and the efficacy of these drugs in this situation is unknown. In patients with HCM who cannot take warfarin, non–vitamin K antagonist oral anticoagulants are reasonable as second-line therapy; however, use of warfarin in this patient is not contraindicated.

Although this patient's calculated CHA_2DS_2-VASc score is low (0 points), initiating aspirin therapy or foregoing therapy would be inappropriate according to current guidelines. The CHA_2DS_2-VASc scoring system is frequently used for decision making with regard to stroke risk-reduction therapy in patients with atrial fibrillation; however, the predictive use of this tool for patients with HCM has not been validated. A low CHA_2DS_2-VASc score may not adequately predict true thromboembolic risk in patients with HCM and should not be used to guide therapy.

KEY POINT

- Patients with atrial fibrillation in the setting of hypertrophic cardiomyopathy should receive warfarin anticoagulation therapy to reduce thromboembolic risk.

Bibliography
Elliott PM, Anastasakis A, Borger MA, Borggrefe M, Cecchi F, Charron P, et al; Authors/Task Force members. 2014 ESC guidelines on diagnosis and management of hypertrophic cardiomyopathy: the Task Force for the Diagnosis and Management of Hypertrophic Cardiomyopathy of the European Society of Cardiology (ESC). Eur Heart J. 2014;35:2733-79. [PMID: 25173338] doi:10.1093/eurheartj/ehu284

Item 66   Answer: A

Educational Objective: Evaluate the severity of aortic stenosis with cardiac catheterization.

The most appropriate next step in management is cardiac catheterization. In patients with symptomatic severe aortic stenosis, surgery with aortic valve replacement is indicated as a life-saving therapy. However, accurate measures of the severity of stenosis are needed to ensure that symptoms are caused by valve obstruction, rather than concurrent coronary, pulmonary, or other systemic disease. The severity of aortic stenosis is determined by Doppler echocardiography and sometimes cardiac catheterization. In some patients, the Doppler echocardiogram may underestimate severity because of the angle-dependent nature of the study. An invasive hemodynamic study is indicated in symptomatic patients being considered for surgery when there are discrepancies between the findings on physical examination and the echocardiographic results. This patient's exertional dyspnea and physical examination findings (carotid tardus, diminished aortic component of S_2, late-peaking systolic murmur) are consistent with severe aortic stenosis; however, the echocardiogram reveals findings of only moderate aortic stenosis. Therefore, further evaluation with cardiac catheterization is needed.

Surgical or transcatheter aortic valve replacement is not indicated in this patient until there is certainty that the aortic valve lesion is severe and can account for the patient's symptoms.

Identification of symptomatic aortic stenosis is crucial; in the absence of symptoms, patients with aortic stenosis–even severe aortic stenosis–have a low risk for mortality, with an estimated risk for sudden death of less than 1%. Although variable, symptoms of heart failure, angina, or syncope generally begin once the valve area is below 1.0 cm². Once symptoms develop, prognosis is poor without valve replacement, with an average survival of less than 10% over the next 2 to 3 years. Therefore, continued clinical observation is not the best option for this patient.

KEY POINT

- In patients with symptoms of aortic stenosis and discrepancies between the physical examination and echocardiographic findings, the severity of stenosis should be established with cardiac catheterization before aortic valve replacement is performed.

Bibliography
Nishimura RA, Otto CM, Bonow RO, Carabello BA, Erwin JP 3rd, Fleisher LA, et al. 2017 AHA/ACC focused update of the 2014 AHA/ACC guideline for the management of patients with valvular heart disease: a report of the American College of Cardiology/American Heart Association Task Force on Clinical Practice Guidelines. J Am Coll Cardiol. 2017;70:252-289. [PMID: 28315732] doi:10.1016/j.jacc.2017.03.011

Item 67   Answer: D

Educational Objective: Manage a patient with a ventricular septal defect.

The most appropriate management for this patient with a small uncomplicated ventricular septal defect (VSD) is follow-up in 3 to 5 years. VSDs are defined by their location on the ventricular septum. The most common type of VSD is perimembranous, making up 80% of cases; these are usually isolated abnormalities. She has no associated symptoms, volume overload of the left heart, pulmonary hypertension, or valve regurgitation; therefore, periodic clinical evaluation and imaging are recommended. If pulmonary vascular disease is present (pulmonary artery systolic pressure >50 mm Hg), patients should be advised against isometric or competitive exercise. In the absence of pulmonary hypertension, pregnancy in women with VSDs is generally well tolerated. It is unnecessary to suggest activity restriction in this patient with a small VSD and normal pulmonary artery pressure, and pregnancy should not be complicated by the VSD.

Cardiac catheterization is not indicated for this patient because her clinical presentation and echocardiogram do not demonstrate features of left heart enlargement or pulmonary hypertension. Cardiac catheterization is primarily performed to delineate the shunt ratio and to determine pulmonary pressures if clinical uncertainty exists regarding the degree or impact of a shunt, or if the VSD is incompletely assessed by echocardiographic measures.

Cardiac magnetic resonance imaging will usually demonstrate a membranous VSD and can quantitate the impact of the shunt on the left heart; however, it is not indicated in this patient because the clinical and echocardiographic assessment are sufficient to suggest that observation is appropriate.

Endocarditis prophylaxis is recommended for patients with unrepaired cyanotic congenital heart disease, including palliative shunts and conduits; a congenital heart defect that has been completely repaired with prosthetic material or device during the first 6 months after the procedure; and repaired congenital heart disease with residual defects. Patients with uncomplicated VSDs without a history of endocarditis do not require endocarditis prophylaxis.

KEY POINT

- Periodic follow-up with clinical evaluation and imaging are appropriate in patients with a small uncomplicated ventricular septal defect.

Bibliography

Penny DJ, Vick GW 3rd. Ventricular septal defect. Lancet. 2011;377:1103-12. [PMID: 21349577] doi:10.1016/S0140-6736(10)61339-6

Item 68   Answer: A

Educational Objective: Diagnose cardiac tamponade.

The most likely diagnosis is cardiac tamponade. Pericarditis is a common cardiac manifestation of systemic lupus erythematosus (SLE), occurring in up to 40% of patients with SLE. Pericarditis may be associated with a neutrophilic pericardial effusion that can rarely lead to tamponade. In this patient, progressive dyspnea, fatigue, chest fullness, and peripheral edema are symptoms consistent with significant cardiac tamponade, and the physical examination findings of jugular venous distention and pulsus paradoxus (fall in systolic pressure of >10 mm Hg with inspiration) are supportive. The chest radiograph demonstrates an enlarged cardiac silhouette ("water-bottle heart"), and the electrocardiogram demonstrates electrical alternans, which may represent swinging of the heart within a large pericardial effusion. This patient also has supraventricular tachycardia.

The pericardium in constrictive pericarditis is rigid and noncompliant, resulting in a total cardiac volume that is largely fixed. Ventricular filling occurs rapidly in early diastole and terminates abruptly near mid-diastole owing to the pericardial restraint. The jugular venous pressure is elevated in nearly all patients, with prominent x and y descents. Physical findings that also may be present include a pericardial knock, pulsus paradoxus, pleural effusion, congestive hepatomegaly, and peripheral edema or ascites. In patients with long-standing constrictive pericarditis, hepatic failure and cirrhosis may be present. Pericardial constriction would not lead to a large cardiac silhouette or electrical alternans, as seen in this patient.

Patients with SLE have increased risk for venous thromboembolic disease. The electrocardiogram in acute pulmonary embolism most commonly demonstrates sinus tachycardia but may also show a new complete or incomplete right bundle branch block or an S1Q3T3 pattern (prominent S wave in lead I, Q wave in lead III, and inverted T wave in lead III). An enlarged globular heart on chest radiograph and electrical alternans on electrocardiogram are not features.

Patients with SLE may have pulmonary thromboembolic disease, pulmonary veno-occlusive disease, or advanced interstitial lung disease with hypoxemia leading to pulmonary hypertension; however, severe symptomatic pulmonary hypertension is more commonly associated with scleroderma or mixed connective tissue disease. An enlarged globular heart on chest radiograph would be unlikely, and the electrocardiogram is likely to demonstrate a right axis deviation and right ventricular hypertrophy but not electrical alternans.

KEY POINT

- Findings of congestion, hypotension, pulsus paradoxus, enlarged cardiac silhouette on chest radiograph, and electrical alternans on electrocardiogram support the diagnosis of cardiac tamponade.

Bibliography

Imazio M. Pericardial involvement in systemic inflammatory diseases. Heart. 2011;97:1882-92. [PMID: 22016400] doi:10.1136/heartjnl-2011-300054

Item 69   Answer: B

Educational Objective: Evaluate a patient with intermediate cardiovascular risk with coronary artery calcium scoring.

This asymptomatic patient at intermediate risk for coronary artery disease can undergo coronary artery calcium (CAC) scoring for further risk stratification. He has an intermediate risk for myocardial infarction and coronary death (5% to less than 7.5% as defined by the Pooled Cohort Equations). Among these patients, further risk stratification can be helpful to identify patients who will benefit from primary prevention, including statin therapy. The evaluation of subclinical disease with CAC scoring is not a component of routine risk assessment, and consideration is reserved for when the result is expected to lead to a change in management based on patient reclassification to a lower- or higher-risk group. A CAC score of 300 Agatston units or higher or a score in the 75th percentile or higher for age, sex, and ethnicity would reclassify this patient as high risk and prompt initiation of primary prevention therapy. Other factors that can help guide risk reclassification are an LDL cholesterol level of 160 mg/dL (4.14 mmol/L) or higher, evidence of other genetic hyperlipidemias, family history of premature coronary artery disease (age <55 years in a first-degree male relative, age <65 years in a first-degree female relative), high-sensitivity C-reactive protein level of 2 mg/L or more, ankle-brachial index less than 0.9, or elevated lifetime risk for cardiovascular disease.

Physiologic tests of coronary perfusion are not indicated because this patient is asymptomatic. Furthermore, adenosine cardiac magnetic resonance imaging, exercise stress echocardiography, and pharmacologic nuclear stress testing are not used to reclassify risk among asymptomatic patients.

Elevated levels of lipoprotein(a), a subtype of LDL cholesterol, have been associated with increased risk for cardiovascular disease, especially coronary artery disease. However, this marker has not been evaluated for purposes of reclassification of asymptomatic, intermediate-risk patients. Additionally, the 2013 American College of Cardiology/American Heart Association cholesterol treatment guideline does not address whether lipoprotein(a) is useful for guiding treatment because evidence is currently insufficient.

KEY POINT

- In patients with an intermediate 10-year risk for atherosclerotic cardiovascular disease, coronary artery calcium scoring may be used to further risk-stratify patients to guide primary prevention therapy.

Bibliography

Nezarat N, Kim M, Budoff M. Role of coronary calcium for risk stratification and prognostication. Curr Treat Options Cardiovasc Med. 2017 Feb; 19(2):8. [PMID: 28275938]

Item 70   Answer: A

Educational Objective: Treat heart failure with reduced ejection fraction with β-blocker therapy.

This patient with heart failure with reduced ejection fraction (HFrEF) should be started on a β-blocker, such as bisoprolol. In patients with heart failure, each follow-up visit should include evaluation for progression of heart failure symptoms, assessment of volume status, and a review of the patient's medications to ensure guideline-directed treatment. Optimal medical therapy includes an ACE inhibitor, β-blocker (specifically, metoprolol succinate, carvedilol, or bisoprolol), and an aldosterone antagonist (in symptomatic patients). β-Blockers improve remodeling, increase ejection fraction, and reduce hospitalization and mortality when added to ACE inhibitor and diuretic therapy. β-Blocker and ACE inhibitor therapies are indicated for all classes of heart failure, including New

York Heart Association functional class I. This patient was discharged from the hospital before initiation of β-blocker therapy, and he should be started on bisoprolol now.

Diltiazem and verapamil are associated with worse outcomes in patients with HFrEF, and these agents should not be used in this population. If calcium channel blockers are necessary for hypertension treatment, amlodipine or felodipine have been shown to be safe in patients with heart failure.

Aldosterone antagonists (spironolactone, eplerenone) have been studied in patients with heart failure and New York Heart Association functional class II to IV symptoms and have been shown to reduce mortality and morbidity. Because of the risk for kidney dysfunction and hyperkalemia, these drugs should be used only in patients with a serum creatinine level below 2.5 mg/dL (221 µmol/L) in men or below 2.0 mg/dL (176.8 µmol/L) in women, and with a serum potassium level below 5.0 mEq/L (5.0 mmol/L). These drugs are not as effective as diuretics at the doses used in heart failure therapy (12.5-25 mg/d for spironolactone, 25-50 mg/d for eplerenone). The patient is asymptomatic now, and spironolactone is not indicated. If it were indicated, it would not be added until after uptitration of the β-blocker and ACE inhibitor doses.

Angiotensin receptor blockers (ARBs), such as losartan, are a suitable alternative to ACE inhibitors for the treatment of HFrEF and offer similar morbidity and mortality benefits. In patients taking an ACE inhibitor, the primary reason to switch to an ARB is ACE inhibitor–induced cough or angioedema. Caution should be exercised when switching patients to an ARB as a result of angioedema because this side effect has been reported with ARB therapy as well. This patient does not have side effects that would prompt switching an ACE inhibitor to an ARB.

KEY POINT

- In patients with heart failure with reduced ejection fraction, β-blockers improve remodeling, increase ejection fraction, and reduce hospitalization and mortality when added to ACE inhibitor and diuretic therapy.

Bibliography

Goldberg LR. In the clinic. Heart failure. Ann Intern Med. 2010;152:ITC61-15; quiz ITC616. [PMID: 20513825] doi:10.7326/0003-4819-152-6-201006010-01006

Item 71   Answer: B

Educational Objective: Treat a patient with multivessel coronary artery disease and left ventricular dysfunction with coronary artery bypass graft surgery.

The most appropriate treatment is coronary artery bypass graft (CABG) surgery. This patient with three-vessel coronary artery disease (CAD), left ventricular dysfunction, and type 2 diabetes mellitus has symptoms of heart failure and angina despite optimal medical therapy. In patients with multivessel coronary artery disease, revascularization with CABG results in decreased recurrence of angina, lower rates of myocardial infarction, and fewer repeat revascularization procedures compared with percutaneous coronary intervention (PCI). Unlike PCI, CABG surgery improves survival in patients with left main or three-vessel CAD and is recommended to reduce mortality in these high-risk patients. CABG surgery has also been shown to improve symptoms and survival in patients with ischemic cardiomyopathy. Long-term follow-up of the STICH trial demonstrated a survival advantage with CABG surgery compared with medical therapy alone among patients with multivessel CAD and severe left ventricular dysfunction. Additionally, CABG surgery has consistently been shown to be the superior revascularization strategy in patients with diabetes and multivessel disease who require revascularization.

Ticagrelor is indicated as a component of dual antiplatelet therapy following acute coronary syndrome, regardless of whether percutaneous coronary intervention is performed. However, there is no clear role for the addition of ticagrelor in this patient.

This patient has two separate indications for CABG surgery: (1) multivessel disease and reduced ejection fraction and (2) diabetes with concomitant multivessel disease. Patients with these indications who undergo CABG have improved survival compared with patients who receive only optimal medical therapy. Therefore, continuing this patient's medical therapy without further intervention would be inappropriate.

KEY POINT

- Coronary artery bypass graft surgery is recommended to improve survival in patients with multivessel coronary artery disease and left ventricular dysfunction and patients with diabetes mellitus and multivessel disease.

Bibliography

Velazquez EJ, Lee KL, Jones RH, Al-Khalidi HR, Hill JA, Panza JA, et al; STICHES Investigators. Coronary-artery bypass surgery in patients with ischemic cardiomyopathy. N Engl J Med. 2016;374:1511-20. [PMID: 27040723] doi:10.1056/NEJMoa1602001

Item 72   Answer: D

Educational Objective: Treat symptomatic premature ventricular contractions.

Catheter ablation is the most appropriate management of this patient with frequent symptomatic premature ventricular contractions (PVCs). PVCs are common and occur in up to 75% of healthy persons. In the absence of high-risk features (syncope, a family history of premature sudden cardiac death, structural heart disease), reassurance is often appropriate management. For patients with bothersome palpitations, the initial diagnostic test is electrocardiography (ECG). If the diagnosis is not established, 24- to 48-hour ambulatory ECG monitoring is used to diagnose and quantify the frequency of PVCs and determine whether they are monomorphic or polymorphic. Symptomatic or frequent monomorphic PVCs (>10,000 PVCs in 24 hours or >10% of all beats) require further

evaluation and treatment. Exercise stress testing can be used to evaluate the patient for ischemia and assess the response of PVCs to exercise. In addition, patients with frequent PVCs or polymorphic PVCs should undergo echocardiography or other cardiovascular imaging (such as cardiac magnetic resonance imaging) to evaluate for the presence of structural heart disease. Up to one third of patients with frequent PVCs can develop PVC-induced cardiomyopathy and progressive left ventricular dysfunction, as documented in this patient. First-line therapy for symptomatic or frequent PVCs includes β-blockers or calcium channel blockers. Patients with continued frequent PVCs despite medical therapy or those who develop left ventricular dysfunction should undergo catheter ablation, which resolves most cases of PVC-induced left ventricular dysfunction.

Amiodarone is usually effective in suppressing PVCs; however, it carries a high risk for adverse effects and end-organ toxicities. Therefore, amiodarone is best avoided in younger patients, such as this one.

This patient had a structurally normal heart and no evidence of ischemia on studies performed 1 year ago, and she has developed no new symptoms. Therefore, cardiac catheterization is not indicated.

Cardiopulmonary exercise testing includes assessment of respiratory gas exchange during treadmill or bicycle exercise for a more detailed assessment of functional capacity and differentiation between potential causes of exercise limitation (cardiac, pulmonary, or deconditioning causes versus volitional causes). It would not be the most appropriate next choice in a patient with a known decrease in left ventricular ejection fraction and frequent PVCs.

KEY POINT

- Patients with premature ventricular contraction–induced cardiomyopathy should be treated with catheter ablation.

Bibliography

Yokokawa M, Good E, Crawford T, Chugh A, Pelosi F Jr, Latchamsetty R, et al. Recovery from left ventricular dysfunction after ablation of frequent premature ventricular complexes. Heart Rhythm. 2013;10:172-5. [PMID: 23099051] doi:10.1016/j.hrthm.2012.10.011

Item 73   Answer: C

Educational Objective: Treat mitral regurgitation with transcatheter mitral valve repair.

The most appropriate next step in management is transcatheter mitral valve repair. Acute severe mitral regurgitation is associated with papillary muscle rupture following acute myocardial infarction, flail mitral valve (dissociation of the valve leaflet from the chordae), and infective endocarditis with leaflet perforation. The sudden large volume in the left atrium and ventricle results in rapid increases in left ventricular end-diastolic pressure and left atrial pressure, which lead to elevated pulmonary artery pressure and pulmonary edema. The diminished left ventricular stroke volume leads to hypotension and shock. Definitive therapy for severe mitral regurgitation is mitral valve surgery. Patients with acute severe mitral regurgitation typically require urgent surgery after hemodynamic stabilization. Positive inotropes, vasodilators, and diuretics are often used for symptom control and as a bridge to cardiac surgery. Mechanical support (for example, with an intra-aortic balloon pump) may be required before or during valve replacement.

Two surgical options are available: mitral valve repair and mitral valve replacement. Mitral valve repair is typically preferred to valve replacement because it is associated with better clinical outcomes. A nonoperative procedure, transcatheter mitral valve repair, is indicated for symptomatic patients with degenerative mitral regurgitation who are at prohibitive surgical risk, such as this patient. With this technique, the mitral valve is plicated using an approach from the femoral vein. In experienced centers, success rates are approximately 90%, with procedural mortality of approximately 2%.

Continuing the patient's current medical therapy is inappropriate. Acute severe mitral regurgitation is an emergency, and prompt mitral valve repair or replacement should be considered for all patients.

KEY POINT

- Transcatheter mitral valve repair is indicated for symptomatic patients with degenerative mitral regurgitation who are not surgical candidates.

Bibliography

Sorajja P, Mack M, Vemulapalli S, Holmes DR Jr, Stebbins A, Kar S, et al. Initial experience with commercial transcatheter mitral valve repair in the United States. J Am Coll Cardiol. 2016;67:1129-40. [PMID: 26965532] doi:10.1016/j.jacc.2015.12.054

Item 74   Answer: C

Educational Objective: Treat a patient with peripheral artery disease with statin therapy.

The most appropriate treatment is high-intensity atorvastatin. This patient with claudication has an ankle-brachial index of less than or equal to 0.90 on the right side, which is diagnostic for peripheral artery disease (PAD). PAD is considered a form of clinical atherosclerotic cardiovascular disease (ASCVD), and as such, this patient should be started on secondary prevention therapy. Additional forms of ASCVD include acute coronary syndrome, history of myocardial infarction, stable or unstable angina, coronary or other arterial revascularization, stroke, or transient ischemic attack. Patients aged 75 years or younger with ASCVD should be started on high-intensity statin therapy, unless a contraindication exists. Options for high-intensity statin therapy include atorvastatin, 40 mg/d or 80 mg/d, and rosuvastatin, 20 mg/d or 40 mg/d.

Proprotein convertase subtilisin/kexin type 9 (PCSK9) inhibitors, such as evolocumab, are a new class of medications that dramatically decrease LDL cholesterol levels. PCSK9 inhibitors are currently approved as adjunctive

therapy to diet and maximally tolerated statin therapy in patients with familial hypercholesterolemia or established ASCVD. Treatment with evolocumab has been associated with a reduction in the composite outcome of cardiovascular death, myocardial infarction, stroke, hospitalization for unstable angina, and coronary revascularization but not cardiovascular mortality or all-cause mortality.

Ezetimibe impairs intestinal cholesterol absorption, resulting in a significant reduction in LDL cholesterol levels. Several trials have shown clinical benefit when ezetimibe is added to statin therapy. However, this patient is not yet taking a statin, and ezetimibe is not appropriate as monotherapy.

Moderate-intensity statin therapy with pravastatin is not the first choice for patients with clinical ASCVD because high-intensity statin therapy offers superior benefits in patients aged 75 years or younger. Patients older than 75 years can be considered for moderate-intensity statin therapy.

Although this patient's 10-year risk for ASCVD, as calculated using the American College of Cardiology/American Heart Association Pooled Cohort Equations, is lower than the threshold of 7.5% for initiation of primary prevention statin therapy, she should be started on high-intensity statin therapy because of her PAD.

KEY POINT

- Patients with peripheral artery disease should be treated statin therapy.

Bibliography

Stone NJ, Robinson JG, Lichtenstein AH, Bairey Merz CN, Blum CB, Eckel RH, et al; American College of Cardiology/American Heart Association Task Force on Practice Guidelines. 2013 ACC/AHA guideline on the treatment of blood cholesterol to reduce atherosclerotic cardiovascular risk in adults: a report of the American College of Cardiology/American Heart Association Task Force on Practice Guidelines. J Am Coll Cardiol. 2014;63:2889-934. [PMID: 24239923] doi:10.1016/j.jacc.2013.11.002

Item 75   Answer: C

Educational Objective: Manage end-stage heart failure with a left ventricular assist device.

The most appropriate management is left ventricular assist device (LVAD) placement. This patient has several signs and symptoms of advanced refractory heart failure, including New York Heart Association (NYHA) functional class IV symptoms despite optimal medical therapy, a low sodium level, worsening kidney function, low pulse pressure, cool extremities, and repeat hospitalizations in the past 6 months. In patients with end-stage heart failure, advanced treatments, including cardiac transplantation or mechanical circulatory support with an LVAD, should be considered. This patient is a good candidate for an LVAD as destination therapy. Placement of a continuous-flow LVAD reduces symptoms and improves survival compared with medical therapy in patients with end-stage heart failure. Although LVADs increase survival rates, they are associated with serious complications, including infection, gastrointestinal bleeding, stroke, and pump thrombus. All patients with progressive heart failure symptoms should be engaged in a discussion about their prognosis, treatment options (including hospice), and the risks and benefits of each therapy.

Cardiac resynchronization therapy is indicated in patients with an ejection fraction less than or equal to 35%, NYHA functional class II to IV heart failure symptoms despite guideline-directed medical therapy, sinus rhythm, and left bundle branch block with a QRS complex of 150 ms or greater. This patient does not meet the electrocardiographic criteria.

Cardiac transplantation remains the gold standard therapy for patients with end-stage heart failure. Indications for cardiac transplantation in these patients include age younger than 65 to 70 years, no medical contraindications (diabetes with end-organ complications, malignancies within 5 years, kidney dysfunction, other chronic illnesses that will decrease survival), and good social support and adherence. Heart transplant is contraindicated in this patient.

This patient has significant mitral regurgitation, most likely secondary to his dilated left ventricle; however, mitral valve repair is unlikely to substantially improve his heart failure symptoms.

KEY POINT

- Patients with end-stage heart failure should be considered for cardiac transplantation or mechanical circulatory support with left ventricular assist device placement.

Bibliography

Stokes MB, Bergin P, McGiffin D. Role of long-term mechanical circulatory support in patients with advanced heart failure. Intern Med J. 2016;46:530–40. [PMID: 26010730] doi:10.1111/imj.12817

Item 76   Answer: C

Educational Objective: Diagnose pulmonary valve regurgitation as a late consequence of tetralogy of Fallot repair.

The most likely diagnosis is pulmonary valve regurgitation, which is the most common structural disorder resulting from tetralogy of Fallot (TOF) repair. Clinical findings include features of right heart volume overload with a parasternal lift and a soft systolic pulmonary outflow murmur. A single S_2 is heard because pulmonary valve function is sacrificed during TOF repair. TOF repair includes closure of the ventricular septal defect and relief of right ventricular outflow tract obstruction, which in turn results in pulmonary regurgitation, causing the diastolic murmur heard at the left sternal border that increases in intensity with inspiration. This patient's chest radiograph demonstrates evidence of previous sternotomy, a clip in the mediastinum from closure of the Blalock-Taussig shunt, a right-sided aortic arch (present in 25% of patients with TOF), and right heart enlargement (indicated by a rounded cardiac border and uplifted cardiac apex as seen on the frontal view and fullness in the retrosternal airspace [*blue arrows*] on lateral view) (see top of next column).

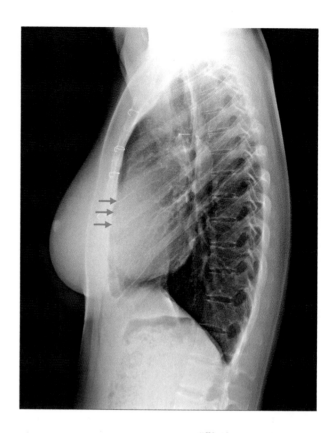

These chest radiograph findings are consistent with repaired TOF with pulmonary regurgitation resulting in right heart enlargement.

Aortic regurgitation infrequently occurs late after TOF repair owing to progressive aortic enlargement. The diastolic murmur of aortic regurgitation is generally heard at the left sternal border and decreases in intensity with inspiration. A right ventricular prominence would not be expected in a patient with aortic regurgitation.

Mitral stenosis is not expected to occur late after TOF repair. Physical examination findings include increased intensity of S_1 and an apical diastolic murmur that increases during expiration.

Recurrent ventricular septal defect can occur in patients following TOF repair. However, the physical examination findings would include a systolic murmur heard at the left sternal border, which often obliterates the S_1 and S_2. Right ventricular prominence would not be expected in a patient with a recurrent ventricular septal defect.

KEY POINT

- Pulmonary regurgitation, presenting with a single S_2, a parasternal lift, and a soft systolic pulmonary outflow murmur, is the most common structural disorder resulting from tetralogy of Fallot repair.

Bibliography

Downing TE, Kim YY. Tetralogy of Fallot: general principles of management. Cardiol Clin. 2015;33:531–41, vii–viii. [PMID: 26471818] doi:10.1016/j.ccl.2015.07.002

Item 77   Answer: C

Educational Objective: Manage an abdominal aortic aneurysm with surveillance.

The most appropriate next step in the management of this patient with an abdominal aortic aneurysm (AAA) is repeat abdominal aortic ultrasonography. The optimal surveillance frequency for abdominal aortic aneurysm is controversial. As aneurysm size increases, risk for rupture also increases. For AAAs with a diameter smaller than 4.0 cm, the 5-year risk for rupture is 2%, and some guidelines recommend a surveillance interval of 24 to 36 months. AAAs with a diameter between 4.0 cm and 5.0 cm have a 5-year risk for rupture of 3% to 12%, and surveillance imaging is recommended more frequently (for example, every 6 to 12 months). AAAs with a diameter between 5.0 and 6.0 cm have a 5-year risk for rupture of 25%. Once an AAA reaches 5.5 cm in maximum diameter, surgical or endovascular repair is warranted, owing to the elevated risk for death due to aortic rupture. Repair is also indicated in patients with symptoms from AAA (abdominal tenderness or pain) and those with rapid expansion in AAA size (>0.5 cm/year). This patient with an AAA with a maximum diameter of 3.5 cm can be managed with surveillance abdominal ultrasonography. Because he is asymptomatic, he does not require surgical repair at this time.

Anatomic imaging tests, such as CT angiography or magnetic resonance angiography, are indicated to determine the exact location of the AAA (suprarenal, juxtarenal, or infrarenal) in planning for aortic repair. When an AAA does not meet the maximum diameter threshold for repair, such as in this patient, anatomic imaging with CT angiography is not indicated. Abdominal ultrasonography is preferred for serial monitoring of an AAA.

Pursuing no further testing or intervention would be inappropriate in this patient. An AAA predisposes the patient to an elevated risk for aortic rupture and death, and surveillance of the aneurysm is recommended.

KEY POINT

- Patients with an abdominal aortic aneurysm smaller than 5.5 cm should undergo surveillance ultrasonography, with frequency determined by aneurysm size.

Bibliography
Chaikof EL, Brewster DC, Dalman RL, Makaroun MS, Illig KA, Sicard GA, et al. SVS practice guidelines for the care of patients with an abdominal aortic aneurysm: executive summary. J Vasc Surg. 2009;50:880-96. [PMID: 19786241] doi:10.1016/j.jvs.2009.07.001

Item 78   Answer: C

Educational Objective: Evaluate for perivalvular abscess in a patient with infective endocarditis.

Transesophageal echocardiography (TEE) is the most appropriate diagnostic test to perform next. According to the modified Duke criteria, this patient has definite endocarditis, with one major criterion (persistently positive blood cultures) and three minor criteria (predisposing valvular abnormality [bicuspid valve], fever with temperature >38 °C [100.4 °F], and a vascular phenomenon [conjunctival hemorrhage]). On physical examination, he has a wide pulse pressure and evidence of a murmur of aortic regurgitation, findings that further support the diagnosis. Additionally, the electrocardiogram shows PR-interval prolongation, which should raise suspicion for the presence of a periaortic abscess that is interfering with the conduction system and causing first-degree atrioventricular block. Perivalvular abscesses may be present in 30% to 40% of patients with infective endocarditis, and the risk may be further increased in those with a bicuspid aortic valve. The preferred imaging modality for evaluating patients with a high pretest probability of infective endocarditis or with potential complications of endocarditis is TEE, as it better visualizes vegetations and abscesses. TEE is also important for surgical planning.

Cardiac magnetic resonance (CMR) imaging is not the most appropriate initial imaging choice for patients with infective endocarditis. CMR imaging is effective in identifying intramyocardial infection, although it is a more complex technology with limited availability in some areas. CMR imaging is often used in situations in which a perivalvular abscess is suspected but transesophageal echocardiographic findings are equivocal.

Coronary CT angiography could be used for evaluation in patients suspected of having perivalvular infections if echocardiography cannot adequately identify the anatomy.

Transthoracic echocardiography can help identify the presence of a vegetation; however, there is an increased likelihood of detecting perivalvular abscess with TEE because of the closer proximity of the ultrasound probe to the valve structures. TEE is preferred to transthoracic echocardiography if this diagnosis is a consideration.

KEY POINT

- The preferred imaging modality for evaluating patients with a high pretest probability of infective endocarditis or with potential complications of endocarditis, such as abscess, is transesophageal echocardiography.

Bibliography
Iung B, Rouzet F, Brochet E, Duval X. Cardiac imaging of infective endocarditis, echo and beyond. Curr Infect Dis Rep. 2017;19:8. [PMID: 28233189] doi:10.1007/s11908-017-0560-2

Item 79   Answer: C

Educational Objective: Treat stable angina with percutaneous coronary intervention.

This patient with diabetes mellitus and single-vessel coronary artery disease should undergo revascularization with percutaneous coronary intervention (PCI) or coronary artery bypass grafting. PCI has not been shown to be superior to optimal medical therapy in patients with stable angina for reduction of cardiovascular endpoints, such as mortality and myocardial infarction. However, PCI has been associated with improvement in quality of life by reducing the severity and frequency of angina. Current guidelines recommend that diagnostic angiography and PCI be reserved for patients with refractory symptoms while receiving optimal medical therapy, those who are unable to tolerate optimal medical therapy owing to side effects, or those with high-risk features on noninvasive exercise and imaging tests. This patient has 90% stenosis of the proximal left anterior descending artery and refractory symptoms; therefore, PCI is a reasonable therapeutic option.

The use of β-carotene, selenium, chromium, vitamin C, vitamin E, and estrogen has not been associated with improved cardiovascular outcomes or relief of symptoms and is not recommended in patients with ischemic heart disease.

Cardiac rehabilitation may be appropriate after revascularization occurs; however, this patient should first undergo revascularization to treat his crescendo angina symptoms.

Aspirin is associated with a decreased risk for myocardial infarction, stroke, and cardiovascular death in patients with coronary artery disease. Aspirin doses of 81 mg to 162 mg daily are recommended in all patients with established coronary artery disease unless contraindicated. In patients allergic to aspirin, clopidogrel is recommended as an alternative. The use of newer antiplatelet agents (prasugrel, ticagrelor) as monotherapy has not been tested in patients with stable angina. Dual antiplatelet therapy for chronic angina in the absence of stent placement is not recommended.

KEY POINT

- In patients with stable angina, diagnostic angiography and percutaneous coronary intervention are reserved for patients with refractory angina symptoms while receiving optimal medical therapy, those who are unable to tolerate optimal medical therapy owing to side effects, or those with high-risk features on noninvasive exercise and imaging tests.

Bibliography

Fihn SD, Gardin JM, Abrams J, Berra K, Blankenship JC, Dallas AP, et al; American College of Cardiology Foundation; American Heart Association Task Force on Practice Guidelines; American College of Physicians; American Association for Thoracic Surgery; Preventive Cardiovascular Nurses Association; Society for Cardiovascular Angiography and Interventions; Society of Thoracic Surgeons. 2012 ACCF/AHA/ACP/AATS/PCNA/SCAI/STS Guideline for the diagnosis and management of patients with stable ischemic heart disease: a report of the American College of Cardiology Foundation/American Heart Association Task Force on Practice Guidelines, and the American College of Physicians, American Association for Thoracic Surgery, Preventive Cardiovascular Nurses Association, Society for Cardiovascular Angiography and Interventions, and Society of Thoracic Surgeons. J Am Coll Cardiol. 2012 Dec 18;60(24):e44-e164. [PMID: 23182125]

Item 80   Answer: A

Educational Objective: Manage anticoagulation therapy in a patient with a mechanical valve prosthesis who is contemplating pregnancy.

The most appropriate anticoagulation regimen to prevent prosthesis thrombosis in this patient is INR-adjusted warfarin.

Pregnant women with a mechanical valve prosthesis represent a high-risk subset of patients; concerns include valve thrombosis with its associated maternal risk, bleeding, and fetal morbidity and mortality. Warfarin anticoagulation appears to be the safest agent to prevent maternal prosthetic valve thrombosis; however, warfarin poses an increased fetal risk, with possible teratogenicity, miscarriage, and fetal loss due to intracranial hemorrhage. Risk to the fetus is dose related, and warfarin is the preferred anticoagulation regimen during the first trimester when the dose is 5 mg daily or less. During the second and early third trimesters, warfarin therapy is the preferred anticoagulation therapy.

Anticoagulation with apixaban is not recommended in patients with a mechanical valve prosthesis because of the potentially increased risk for valve thrombosis. In addition, its use has not been demonstrated to be safe during pregnancy.

In patients who prefer not to take warfarin during the first trimester of pregnancy, dose-adjusted intravenous unfractionated heparin can be used; however, 5000 units of unfractionated heparin will not provide adequate anticoagulation coverage for a patient with a mechanical prosthetic valve. Dose-adjusted, intravenous unfractionated heparin is an appropriate therapeutic option during the first trimester of pregnancy if the warfarin dose is more than 5 mg daily. Intravenous unfractionated heparin is the drug of choice for patients with a mechanical valve prosthesis around the time of delivery.

Weight-based low-molecular-weight heparin does not provide adequate anticoagulation coverage for a pregnant patient with a mechanical valve prosthesis and should not be used in this patient. Dose-adjusted low-molecular-weight heparin administered subcutaneously is appropriate during the first trimester if the warfarin dose is more than 5 mg daily.

KEY POINT

- In pregnant patients with a mechanical valve prosthesis, warfarin is the preferred anticoagulation therapy during the first trimester if the dose is 5 mg daily or less; warfarin is preferred to all other anticoagulants during the second and early third trimesters.

Bibliography

Nishimura RA, Otto CM, Bonow RO, Carabello BA, Erwin JP 3rd, Guyton RA, et al; American College of Cardiology/American Heart Association Task Force on Practice Guidelines. 2014 AHA/ACC guideline for the management of patients with valvular heart disease: executive summary: a report of the American College of Cardiology/American Heart Association Task Force on Practice Guidelines. J Am Coll Cardiol. 2014;63:2438-88. [PMID: 24603192] doi:10.1016/j.jacc.2014.02.537

Item 81   Answer: B

Educational Objective: Manage acquired QT-interval prolongation.

Moxifloxacin should be discontinued in this patient who had an episode of nonsustained polymorphic ventricular tachycardia

(VT). VT is subdivided into sustained VT and nonsustained VT. VT is sustained when it persists for longer than 30 seconds or requires termination because of hemodynamic collapse. Nonsustained VT has three or more beats but lasts for less than 30 seconds. VT is also categorized by the morphology of the QRS complexes. VT is monomorphic if QRS complexes in the same leads do not vary in contour or polymorphic if the QRS complexes in the same leads vary in contour. In this patient, the electrocardiogram obtained after the episode of VT also demonstrates QT-interval prolongation, which is consistent with the diagnosis of torsades de pointes. Torsades de pointes is a special subset of polymorphic VT; the ventricular rate ranges from 200/min to 300/min and is associated with long QT syndrome, which may be congenital or acquired. The patient's electrocardiogram was normal upon admission, and her corrected QT interval is greater than 550 ms following the arrhythmic event, suggesting an acquired long QT interval. Causes of acquired QT-interval prolongation include medications such as antiarrhythmic agents, antibiotics (macrolides and fluoroquinolones), antipsychotic drugs, and antidepressants; structural heart disease; and electrolyte abnormalities.

Although carvedilol slows the heart rate and can increase the risk for bradycardia-dependent arrhythmias in patients with acquired QT-interval prolongation, discontinuing the offending QT-prolonging agents is the most important intervention in this patient.

Simvastatin is a statin used in the treatment of dyslipidemia. It has no effect on the QT interval and does not need to be discontinued.

Venlafaxine is a serotonin-norepinephrine reuptake inhibitor that is used to treat depression and anxiety disorders. There is a possible risk for QT-interval prolongation with venlafaxine, but there is no evidence that this occurs when the medication is taken as recommended. Therefore, discontinuation of venlafaxine is unnecessary.

KEY POINT

- QT-interval prolongation has many causes, including medications such as antiarrhythmic agents, antibiotics (macrolides and fluoroquinolones), antipsychotic drugs, and antidepressants; structural heart disease; and electrolyte abnormalities.

Bibliography

Isbister GK, Page CB. Drug induced QT prolongation: the measurement and assessment of the QT interval in clinical practice. Br J Clin Pharmacol. 2013;76:48-57. [PMID: 23167578] doi:10.1111/bcp.12040

Item 82   Answer: A

Educational Objective: Treat chronic aortic regurgitation with aortic valve and root replacement.

The most appropriate management is aortic valve and root replacement. This young, asymptomatic patient with a bicuspid aortic valve has significant aortic regurgitation. The transthoracic echocardiogram demonstrates a dilated left ventricle, mildly decreased systolic function, and a moderately dilated ascending aorta. Asymptomatic patients with severe aortic regurgitation who develop left ventricular dilatation or systolic dysfunction are at increased risk for sudden cardiac death, death, and heart failure. Therefore, these patients should be referred for aortic valve replacement. The prognosis of asymptomatic patients with severe aortic regurgitation but with normal left ventricular size and function is excellent. The American College of Cardiology/American Heart Association valvular heart disease guidelines recommend surgery in asymptomatic patients with severe aortic regurgitation when the left ventricular end-systolic dimension reaches 50 mm or the ejection fraction is less than 50%. In patients undergoing cardiac surgery, repair of the ascending aorta is indicated when the diameter exceeds 45 mm; thus, concomitant aortic root replacement, in addition to aortic valve replacement, is indicated in this patient.

In asymptomatic patients who do not meet surgical criteria, serial echocardiography is warranted to assess for disease progression. Patients with mild regurgitation should receive an annual clinical evaluation and echocardiography every 3 to 5 years, whereas patients with severe regurgitation should undergo clinical evaluation and echocardiography every 6 to 12 months.

For asymptomatic patients with normal systolic function and mild regurgitation, vasodilator therapy with nifedipine or ACE inhibitors is not recommended. For asymptomatic patients with normal systolic function and severe regurgitation, vasodilator therapy may be considered, but medical therapy does not supplant surgical intervention in these patients.

In patients with significant aortic regurgitation and equivocal symptoms, exercise-induced increases in pulmonary systolic pressure to more than 60 mm Hg (or a 25-mm Hg increase above baseline) identified during treadmill stress echocardiography suggest hemodynamic significance and may lead to earlier referral for surgical intervention. In this patient, however, ventricular dilatation and decreased ejection fraction are adequate criteria for recommending surgery.

KEY POINT

- Valve replacement surgery is recommended for asymptomatic patients with a bicuspid aortic valve and severe aortic regurgitation when the left ventricular end-systolic diameter reaches 50 mm or the left ventricular ejection fraction is less than 50%.

Bibliography

Enriquez-Sarano M, Tajik AJ. Clinical practice. Aortic regurgitation. N Engl J Med. 2004;351:1539-46. [PMID: 15470217]

Item 83   Answer: D

Educational Objective: Prevent heart failure readmission with early physician follow-up.

The most appropriate management is to schedule follow-up within 1 week of discharge. This patient was hospitalized for

CONT.

a heart failure exacerbation. Before discharge, it is important to initiate several strategies to prevent readmission. First, the reason for the heart failure exacerbation should be identified. Often, it is impossible to determine a cause; however, in a situation such as this one, addressing the reasons for the patient's nonadherence might prevent readmission. Second, patients should be receiving optimal doses of evidence-based medications before discharge. When medications, especially β-blockers, are restarted, it is important to begin at a low dose and slowly uptitrate over time. Third, patients should not be discharged until they have achieved euvolemia with diuresis, and their electrolyte levels and kidney function are optimized. Finally, appropriate follow-up should be scheduled. Studies have shown that patients seen within 1 week of a heart failure discharge have reduced admissions compared with those with later outpatient contact. The purpose of an early visit is to reinforce heart failure education, ensure proper medication use, evaluate volume status, and uptitrate or initiate medications as needed. This patient is euvolemic and is taking appropriate medications, and he should be scheduled for a follow-up visit within 1 week to prevent readmission.

Ivabradine reduces heart failure–associated hospitalizations in patients with chronic symptomatic heart failure with left ventricular ejection fraction less than or equal to 35% who are in sinus rhythm and taking guideline-directed medical therapy. This patient has atrial fibrillation, and ivabradine is not indicated.

ACE inhibitor and β-blocker therapies should be uptitrated to maximally tolerated doses before initiation of spironolactone. It is important to add an aldosterone antagonist later, but the dosage of the other agents should be maximized first.

There is no evidence of a survival advantage or reduction in stroke with cardioversion and maintenance of sinus rhythm in patients with atrial fibrillation, including those with heart failure. Therefore, the decision to institute a rate or rhythm control strategy largely depends on symptoms and patient preference. Patients who are asymptomatic can be managed with rate control only, with a resting heart rate goal of less than 110/min. Patients with tachycardia-induced cardiomyopathy, heart failure, or left ventricular ejection fraction of less than 40% may require more stringent rate control (heart rate of 60/min to 80/min at rest).

KEY POINT

- Following heart failure hospitalization, early follow-up (within 1 week) should be scheduled to reinforce heart failure education, ensure proper medication use, evaluate volume status, and uptitrate or initiate medications as needed.

Bibliography

Lee KK, Yang J, Hernandez AF, Steimle AE, Go AS. Post-discharge follow-up characteristics associated with 30-day readmission after heart failure hospitalization. Med Care. 2016;54:365-72. [PMID: 26978568] doi: 10.1097/MLR.0000000000000492

Item 84   Answer: D

Educational Objective: Evaluate a patient for hypertrophic cardiomyopathy with genetic counseling and testing.

The most appropriate management of the patient's 16-year-old daughter is genetic counseling and testing. Hypertrophic cardiomyopathy (HCM) is an autosomal dominant heritable disorder characterized by the presence of increased left ventricular wall thickness in the absence of loading conditions or other underlying causes. In patients with HCM and a known pathogenic mutation, genetic counseling and testing is recommended for all first-degree family members, regardless of the presence or absence of symptoms. In this case, genetic testing of the index patient has revealed a mutation known to be associated with HCM. Mutation-negative family members do not require further evaluation and have no increased risk for future development of HCM. Family members who test positive for an HCM-related genetic mutation should be further evaluated with physical examination, 12-lead electrocardiography, and echocardiography (or cardiac magnetic resonance imaging). Genetic counseling is an important facet of care for patients with HCM, regardless of whether genetic testing is performed. Counseling enables informed decision making about the risks and benefits of testing and facilitates interpretation of the results.

The development of HCM is a dynamic process, and phenotypic expression may change as a patient ages. Because of this, if the daughter tests positive for the mutated gene but the electrocardiogram and echocardiogram are normal, she may still require repeated screening because of the possibility of phenotypic disease expression at any age. In that case, screening with physical examination, echocardiography, and 12-lead electrocardiography is recommended annually starting at age 12 years until adulthood. For adults who are genotype-positive and phenotype-negative, screening should be performed every 5 years or with a change in clinical status.

Mutation carriers with phenotypic expression of HCM should undergo further risk stratification for sudden cardiac death.

KEY POINT

- Genetic counseling and testing are recommended for patients with hypertrophic cardiomyopathy (HCM) and for all first-degree family members of patients with HCM who have an identified genetic mutation, regardless of the presence or absence of symptoms.

Bibliography

Gersh BJ, Maron BJ, Bonow RO, Dearani JA, Fifer MA, Link MS, et al; American College of Cardiology Foundation/American Heart Association Task Force on Practice Guidelines. 2011 ACCF/AHA guideline for the diagnosis and treatment of hypertrophic cardiomyopathy: a report of the American College of Cardiology Foundation/American Heart Association Task Force on Practice Guidelines. Developed in collaboration with the American Association for Thoracic Surgery, American Society of Echocardiography, American Society of Nuclear Cardiology, Heart Failure Society of America, Heart Rhythm Society, Society for Cardiovascular Angiography and Interventions, and Society of Thoracic Surgeons. J Am Coll Cardiol. 2011;58:e212-60. [PMID: 22075469] doi:10.1016/j.jacc.2011.06.011

Item 85   Answer: D

Educational Objective: Identify inflammatory disease as a risk factor for coronary artery disease.

This patient's most significant risk factor for cardiovascular disease (CVD) is the presence of rheumatoid arthritis. Patients with systemic inflammatory conditions, such as systemic lupus erythematosus and rheumatoid arthritis, have an increased risk for CVD. Patients with rheumatoid arthritis have a 1.5- to 2-fold elevated risk for coronary artery disease compared with the general population. Most deaths in patients with SLE and nearly 40% of deaths in patients with rheumatoid arthritis are cardiovascular and, in particular, heart failure related. The risk for CVD increases with the duration of the underlying inflammatory condition. In patients with rheumatoid arthritis, the risk for CVD increases from two times to three times that of the general population after 10 years' duration of rheumatoid arthritis. The increased atherosclerotic burden is likely a result of both the inflammatory process of the systemic disease, including a prothrombotic state, and the presence of traditional cardiovascular risk factors. The risk for future atherosclerotic CVD is typically calculated by using the American College of Cardiology/American Heart Association CVD risk calculator based on the Pooled Cohort Equations; however, this calculator underestimates risk in patients with nontraditional risk factors, as in this patient with rheumatoid arthritis.

Sedentary lifestyle, poor diet, and obesity contribute to increased cardiovascular risk and increased risk for diabetes mellitus. Moderate-intensity exercise for 30 minutes or longer on 5 to 7 days per week is recommended for nearly all persons and is being achieved by this patient.

Regular moderate alcohol consumption (one to two drinks daily for men, one drink daily for women) has been associated with a decreased incidence of CVD. Because of the known deleterious effects of drinking, the American Heart Association does not recommend that nondrinking patients consume moderate amounts of alcohol as a measure to decrease the risk for CVD. This patient has one drink per day, which is likely beneficial in reducing her CVD risk.

The prevalence of CVD and CVD risk factors in the United States varies by ethnicity. Hawaiians and Pacific Islanders have the highest rate of heart disease (19.1%), followed by American Indians and Alaska Natives (13.7%), non-Hispanic whites (11.1%), blacks (10.3%), Hispanics and Latinos (7.8%), and Asians (6.0%). This patient's ethnicity places her in the lowest risk category for CVD.

KEY POINT

- Patients with rheumatoid arthritis have a 1.5- to 2-fold elevated risk for coronary artery disease compared with the general population.

Bibliography
Crowson CS, Liao KP, Davis JM 3rd, Solomon DH, Matteson EL, Knutson KL, et al. Rheumatoid arthritis and cardiovascular disease. Am Heart J. 2013;166:622-628.e1. [PMID: 24093840] doi:10.1016/j.ahj.2013.07.010

Item 86   Answer: B

Educational Objective: Diagnose inappropriate sinus tachycardia.

This patient with sinus tachycardia and a structurally normal heart has symptoms, electrocardiographic features, and ambulatory electrocardiographic findings consistent with the diagnosis of inappropriate sinus tachycardia (IST). IST is characterized by elevated resting heart rate, with exaggerated increases in heart rate with light activity. The sinus rates typically decrease during sleep, as identified on this patient's ambulatory electrocardiographic monitor. IST frequently presents in women in their second to fourth decades and appears to be more common in health care professionals. Symptoms vary and can include palpitations, lightheadedness, syncope or near-syncope, dyspnea, and fatigue. Emotional manifestations, such as anxiety or depression, may also be present. Diagnosis of IST is based on the exclusion of other causes of tachycardia, such as hyperthyroidism, anemia, pheochromocytoma, and structural heart disease. First-line therapy is removal of aggravating factors and exercise therapy. In patients with bothersome and persistent symptoms, pharmacologic therapy with β-blockers or calcium channel blockers can be considered. Ivabradine is a relatively new drug that impairs the I_f or "I-funny" current and may play a role in the treatment of IST refractory to standard therapy.

The diagnostic criteria for generalized anxiety disorder are as follows: (1) excessive anxiety or worry about a number of events or activities occurring for 6 months or longer; (2) the patient recognizes it is difficult to control the worry; (3) the anxiety or worry is associated with three or more of the following symptoms: restlessness, easy fatigability, difficulty concentrating, irritability, muscle tension, and sleep disturbance; (4) the anxiety, worry, or symptoms cause impairment at school, work, or other settings and cannot be attributable to medical or other psychiatric conditions, medications, or substance use. Diagnostic criteria for somatic symptom disorder include at least one somatic symptom causing distress or interference with daily life; excessive thoughts, behaviors, and feelings related to the somatic symptom(s); and persistent somatic symptoms for at least 6 months. This patient does not fulfill the diagnostic criteria for generalized anxiety disorder or somatic symptom disorder.

Subclinical hyperthyroidism is a laboratory-based diagnosis, defined as the presence of a suppressed thyroid-stimulating hormone level with normal triiodothyronine and thyroxine levels. Symptoms of thyrotoxicosis are typically mild; most patients are asymptomatic. This patient's normal thyroid-stimulating hormone level argues against this diagnosis.

KEY POINT

- Diagnosis of inappropriate sinus tachycardia is based on symptoms and findings on ambulatory electrocardiographic monitoring after the exclusion of other causes of tachycardia, such as hyperthyroidism, anemia, pheochromocytoma, and structural heart disease.

Bibliography

Olshansky B, Sullivan RM. Inappropriate sinus tachycardia. J Am Coll Cardiol. 2013;61:793-801. [PMID: 23265330] doi:10.1016/j.jacc.2012.07.074

Item 87   Answer: A

Educational Objective: Evaluate for coronary artery disease in a patient with left bundle branch block on a baseline electrocardiogram.

Adenosine single-photon emission CT is the most appropriate next diagnostic test. This patient with several cardiovascular risk factors has exertional dyspnea, which may be an angina equivalent, and he should undergo stress testing to evaluate for coronary artery disease (CAD). Because his electrocardiogram (ECG) shows left bundle branch block, ST-segment changes with exercise cannot be used to evaluate for the presence of obstructive CAD. He must undergo stress testing with additional imaging, such as nuclear perfusion imaging or stress echocardiography. Exercise is typically the preferred mode of stress because of the additional functional information it provides. However, in the case of left bundle branch block, myocardial perfusion imaging with exercise or dobutamine stress may result in a false-positive perfusion defect in the basilar septum, and these stressors should be avoided. Instead, vasodilator stress testing should be used. Vasodilators, such as dipyridamole, regadenoson, and adenosine, produce hyperemia and a flow disparity between myocardium supplied by unobstructed vessels and myocardium supplied by the stenotic vessel (due to the inability of the distal vasculature to dilate).

Coronary artery calcium scoring, which quantifies the amount of calcium in the walls of the coronary arteries, would document the presence of atherosclerotic disease in this symptomatic patient with risk factors, but it would not determine whether there is obstructive CAD. Although the absence of any coronary artery calcification has been shown to have a high specificity for the absence of obstructive CAD, trials evaluating coronary artery calcium scoring have typically focused on primary prevention in asymptomatic patients.

KEY POINT

- In patients with left bundle branch block, the preferred diagnostic test for coronary artery disease is a vasodilator stress test because myocardial perfusion imaging with exercise or dobutamine stress may result in a false-positive perfusion defect in the basilar septum.

Bibliography

Hendel RC, Berman DS, Di Carli MF, Heidenreich PA, Henkin RE, Pellikka PA, et al; American College of Cardiology Foundation Appropriate Use Criteria Task Force. ACCF/ASNC/ACR/AHA/ASE/SCCT/SCMR/SNM 2009 appropriate use criteria for cardiac radionuclide imaging: a report of the American College of Cardiology Foundation Appropriate Use Criteria Task Force, the American Society of Nuclear Cardiology, the American College of Radiology, the American Heart Association, the American Society of Echocardiography, the Society of Cardiovascular Computed Tomography, the Society for Cardiovascular Magnetic Resonance, and the Society of Nuclear Medicine. J Am Coll Cardiol. 2009;53:2201-29. [PMID: 19497454] doi:10.1016/j.jacc.2009.02.013

Item 88   Answer: D

Educational Objective: Evaluate a patient with new-onset heart failure.

Thyroid studies should be performed next in this patient with new-onset heart failure. Once a diagnosis of heart failure is suspected, echocardiography should be performed to ascertain the left ventricular ejection fraction and to potentially determine the cause and chronicity of the patient's heart failure. A large, dilated left ventricle suggests a chronic process with less chance of recovery. The initial laboratory evaluation of patients with new-onset heart failure should include a B-type natriuretic peptide or N-terminal pro–B-type natriuretic peptide assay, complete blood count, serum electrolyte measurement, kidney function tests, liver chemistry tests, glucose and lipid levels, and serum thyroid-stimulating hormone measurement. Specifically, thyroid-stimulating hormone measurement is indicated to evaluate for occult hypo- or hyperthyroidism as a reversible cause of heart failure. In hyperthyroidism in particular, the predominant manifestation of thyroid dysfunction may be cardiac symptoms, which will abate when the hyperthyroidism is treated.

The classic presentation of viral myocarditis includes a viral prodrome with fever, myalgia, and upper respiratory tract symptoms, but a prodrome does not always occur. Patients present with dyspnea, chest pain, and arrhythmias. Electrocardiographic abnormalities are often observed. This patient's presentation is not typical for viral myocarditis, and viral studies are not indicated at this time.

Although coronary artery disease is the most common cause of heart failure, the investigation for coronary artery disease by stress testing or cardiac catheterization is not considered part of the routine evaluation of all patients with newly diagnosed heart failure, owing to expense and radiation exposure. Cardiac catheterization should be performed in patients presenting with angina or significant ischemia.

Hereditary hemochromatosis results from an autosomal recessive defect in the *HFE* gene, which leads to increased absorption of dietary iron. Patients may present with heart failure or arrhythmias. However, women do not develop overt iron overload until after menopause, and serum iron and ferritin studies are not indicated in this young woman.

KEY POINT

- The initial laboratory evaluation of patients with new-onset heart failure should include a B-type natriuretic peptide or N-terminal pro–B-type natriuretic peptide assay, complete blood count, serum electrolyte measurement, kidney function tests, liver chemistry tests, and serum thyroid-stimulating hormone measurement.

Bibliography

Yancy CW, Jessup M, Bozkurt B, Butler J, Casey DE Jr, Drazner MH, et al; American College of Cardiology Foundation. 2013 ACCF/AHA guideline for the management of heart failure: a report of the American College of Cardiology Foundation/American Heart Association Task Force on Practice Guidelines. J Am Coll Cardiol. 2013;62:e147-239. [PMID: 23747642] doi:10.1016/j.jacc.2013.05.019

Item 89   Answer: C

Educational Objective: Diagnose acute mitral regurgitation due to papillary muscle rupture.

The most likely diagnosis is acute mitral regurgitation. This patient has evidence of a recent inferolateral myocardial infarction and decompensated heart failure. The mitral regurgitation is likely secondary to papillary muscle dysfunction (or rupture) and/or ventricular dysfunction. In acute mitral regurgitation, heart failure symptoms may occur abruptly because there has not been time for adaptive chamber dilatation. The murmur of acute mitral regurgitation may be present only in early diastole, owing to rapid diastolic equalization of ventricular and atrial pressures caused by the high volume overload. In cases of severe mitral regurgitation, a diastolic rumble occurs because of the large regurgitant volume during diastole. If present, the systolic murmur of acute mitral regurgitation is typically soft and ends before A_2. It is best heard along the left sternal border and base of the heart, generally without a thrill.

In patients with aortic stenosis, the murmur characteristically gets louder and then softer (crescendo-decrescendo) during systole; it is loudest at the second right intercostal space, with radiation to the carotid arteries. These findings are not present in this patient.

Left ventricular free wall rupture is an often fatal complication of myocardial infarction that occurs 3 to 7 days after the initial event. Patients most commonly present with cardiac tamponade (due to hemopericardium), pulseless electrical activity, and death. Patients with cardiac tamponade typically do not have a heart murmur or a preserved or exaggerated x descent in the jugular venous pulse, as seen in this patient.

Most patients with mild to moderate tricuspid regurgitation are asymptomatic. Examination reveals a systolic murmur that is loudest at the left lower sternal border and increases with inspiration. Symptoms and signs of right-sided heart failure, such as fatigue, elevated jugular venous pulse, and lower extremity edema, may be found; however, tricuspid regurgitation does not cause volume overload in the lungs, as was observed in this patient.

KEY POINT

- Acute severe mitral regurgitation is associated with papillary muscle rupture following acute myocardial infarction.

Bibliography

Kutty RS, Jones N, Moorjani N. Mechanical complications of acute myocardial infarction. Cardiol Clin. 2013;31:519-31, vii-viii. [PMID: 24188218] doi:10.1016/j.ccl.2013.07.004

Item 90   Answer: B

Educational Objective: Manage dual antiplatelet therapy in a patient with non–ST-elevation myocardial infarction.

This patient with a non–ST-elevation myocardial infarction (NSTEMI) should receive low-dose aspirin indefinitely and ticagrelor for 1 year. Dual antiplatelet therapy, composed of aspirin and a $P2Y_{12}$ inhibitor, is indicated in all patients following acute coronary syndrome (ACS) for the prevention of vascular ischemic events. Aspirin should be continued indefinitely, and in patients with ACS treated with medical therapy alone, the optimal duration for $P2Y_{12}$ inhibitor therapy (clopidogrel or ticagrelor) is at least 12 months. Although clopidogrel is an option in this patient, in the PLATO trial, the combination of low-dose aspirin and ticagrelor was superior to aspirin and clopidogrel in reducing the incidence of cardiovascular death, myocardial infarction, and stroke following ACS; the effect size was identical in medically treated patients and those who underwent early invasive treatment. The American College of Cardiology and American Heart Association prefer ticagrelor to clopidogrel (class IIa, level B recommendation) but caution that additional studies with focused objectives are needed.

Prasugrel, another $P2Y_{12}$ inhibitor, is recommended for use only in patients with ACS who undergo percutaneous coronary intervention. Prasugrel is no more effective than clopidogrel in comparison studies of medically treated patients with ACS, and it carries a higher risk for bleeding than does clopidogrel.

Anticoagulation with warfarin is not routinely recommended following ACS unless there is another indication for its use, such as venous thromboembolic disease or atrial fibrillation.

Aspirin therapy alone would not offer adequate protection against cardiovascular events in this patient with NSTEMI.

KEY POINT

- Dual antiplatelet therapy, composed of aspirin and a $P2Y_{12}$ inhibitor, is indicated in all patients following acute coronary syndrome for the prevention of vascular ischemic events.

Bibliography

Wallentin L, Becker RC, Budaj A, Cannon CP, Emanuelsson H, Held C, et al; PLATO Investigators. Ticagrelor versus clopidogrel in patients with acute coronary syndromes. N Engl J Med. 2009;361:1045-57. [PMID: 19717846] doi:10.1056/NEJMoa0904327

Item 91   Answer: B

Educational Objective: Diagnose constrictive pericarditis.

The most likely diagnosis in this patient with a history of chest radiotherapy is constrictive pericarditis. Constrictive pericarditis is characterized by pericardial thickening, fibrosis, and sometimes calcification that impair diastolic filling and limit total cardiac volume. Most cases are viral or idiopathic in origin; however, cardiac surgery, chest irradiation, autoimmune disease, and tuberculosis or other bacterial infections may be causes. Patients with constrictive pericarditis most commonly present with indolent progression of right-sided heart failure symptoms, including peripheral edema, ascites, and fatigue.

In this patient, signs of venous congestion predominate, pericardial calcification is present on the chest radiograph, and the serum B-natriuretic peptide level is low and does not suggest greatly increased wall tension. The echocardiographic findings of respiratory variation in filling of right and left ventricles, ventricular septal shift during respiration, and dilation of the inferior vena cava are characteristic of constrictive pericarditis.

Cardiac amyloidosis and restrictive cardiomyopathy are not associated with pericardial calcification, and patients with these conditions more commonly present with moderate to severe pulmonary hypertension rather than the mild pulmonary hypertension seen in this patient. Respiratory variation in filling of the right and left ventricles and ventricular septal shift during respiration are characteristic of pericardial constraint rather than myocardial disease.

Patients with heart failure with preserved ejection fraction will present with edema, exertional dyspnea, and fatigue. Normal systolic contraction and abnormal diastolic relaxation are present on echocardiogram and result in restricted filling and high filling pressures. Patients with heart failure typically have an elevated B-type natriuretic peptide level, often greater than of 600 pg/mL (600 ng/L), which is not found in this patient.

KEY POINT

- Constrictive pericarditis is commonly characterized by symptoms of right-sided heart failure, low or normal B-type natriuretic peptide level, and the finding of pericardial thickening or calcification on imaging studies.

Bibliography

Jaworski C, Mariani JA, Wheeler G, Kaye DM. Cardiac complications of thoracic irradiation. J Am Coll Cardiol. 2013;61:2319-28. [PMID: 23583253] doi:10.1016/j.jacc.2013.01.090

Item 92   Answer: A

Educational Objective: Diagnose ostium secundum atrial septal defect.

An ostium secundum atrial septal defect (ASD) is the most likely diagnosis in this patient. Adults with an ASD most often present with dyspnea or atrial arrhythmias; elevated central venous pressure, fixed splitting of the S_2, and a right ventricular heave are characteristic findings. The fixed splitting of the S_2 in patients with an ostium secundum ASD results from prolongation of right ventricular systole and lack of respiratory change in the right ventricular stroke volume. With expiration, the decrease in venous return is counteracted by an increase in left-to-right shunting, resulting in a fixed right ventricular preload. A large left-to-right shunt causes a pulmonary midsystolic flow murmur and a tricuspid diastolic flow rumble owing to increased flow. In ostium secundum ASD, the electrocardiogram (ECG) demonstrates right-axis deviation and incomplete right bundle branch block.

Aortic stenosis due to a bicuspid aortic valve causes a systolic murmur at the second right intercostal space. The central venous pressure is normal in aortic stenosis, and a right ventricular impulse would not be expected. A systolic ejection click is often heard in patients with bicuspid aortic valve, but fixed splitting of the S_2 is not heard. The ECG typically demonstrates a normal axis and features of left ventricular hypertrophy.

Pulmonary stenosis is usually congenital, and severe obstruction can cause exertional dyspnea. Physical examination features depend on the severity of obstruction and associated elevation of right heart pressure; these include central venous pressure elevation with a prominent a wave and a parasternal impulse. The systolic murmur of pulmonary stenosis is generally heard at the second left intercostal space, and the timing of the murmur is related to stenosis severity. An ejection click is often heard; the proximity of the click to the S_2 varies depending on the severity of stenosis. S_2 becomes fixed in severe pulmonary stenosis. The ECG demonstrates right axis deviation and features of right ventricular hypertrophy.

Patients with mitral stenosis might present with symptoms of dyspnea. A right ventricular impulse can occur, and the central venous pressure might be elevated with associated pulmonary hypertension or tricuspid regurgitation. The murmur of mitral stenosis is generally best heard at the apex. An opening snap might be heard, followed by a diastolic murmur. Fixed splitting of the S_2 is not heard. The ECG typically demonstrates left atrial enlargement.

KEY POINT

- Elevated central venous pressure, fixed splitting of the S_2, a right ventricular heave, and right-axis deviation and incomplete right bundle branch block on electrocardiogram are characteristic findings in patients with ostium secundum atrial septal defect.

Bibliography

Baumgartner H, Bonhoeffer P, De Groot NM, de Haan F, Deanfield JE, Galie N, et al; Task Force on the Management of Grown-up Congenital Heart Disease of the European Society of Cardiology (ESC). ESC guidelines for the management of grown-up congenital heart disease (new version 2010). Eur Heart J. 2010;31:2915-57. [PMID: 20801927] doi:10.1093/eurheartj/ehq249

Item 93   Answer: C

Educational Objective: Diagnose the cause of cryptogenic stroke.

The most appropriate diagnostic testing option is 30-day event-triggered loop recording. This patient had a cryptogenic stroke given the absence of an apparent vascular, structural, or thromboembolic cause for her ischemic event. Among patients aged 55 years and older who have a cryptogenic ischemic neurologic event, such as a stroke or transient ischemic attack, occult intermittent atrial fibrillation is thought to be present in up to 25% of cases. These patients have a high risk for recurrent stroke, and efforts should be made to detect and treat atrial fibrillation for stroke prevention. Non-invasive ambulatory electrocardiographic (ECG) monitoring for 30 days improves the detection of atrial fibrillation by fivefold compared with short-term ECG monitoring. Patients who have premature atrial contractions and other findings of ectopy on short-term telemetry may be more likely to have paroxysmal atrial fibrillation. Patients who undergo longer-term ECG monitoring and are subsequently diagnosed with atrial fibrillation are also more likely to receive appropriate secondary prevention stroke therapy with oral anticoagulants.

Antiphospholipid antibodies are acquired autoantibodies against phospholipids and phospholipid-binding proteins, such as cardiolipin and β_2-glycoprotein I. In vitro, they can prolong clotting tests, but in vivo, they increase the risk for venous and arterial thrombosis and are associated with increased fetal loss. Testing for autoimmune and hypercoagulable disorders, such as antiphospholipid antibody syndrome, can be considered in young patients with otherwise unexplained stroke. Aside from stroke, this patient does not have any features concerning for a prothrombotic state or autoimmune disease. Therefore, testing for antiphospholipid antibodies is not appropriate.

Cardiac catheterization is not indicated in this patient. Because she had a normal transesophageal echocardiogram, there is no concern for a structural abnormality, such as an intracardiac shunt.

Short-term ECG monitoring (24-48 hours) with an ambulatory ECG monitor is inferior to extended ECG monitoring in the detection of paroxysmal atrial fibrillation.

KEY POINT

- In the evaluation of cryptogenic stroke, noninvasive ambulatory electrocardiographic (ECG) monitoring for 30 days improves the detection of atrial fibrillation by fivefold compared with short-term ECG monitoring.

Bibliography
Gladstone DJ, Spring M, Dorian P, Panzov V, Thorpe KE, Hall J, et al; EMBRACE Investigators and Coordinators. Atrial fibrillation in patients with cryptogenic stroke. N Engl J Med. 2014;370:2467-77. [PMID: 24963566] doi:10.1056/NEJMoa1311376

Item 94   Answer: B

Educational Objective: Treat acute decompensated heart failure with intravenous furosemide.

The most appropriate treatment is administration of intravenous furosemide. This patient with a history of heart failure has signs and symptoms of an acute exacerbation, with volume overload and possibly reduced kidney function. The mainstay of therapy for acute heart failure is intravenous diuretics. The intravenous diuretic dose should equal or exceed the patient's oral dose for chronic heart failure. If the patient does not respond appropriately to that dose, rapid uptitration should be performed to assist in fluid removal.

A recent study assessing different diuretic strategies (normal versus high dose, bolus versus continuous infusion) in patients with acute decompensated heart failure showed no difference in the outcomes of length of stay, readmission, or kidney function between groups. The patient's usual outpatient medications should be cautiously continued unless the patient is hypotensive or demonstrates signs of poor perfusion (worsening kidney or liver function, cool extremities), in which case dose reduction or discontinuation of both the ACE inhibitor and β-blocker should be considered.

Low-dose dopamine plus diuretic therapy was studied in the ROSE trial to determine whether dopamine improves diuresis and preserves kidney function in patients with acute heart failure. Compared with placebo, there was no difference in patient symptoms, urine output at 72 hours, or kidney function. Intravenous dopamine would not benefit this patient.

Intravenous inotropes, such as milrinone or dobutamine, should be considered in patients with signs of poor perfusion to improve cardiac function; however, this patient has no signs of hypoperfusion to suggest that this exacerbation is related to low cardiac output. Additionally, the PROMISE study showed no benefit of routine inotropic therapy in patients admitted with a heart failure exacerbation.

The vasodilator nesiritide has not been shown to improve diuresis, reduce length of stay, or prevent readmissions when used routinely for patients hospitalized for a heart failure exacerbation. Nitroglycerin or nitroprusside is occasionally used in patients who are hypertensive or who have high systemic vascular resistance, but usually only in a closely monitored setting, such as the coronary care unit.

KEY POINT

- The mainstay of therapy for acute decompensated heart failure is intravenous diuretics.

Bibliography
Chen HH, Anstrom KJ, Givertz MM, Stevenson LW, Semigran MJ, Goldsmith SR, et al; NHLBI Heart Failure Clinical Research Network. Low-dose dopamine or low-dose nesiritide in acute heart failure with renal dysfunction: the ROSE acute heart failure randomized trial. JAMA. 2013;310:2533-43. [PMID: 24247300] doi:10.1001/jama.2013.282190

Item 95   Answer: D

Educational Objective: Evaluate suspected infective endocarditis with transthoracic echocardiography.

The most appropriate next step in management is transthoracic echocardiography (TTE). This patient has symptoms and signs that are suspicious for infective endocarditis. According to the modified Duke criteria for infective endocarditis, he meets three minor criteria (injection drug use, fever with temperature >38 °C [100.4 °F], and vascular phenomena [in this case, erythematous nonpainful macular lesions known as Janeway lesions]), which indicates a possible diagnosis of infective endocarditis. A definitive diagnosis may be made with positive blood cultures and characteristic echocardiographic findings. TTE, as a first-line imaging modality, is indicated to identify vegetations or abscesses (diagnostic for infective endocarditis), determine the severity of valvular lesions, assess ventricular function, and detect complications. The sensitivity of TTE is approximately 75%; therefore, a negative imaging test result does not rule out the presence of infective endocarditis, and other imaging modalities should be used.

When the TTE findings are normal or inadequate in patients with a high pretest probability of infective endocarditis, or suspicion remains for undetected complications, further examination with TEE, cardiac CT, or MRI should be considered. The diagnostic sensitivity of TEE for infective endocarditis is approximately 90%. TEE is also superior to TTE in the detection of perivalvular abscesses, leaflet perforation, and other complications. Cardiac CT and chest MRI can be helpful in assessing for the presence of aortic root abscess when TEE is inconclusive, and CT is helpful to identify areas of peripheral embolization, such as in the kidney, spine, spleen, and brain. However, because of cost, accessibility, and invasiveness, TEE, chest MRI, and cardiac CT are not the best initial imaging choices.

KEY POINT

- Transthoracic echocardiography is the first-line imaging modality in patients suspected of having infective endocarditis to identify vegetations, determine the severity of valvular lesions, assess ventricular function, and detect complications.

Bibliography

Baddour LM, Wilson WR, Bayer AS, Fowler VG Jr, Tleyjeh IM, Rybak MJ, et al; American Heart Association Committee on Rheumatic Fever, Endocarditis, and Kawasaki Disease of the Council on Cardiovascular Disease in the Young, Council on Clinical Cardiology, Council on Cardiovascular Surgery and Anesthesia, and Stroke Council. Infective endocarditis in adults: diagnosis, antimicrobial therapy, and management of complications: a scientific statement for healthcare professionals from the American Heart Association. Circulation. 2015;132:1435-86. [PMID: 26373316] doi:10.1161/CIR.0000000000000296

Item 96   Answer: C

Educational Objective: Manage non–ST-elevation acute coronary syndrome with an ischemia-guided approach.

Exercise stress testing is the most appropriate management of this patient with a non–ST-elevation acute coronary syndrome (NSTE-ACS). Many treatment options are available for patients with a NSTE-ACS, and risk stratification tools, such as the TIMI or GRACE risk scores, can be used to aid in diagnostic and therapeutic decision making. An ischemia-guided approach is appropriate in low-risk patients (TIMI score <2 or GRACE score <109), whereas intermediate- and high-risk patients should be treated with an early invasive strategy. With an ischemia-guided approach, cardiac catheterization is reserved for patients at very high clinical risk based on risk score and patients with active or intermittent ischemia, including those with angina despite medical therapy or evidence of ischemia on stress testing. Given this patient's ST-segment depression on electrocardiogram, her TIMI risk

score is 1, or low risk. Stress testing is indicated to guide further management.

Amlodipine may be used to treat patients suspected of having coronary vasospasm. Although this patient's symptoms could be caused by coronary vasospasm, it would be prudent to exclude ischemic heart disease before initiating this treatment.

The benefit of glycoprotein IIb/IIIa inhibitors, such as eptifibatide, appears to be isolated to certain high-risk patients and those undergoing percutaneous coronary intervention, although use of these drugs has been declining in those settings. There is no role for glycoprotein IIb/IIIa blockade in this patient with a low TIMI risk score and normal cardiac enzyme levels.

In patients with NSTE-ACS who have an elevated clinical risk score, significant ST-segment deviation, or elevated cardiac biomarkers, cardiac catheterization is usually performed within 24 hours of presentation. However, an early invasive strategy is not indicated in this patient given her low TIMI risk score.

KEY POINT

- In patients with non–ST-elevation acute coronary syndrome, an ischemia-guided approach is appropriate for patients at low risk based on clinical risk score.

Bibliography

Amsterdam EA, Wenger NK, Brindis RG, Casey DE Jr, Ganiats TG, Holmes DR Jr, et al; ACC/AHA Task Force Members. 2014 AHA/ACC guideline for the management of patients with non–ST-elevation acute coronary syndromes: executive summary: a report of the American College of Cardiology/American Heart Association Task Force on Practice Guidelines. Circulation. 2014;130:2354-94. [PMID: 25249586] doi:10.1161/CIR.0000000000000133

Item 97   Answer: C

Educational Objective: Treat a patient with intermittent claudication with cilostazol.

The most appropriate next step in management is to initiate cilostazol. In patients with intermittent claudication and confirmed lower extremity peripheral artery disease (PAD) with an abnormal ankle-brachial index (≤0.9), American College of Cardiology/American Heart Association guidelines recommend exercise training and medical therapy (cilostazol) to improve limb symptoms. In a meta-analysis of 15 studies, cilostazol, a phosphodiesterase inhibitor with antiplatelet and vasodilator activity, was shown to improve symptoms and walking distance in patients with claudication when compared with placebo. As with other oral phosphodiesterase inhibitors (such as milrinone), the FDA has placed a black box warning on the use of cilostazol in patients with heart failure. This patient with established PAD (left ankle-brachial index of 0.67) has been enrolled in a supervised exercise program but has progressive symptoms, and the next most appropriate step in his management is to add cilostazol to his medication regimen.

PAD is considered a coronary artery disease risk equivalent, and patients with PAD should be treated with a high-intensity statin to prevent cardiovascular events. However, no evidence supports switching atorvastatin to rosuvastatin to reduce limb symptoms in these patients.

Guidelines recommend antiplatelet therapy for patients with PAD to reduce risk for myocardial infarction, stroke, or vascular death. However, in the absence of a specific indication, dual antiplatelet therapy has not been shown to have greater benefit than antiplatelet monotherapy in patients with PAD. Adding clopidogrel to aspirin would not relieve this patient's limb symptoms.

If this patient does not have improvement in his symptoms with cilostazol or cannot tolerate cilostazol therapy, he should be referred for invasive management (endovascular or surgical revascularization).

KEY POINT

- Smoking cessation, exercise training, and medical therapy (cilostazol) are recommended to improve limb symptoms in patients with peripheral artery disease and intermittent claudication.

Bibliography

Gerhard-Herman MD, Gornik HL, Barrett C, Barshes NR, Corriere MA, Drachman DE, et al. 2016 AHA/ACC guideline on the management of patients with lower extremity peripheral artery disease: executive summary: a report of the American College of Cardiology/American Heart Association Task Force on Clinical Practice Guidelines. J Am Coll Cardiol. 2017;69:1465-1508. [PMID: 27851991] doi:10.1016/j.jacc.2016.11.008

Item 98   Answer: A

Educational Objective: Treat supraventricular tachycardia.

The most appropriate next step in treatment is administration of adenosine. This patient, who is symptomatic but hemodynamically stable, has supraventricular tachycardia (SVT). Because supraventricular impulses below the atrioventricular (AV) node are conducted normally, the electrocardiogram in SVT usually reveals narrow-complex tachycardia; however, the QRS complexes can be wide (>120 ms) in the presence of bundle branch block, aberrancy, pacing, or anterograde accessory pathway conduction (antidromic tachycardia). This patient's rhythm is consistent with the presence of an accessory pathway (orthodromic atrioventricular reciprocating tachycardia [AVRT]). Orthodromic AVRT is the most common type of AVRT, accounting for more than 90% to 95% of cases. This type of AVRT has a narrow QRS complex owing to conduction over the AV node and the His-Purkinje system. Vagal maneuvers, such as the Valsalva maneuver (bearing down), are first-line therapy for termination of SVT. Adenosine can be used to interrupt AV conduction if vagal maneuvers are ineffective, such as in this patient. Adenosine may also help ascertain the nature of an arrhythmia. For example, when adenosine is administered to patients with atrial tachycardia and rapid 1:1 conduction, it demonstrates persistent rapid P waves despite AV block, which indicates the presence of an atrial tachycardia. Adenosine is metabolized by adenosine deaminase in the blood and has a very short half-life

(6 seconds). It is contraindicated in preexcited atrial fibrillation with antidromic tachycardia, which presents with a QRS duration greater than 120 ms due to conduction down the accessory pathway.

Amiodarone is frequently used to treat patients with recurrent ventricular tachycardia or maintain sinus rhythm after conversion from atrial fibrillation. It is not a guideline-recommended agent for the treatment of SVT.

Ibutilide is an intravenous antiarrhythmic drug approved for pharmacologic cardioversion of atrial fibrillation and atrial flutter of recent onset (within 7 days). Ibutilide is associated with an increased risk for polymorphic and monomorphic ventricular tachycardia, and several hours of electrocardiographic monitoring is required following administration.

Synchronized cardioversion should be reserved for patients who are hemodynamically unstable or those with continued SVT despite vagal maneuvers and adenosine.

KEY POINT

- Hemodynamically stable patients with supraventricular tachycardia refractory to vagal maneuvers should be given adenosine.

Bibliography

Page RL, Joglar JA, Caldwell MA, Calkins H, Conti JB, Deal BJ, et al; Evidence Review Committee Chair. 2015 ACC/AHA/HRS guideline for the management of adult patients with supraventricular tachycardia: a report of the American College of Cardiology/American Heart Association Task Force on Clinical Practice Guidelines and the Heart Rhythm Society. Circulation. 2016;133:e506-74. [PMID: 26399663] doi:10.1161/CIR.0000000000000311

Item 99   Answer: A

Educational Objective: Diagnose amyloid cardiomyopathy.

The most likely diagnosis is cardiac amyloidosis. This patient has heart failure, elevated right heart pressure, and severe concentric wall thickening with preserved systolic function and severe pulmonary hypertension. The electrocardiogram paradoxically demonstrates low QRS voltage and a "pseudoinfarct" pattern: Q waves in the anteroseptal leads without regional wall motion abnormalities on echocardiogram. The most likely diagnosis is cardiac amyloidosis, likely related to a Val122Ile mutation in transthyretin (*TTR*), which is present in 3% to 4% of the black population. Cardiac amyloidosis should be suspected in black patients older than 50 years who have left ventricular wall thickening that is not explained by loading conditions (for example, hypertension or aortic stenosis) and present with heart failure or features of diastolic dysfunction. Although a monoclonal gammopathy is present in immunoglobulin light-chain (AL) amyloidosis, this is not a feature of TTR amyloidosis. Diagnosis is established by histopathology; endomyocardial biopsy is more sensitive than abdominal fat pad biopsy.

Patients with constrictive pericarditis usually have normal or only mildly increased left ventricular wall thickness. Severe pulmonary hypertension is usually not present.

Amyloidosis may be mistaken for hypertensive heart disease; however, the left ventricular wall thickness in this patient is greater than expected for a patient without hypertensive heart disease. Additionally, electrocardiographic features of left ventricular hypertrophy (increased voltage) would be expected.

Hypertrophic cardiomyopathy may be symmetric and nonobstructive and may demonstrate a restrictive filling pattern on echocardiogram. However, in most cases, the QRS voltage on electrocardiogram is congruent with the degree of hypertrophy.

KEY POINT

- Cardiac amyloidosis should be suspected in black patients older than 50 years who have left ventricular wall thickening that is not explained by loading conditions (for example, hypertension or aortic stenosis) and present with heart failure or features of diastolic dysfunction.

Bibliography

Shah KB, Mankad AK, Castano A, Akinboboye OO, Duncan PB, Fergus IV, et al. Transthyretin cardiac amyloidosis in black Americans. Circ Heart Fail. 2016;9:e002558. [PMID: 27188913] doi:10.1161/CIRCHEART FAILURE.115.002558

Item 100   Answer: A

Educational Objective: Diagnose aortic stenosis associated with repaired aortic coarctation.

This patient most likely has a bicuspid aortic valve with associated aortic stenosis. A bicuspid aortic valve is present in more than 50% of patients with aortic coarctation. The systolic ejection click at the left sternal border suggests a bicuspid aortic valve. The murmur is mid peaking instead of late peaking, and the S_2 is still audible, suggesting mild to moderate aortic stenosis. A bicuspid aortic valve may occur with other cardiovascular and systemic abnormalities, such as aneurysm of the sinuses of Valsalva and patent ductus arteriosus. Patients with a bicuspid aortic valve are predisposed to aortic aneurysm and dissection owing to aortic connective tissue abnormalities. In patients with bicuspid aortic valve, the ascending aortic diameter should be assessed by echocardiography, with the evaluation interval determined by degree and rate of aortic dilation.

Hypertrophic cardiomyopathy is not an expected sequela of aortic coarctation or previous repair. The murmurs in hypertrophic cardiomyopathy characteristically include an ejection-quality systolic murmur at the left sternal border related to outflow obstruction and a late systolic murmur at the apex related to mitral regurgitation from systolic anterior motion of the mitral valve. An ejection click is not heard in patients with hypertrophic cardiomyopathy.

Mitral regurgitation is not an expected finding in a patient with aortic coarctation, with or without previous repair. Clinical features in patients with mitral regurgitation include a holosystolic murmur, heard best at the apex and generally radiating to the axilla.

Recurrent coarctation occurs in approximately 20% of patients with previous coarctation repair. Clinical features include hypertension that is difficult to control with medical therapy and occasional claudication. Other features of recurrent coarctation not demonstrated in this patient include a radial artery–to–femoral artery pulse delay and a systolic murmur over the left anterior or posterior chest.

KEY POINT

- A bicuspid aortic valve is present in more than 50% of patients with aortic coarctation.

Bibliography

Phillips SD, Bonnichsen CR, McLeod CJ, Ammash NM, Burkhart HM, Connolly HM. Adults with congenital heart disease and previous intervention. Curr Probl Cardiol. 2013;38:293-357. [PMID: 23906039] doi:10.1016/j.cpcardiol.2013.05.002

Item 101   Answer: C

Educational Objective: Treat new-onset heart failure with maximal β-blocker therapy.

The dosage of carvedilol should be increased in this patient with new-onset heart failure who is symptomatically improving with standard heart failure therapy. All patients with heart failure with reduced ejection fraction should be treated with an ACE inhibitor and a β-blocker, such as carvedilol, to control heart failure symptoms, improve left ventricular ejection fraction, and decrease mortality. Data suggest improved outcomes with higher dosages of β-blockers. Therefore, in patients with new-onset heart failure, it is generally reasonable to increase the β-blocker dosage every 2 to 4 weeks until the patient achieves a heart rate of approximately 60/min or has symptomatic hypotension. Volume status should always be assessed before initiation and uptitration of a β-blocker because patients with volume overload will experience dyspnea if the dosage is increased. Because this patient has a systolic blood pressure of 120 mm Hg, a heart rate of 84/min, and no evidence of volume overload, he should be able to tolerate an increase in the β-blocker dosage. Repeat echocardiography should be performed to assess for improvement or recovery of ejection fraction once the ACE inhibitor and β-blocker have been uptitrated to maximally tolerated dosages.

Digoxin reduces the incidence of hospitalizations in patients with symptomatic heart failure. This patient is asymptomatic; therefore, there is no reason to start digoxin at this time.

Hydralazine and isosorbide dinitrate improve survival in patients who are black and are already receiving maximal therapy for New York Heart Association functional class III or IV heart failure symptoms. This patient has New York Heart Association functional class I symptoms and is not yet taking optimal dosages of medical therapy; both the ACE inhibitor and β-blocker dosages should be uptitrated before other therapies are added to this patient's medication regimen.

Diuretics are the primary treatment for symptoms of heart failure associated with volume overload. In general, the lowest diuretic dosage that achieves euvolemia should be used. In this patient without evidence of fluid overload, there is no reason to increase the furosemide dosage.

KEY POINT

- All patients with heart failure with reduced ejection fraction should be treated with an ACE inhibitor and a β-blocker; β-blocker dosage should be uptitrated every 2 to 4 weeks until the patient achieves a heart rate of approximately 60/min or has symptomatic hypotension.

Bibliography

Okwuosa IS, Princewill O, Nwabueze C, Mathews L, Hsu S, Gilotra NA, et al. The ABCs of managing systolic heart failure: past, present, and future. Cleve Clin J Med. 2016;83:753-765. [PMID: 27726827] doi:10.3949/ccjm.83a.16006

Item 102   Answer: D

Educational Objective: Treat Mobitz type 2 second-degree atrioventricular block following ST-elevation myocardial infarction.

This patient with Mobitz type 2 second-degree atrioventricular (AV) block following a large anterior myocardial infarction requires temporary pacing. In the peri-infarct setting, arrhythmias are common, and benign forms of vagally mediated heart block must be differentiated from more serious conduction abnormalities. Second-degree AV block is frequently seen with acute myocardial infarction. When progressive PR prolongation is observed before a blocked beat, second-degree Mobitz type 1 (Wenckebach) block is present. When the PR interval is constant before nonconducted P waves, the second-degree block is termed Mobitz type 2 block. When 2:1 block is present, Mobitz type 1 versus type 2 block may not be distinguishable with surface electrocardiography. Mobitz type 2 second-degree AV block is an uncommon but potentially life-threatening electrical complication of an anterior myocardial infarction. It usually represents a block lower in the conduction system and suggests significant conduction disease, likely resulting from ischemia and necrosis of the septum (along which the His-Purkinje system is located). Because of the high risk for progression to complete heart block, prompt implantation of a temporary or permanent pacemaker is indicated.

Atropine improves AV nodal conduction and quickens the sinus rate. In patients with Mobitz type 2 block, atropine may not alter conduction, and the degree of heart block may paradoxically worsen. Furthermore, this agent has a relatively short-lived effect and will not address the underlying pathology.

Cessation of β-blocker therapy alone will not improve conduction in this patient, as the pathology of Mobitz type 2 block is beyond the AV node. In contrast, Mobitz type 1 second-degree AV block is frequently seen with acute inferior myocardial infarction and may be associated with periods of complete heart block. Observation and withholding of AV

nodal blocking agents is appropriate in that context, as the need for permanent pacing is extremely low with inferior myocardial infarction.

In the absence of chest pain or ST-segment elevations on electrocardiogram, urgent angiography is not indicated.

KEY POINT

- Mobitz type 2 second-degree atrioventricular block is an uncommon but potentially life-threatening electrical complication of anterior myocardial infarction; temporary or permanent pacing is indicated in this setting.

Bibliography

Epstein AE, DiMarco JP, Ellenbogen KA, Estes NA 3rd, Freedman RA, Gettes LS, et al; American College of Cardiology/American Heart Association Task Force on Practice Guidelines (Writing Committee to Revise the ACC/AHA/NASPE 2002 Guideline Update for Implantation of Cardiac Pacemakers and Antiarrhythmia Devices). ACC/AHA/HRS 2008 guidelines for device-based therapy of cardiac rhythm abnormalities: a report of the American College of Cardiology/American Heart Association Task Force on Practice Guidelines (Writing Committee to Revise the ACC/AHA/NASPE 2002 Guideline Update for Implantation of Cardiac Pacemakers and Antiarrhythmia Devices) developed in collaboration with the American Association for Thoracic Surgery and Society of Thoracic Surgeons. J Am Coll Cardiol. 2008;51:e1-62. [PMID: 18498951] doi:10.1016/j.jacc.2008.02.032

Item 103   Answer: B

Educational Objective: Diagnose aortopathy in a patient with a bicuspid aortic valve.

The most appropriate next step in management is CT angiography of the aorta. Bicuspid aortic valve is a common congenital heart abnormality, occurring in 1% to 2% of the general population. It is also heritable, and screening of first-degree relatives is recommended. Aortopathy commonly accompanies bicuspid aortic valve disease and may be associated with aortic aneurysm, dissection, and coarctation. Owing to the life-threatening nature of these abnormalities, all patients with a bicuspid aortic valve should be evaluated for possible aortopathy. This patient's severe hypertension suggests the possibility of aortic coarctation. Without a diagnosis and therapeutic intervention, the mean life expectancy of unoperated patients with coarctation of the aorta is only 35 years; major complications consist of early coronary atherosclerosis, stroke, aortic dissection, systemic hypertension, and heart failure. The presence of a radial artery–to–femoral artery pulse delay may be helpful in diagnosis at the bedside, but the definitive study is an imaging evaluation (CT or cardiac magnetic resonance imaging).

Patients with a bicuspid aortic valve and severe aortic stenosis or regurgitation require echocardiography every 6 to 12 months; those with mild stenosis or regurgitation should have echocardiography every 3 to 5 years. This patient does not require annual echocardiography; rather, he should be promptly evaluated for abnormalities of the aorta because of the presence of a bicuspid aortic valve.

Bicuspid aortic valve carries an increased risk for infective endocarditis, and good dental care is important in these patients. However, guidelines no longer recommend antibiotic prophylaxis for this patient population.

Surgical aortic valve replacement is not indicated for mild aortic regurgitation. In general, indications for aortic valve intervention include the presence of symptoms, left ventricular ejection fraction of 50% or less, moderate or severe aortic regurgitation at the time of other cardiac surgery, and significant left ventricular dilatation (end-systolic dimension >50 mm or indexed end-systolic dimension >25 mm/m^2).

KEY POINT

- Bicuspid valve disease is commonly associated with abnormalities of the aorta, including aneurysm, dissection, and coarctation; therefore, all patients with a bicuspid aortic valve should be evaluated for possible aortopathy with CT or cardiac magnetic resonance imaging.

Bibliography

Warnes CA, Williams RG, Bashore TM, Child JS, Connolly HM, Dearani JA, et al. ACC/AHA 2008 guidelines for the management of adults with congenital heart disease: executive summary: a report of the American College of Cardiology/American Heart Association Task Force on Practice Guidelines (writing committee to develop guidelines for the management of adults with congenital heart disease). Circulation. 2008;118:2395-451. [PMID: 18997168] doi:10.1161/CIRCULATIONAHA.108.190811

Item 104   Answer: A

Educational Objective: Identify the impact of diabetes mellitus on risk for atherosclerotic cardiovascular disease.

The factor associated with the highest risk for atherosclerotic cardiovascular disease (ASCVD) is the diagnosis of diabetes mellitus. The presence of diabetes is associated with increased cardiovascular risk, particularly among women. Patients with diabetes have a two to four times increased risk for cardiovascular disease, with more than two thirds of patients with diabetes eventually dying of heart disease. The risk for stroke is increased 1.8- to 6-fold in patients with diabetes. Additionally, patients with diabetes are more likely to have undiagnosed coronary artery disease and have worse outcomes when hospitalized for other cardiovascular diseases, such as heart failure. In this patient, the development of diabetes alone (with all other risk factors held constant) nearly doubled her 10-year risk for ASCVD. Her current 10-year risk, including diabetes, changes in her age, and blood pressure and lipid levels, is 19.4%. Appropriate treatment of cardiovascular risk factors in patients with diabetes is associated with reduced cardiovascular risk. The most recent American College of Cardiology/American Heart Association cholesterol treatment guideline recommends that patients aged 40 to 75 years with diabetes and a 10-year ASCVD risk greater than or equal to 7.5% should receive high-intensity statin therapy. In patients in this age group with diabetes and a 10-year risk less than 7.5%, moderate-intensity statin therapy is recommended.

A diastolic blood pressure of 90 mm Hg, HDL cholesterol level of 30 mg/dL (0.78 mmol/L), systolic blood pressure of 140 mm Hg, and total cholesterol level of 250 mg/dL (6.47 mmol/L) have a relatively small effect on 10-year ASCVD risk compared with the presence of diabetes.

KEY POINT

- Patients with diabetes mellitus have a two to four times increased risk for cardiovascular disease, with more than two thirds of patients with diabetes eventually dying of heart disease.

Bibliography

Lloyd-Jones DM, Huffman MD, Karmali KN, Sanghavi DM, Wright JS, Pelser C, et al. Estimating longitudinal risks and benefits from cardiovascular preventive therapies among Medicare patients: the Million Hearts Longitudinal ASCVD Risk Assessment Tool: a special report from the American Heart Association and American College of Cardiology. J Am Coll Cardiol. 2017;69:1617-1636. [PMID: 27825770] doi:10.1016/j.jacc.2016.10.018

Item 105   Answer: A

Educational Objective: Diagnose infection of a cardiac implanted electronic device.

The most appropriate management of this patient is to obtain a complete blood count, erythrocyte sedimentation rate, and two sets of blood cultures. Patients with a cardiac implanted electronic device can develop a localized tissue infection at the implant site (pocket infection) or a systemic infection with bacteremia (such as endocarditis). These infections can occur after initial implantation, late after implantation, or after a battery replacement or revision. The most common pathogens are skin colonizers, such as the coagulase-negative *Staphylococcus* spp. and *S. aureus*. Symptoms of cardiac device infection include fever, chills, malaise, lassitude, or failure to thrive, especially in the elderly. There may also be local findings suggestive of infection, such as redness or warmth at the pacemaker pocket. These patients should undergo laboratory evaluation for signs of infection. An elevated erythrocyte sedimentation rate, leukocytosis with a left shift, and anemia all suggest infection of a cardiac implanted electronic device. All patients suspected of having infection (with or without fever) should have a minimum of two blood cultures drawn from separate sites. Once there is suspicion for infection of a cardiac implanted electronic device, referral to an electrophysiologist or an infectious disease specialist is mandatory.

Empiric antibiotic therapy without first identifying the presence and cause of the infection is not best medical practice. In addition, antibiotic therapy for a confirmed infection without removal of the device is not curative and is associated with a high fatality rate.

Pacemaker pocket aspiration should never be performed because it can seed a sterile pocket and lead to infection, especially if there is superficial cellulitis without deeper tissue involvement.

In patients with high suspicion of infection despite equivocal laboratory findings, PET/CT can help determine whether there is evidence of local tissue inflammation consistent with a device infection. However, the basic evaluation for infection should be completed and analyzed first.

- In all patients suspected of having infection of a cardiac implanted electronic device, a minimum of two blood cultures should be drawn from separate sites.

Bibliography

Harrison JL, Prendergast BD, Sandoe JA. Guidelines for the diagnosis, management and prevention of implantable cardiac electronic device infection [Editorial]. Heart. 2015;101:250-2. [PMID: 25550318] doi:10.1136/heartjnl-2014-306873

Item 106   Answer: B

Educational Objective: Diagnose an acute exacerbation of heart failure in a patient with COPD.

The most likely cause of this patient's symptoms is an exacerbation of heart failure. He demonstrates the classic heart failure symptoms of dyspnea, orthopnea, and peripheral edema. In particular, the patient's orthopnea, as evidenced by his sleeping in a recliner, correlates with a pulmonary capillary wedge pressure greater than 20 mm Hg, which is suggestive of left-sided heart failure. Other features that increase the likelihood of heart failure include the presence of paroxysmal nocturnal dyspnea (greater than twofold increased likelihood) and the presence of an S_3 (11 times greater likelihood). Factors that would decrease the likelihood of heart failure are the absence of dyspnea on exertion (50% decreased likelihood) and the absence of crackles on pulmonary auscultation. A recently enlarged cardiac silhouette also supports a cardiac process.

An exacerbation of COPD is less likely to be the cause of this patient's dyspnea because the patient has no productive cough. Additionally, exacerbations are commonly precipitated by a respiratory infection, which is absent in this patient.

If clinical findings suggest pneumonia, chest radiography should be performed. The chest radiograph must show an infiltrate for pneumonia to be diagnosed. When clinical symptoms and examination findings otherwise support the diagnosis of pneumonia, a false-negative chest radiograph is a possibility; volume depletion can cause an initial negative finding on chest radiograph that, upon rehydration and repeat imaging, may become positive. The absence of an infiltrate, fever, and lung findings make pneumonia an unlikely cause of the patient's dyspnea.

Deep venous thrombosis with a resultant pulmonary embolism is always a concern in patients with new-onset dyspnea. However, he reports no chest pain, and his dyspnea was slow in onset (over the course of 1 week) rather than an acute process. A pulmonary embolism should be considered in the differential diagnosis, but heart failure is the more likely cause.

- Patients with heart failure classically present with symptoms of dyspnea, paroxysmal nocturnal dyspnea, orthopnea, and peripheral edema.

Bibliography

Wang CS, FitzGerald JM, Schulzer M, Mak E, Ayas NT. Does this dyspneic patient in the emergency department have congestive heart failure? JAMA. 2005;294:1944-56. [PMID: 16234501]

Item 107   Answer: B

Educational Objective: Treat ST-elevation myocardial infarction complicated by ventricular fibrillation.

Primary percutaneous coronary intervention (PCI) is the most appropriate next step in management. ST-elevation myocardial infarction (STEMI) is caused by a complete occlusion of an epicardial coronary artery by a thrombus at the site of plaque disruption. It is defined by the presence of ischemic chest pain (or an equivalent) and the presence of greater than 1-mm ST-segment elevation in two or more consecutive leads or new left bundle branch block on electrocardiogram. This patient presumably has an anterior myocardial infarction, which is complicated by ventricular fibrillation arrest. The electrocardiogram demonstrates left bundle branch block and is assumed to be new in onset. In some cases, ventricular arrhythmias may signify spontaneous reperfusion events, but the new left bundle branch block is worrisome for persistent left anterior descending artery occlusion, which remains the obvious culprit for the patient's presentation. Prompt reperfusion is required. Primary PCI is the preferred method of reperfusion in patients with STEMI.

Amiodarone may be necessary if this patient has recurrent ventricular fibrillation or ventricular tachycardia; however, amiodarone alone is unlikely to control his ischemic-related arrhythmias, and reperfusion is the foremost priority. Furthermore, intravenous amiodarone may precipitate hypotension and shock owing to its acute β-blocking activity, and it must be used carefully in patients with STEMI.

Therapeutic hypothermia is an important adjunct therapy to improve outcomes of patients experiencing out-of-hospital cardiac arrest, although hypothermia protocols are not indicated in noncomatose patients. This patient's arrest was a witnessed arrest, and the patient is awake and conversant.

Coronary artery bypass graft (CABG) surgery is not commonly performed for STEMI. Urgent CABG surgery is typically reserved for patients in whom thrombolytic therapy or PCI has failed, or for those who develop life-threatening mechanical complications, such as ventricular free wall rupture. Compared with PCI and thrombolytic therapy, urgent CABG surgery is associated with an increased death rate in the first 3 to 7 days after STEMI, and this potential harm must be carefully weighed against the potential benefits.

Bibliography

Callaway CW, Donnino MW, Fink EL, Geocadin RG, Golan E, Kern KB, et al. Part 8: Post-cardiac arrest care: 2015 American Heart Association guidelines update for cardiopulmonary resuscitation and emergency cardiovascular care. Circulation. 2015;132:S465-82. [PMID: 26472996] doi:10.1161/CIR.0000000000000262

Item 108   Answer: D

Educational Objective: Diagnose upper extremity peripheral artery disease.

CT angiography is indicated in this patient suspected of having upper extremity peripheral artery disease (PAD). Upper extremity PAD is characterized by atherosclerotic narrowing of the arteries in the upper extremities. Most patients with upper extremity PAD have no symptoms, although patients may present with arm claudication, arm ischemia, or dizziness with arm activity (subclavian steal syndrome). In patients at risk for atherosclerotic cardiovascular disease, measurement of bilateral arm pressures is indicated in asymptomatic and symptomatic patients to assess for upper extremity PAD. A characteristic finding on physical examination is a difference in systolic blood pressures between the arms, typically more than 15 mm Hg. In this patient with exercise-induced arm pain and a systolic blood pressure differential of 35 mm Hg between arms, imaging of the innominate and subclavian arteries with CT angiography is appropriate to confirm the diagnosis of upper extremity PAD and plan for intervention, such as revascularization.

The Adson maneuver (or thoracic outlet maneuver) is used to evaluate for neurovascular impingement at the point where the subclavian vessels and brachial plexus pass the first rib and exit the thoracic cavity. Although thoracic outlet syndrome could account for this patient's arm fatigue, he does not have other symptoms or signs suggestive of this condition (for example, arm edema, numbness/tingling), and thoracic outlet syndrome does not explain his dizziness.

The ankle-brachial index is most useful in diagnosing lower extremity PAD. In this patient with upper extremity symptoms, an ankle-brachial index would not be helpful in confirming a diagnosis of innominate or subclavian stenosis.

Although bilateral carotid artery stenosis has been associated with dizziness or syncope in some patients, the systolic blood pressure differential in the upper limbs and diminished ipsilateral carotid pulsation make this diagnosis unlikely. Therefore, carotid duplex ultrasonography is not the most appropriate next step.

KEY POINT

- Symptoms of upper extremity peripheral artery disease may include arm claudication, arm ischemia, or dizziness with arm activity; CT angiography is useful to confirm the diagnosis and plan for intervention.

Bibliography

Ochoa VM, Yeghiazarians Y. Subclavian artery stenosis: a review for the vascular medicine practitioner. Vasc Med. 2011;16:29-34. [PMID: 21078767] doi:10.1177/1358863X10384174

Item 109   Answer: C

Educational Objective: Treat type A aortic dissection.

The most appropriate next step in the management of this patient with an acute type A aortic dissection is emergent open surgical aortic repair. This patient's CT scan (shown) reveals a dissection plane extending through the aortic arch (*arrow*). Acute aortic dissection classically manifests as sudden-onset chest or back pain that has a tearing or ripping quality, such as in this patient; however, patients may present with hypertension, syncope, a murmur of aortic regurgitation, or heart failure in the setting of sudden aortic insufficiency. Unequal blood pressures in the upper extremities and asymmetric pulses further raise the suspicion for acute aortic dissection. Stanford type A aortic dissections, which originate within the ascending aorta or arch, confer a high risk for death and complications. The early mortality rate is approximately 1% per hour after symptom onset; therefore, patients with acute type A aortic dissection should be evaluated emergently for open surgical repair.

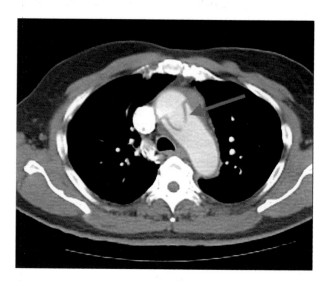

In patients with acute aortic dissection, performing coronary angiography before aortic repair has not been shown to alter in-hospital survival or the need for coronary artery bypass surgery at the time of aortic repair. Furthermore, coronary angiography often delays surgical repair.

Medical therapy for acute aortic dissection includes β-blockers, intravenous nitroprusside, and opioid analgesia. Surgery provides a survival benefit over medical therapy alone and is the definitive treatment.

Emergency surgery is recommended for all patients with type A aortic dissection. Concomitant aortic arch

CONT.

reconstruction, coronary artery reimplantation, aortic valve repair or replacement, or branch vessel repair may be required depending on the anatomy and pathology of the lesion. This patient has evidence of compromise of his right innominate artery with diminished right arm blood pressure and pulses and requires branch vessel repair, not endovascular stenting.

> **KEY POINT**
>
> - Patients with acute type A aortic dissection should be treated emergently with open surgical repair.

Bibliography

Erbel R, Aboyans V, Boileau C, Bossone E, Bartolomeo RD, Eggebrecht H, et al; ESC Committee for Practice Guidelines. 2014 ESC Guidelines on the diagnosis and treatment of aortic diseases: document covering acute and chronic aortic diseases of the thoracic and abdominal aorta of the adult. The Task Force for the Diagnosis and Treatment of Aortic Diseases of the European Society of Cardiology (ESC). Eur Heart J. 2014;35:2873-926. [PMID: 25173340] doi:10.1093/eurheartj/ehu281

Item 110   Answer: C

Educational Objective: Evaluate an asymptomatic murmur with transthoracic echocardiography.

The most appropriate management of this asymptomatic patient with a heart murmur is transthoracic echocardiography (TTE). Diastolic murmurs are always considered abnormal and require further structural evaluation. Systolic murmurs may be either innocent or indicative of significant valve disease. Some murmurs are associated with normal valves but abnormal systemic processes (for example, anemia and other high-output states, such as hyperthyroidism or pregnancy) or increased flow (for example, a systolic murmur in the setting of aortic regurgitation). Innocent murmurs are characteristically brief, are often midsystolic, do not radiate, and are associated with normal heart sounds and no hemodynamic abnormalities. Patients with grade 1 or 2 midsystolic murmurs (grade 1, faintest murmur that can be heard; grade 2, faint murmur but can be identified immediately) who are asymptomatic with no associated findings and those with continuous murmurs suggestive of a venous hum or mammary souffle (a continuous murmur heard over the breast in lactating women) do not warrant echocardiographic evaluation. TTE is indicated for patients with the following findings: (1) a systolic murmur grade 3/6 or higher (grade 3, moderately loud murmur; grade 4, loud murmur associated with a palpable thrill; grade 5, very loud murmur but cannot be heard without the stethoscope; and grade 6, can be heard without a stethoscope); (2) late or holosystolic murmurs; (3) diastolic or continuous murmurs; or (4) murmurs with accompanying symptoms. This patient with a holosystolic murmur that radiates to the axilla needs further evaluation with TTE.

Transesophageal echocardiography (TEE) provides improved image quality over TTE because the probe has only the thin tissue of the esophagus through which to image. TEE is indicated for patients with severe disease who need further quantification, for better identification of leaflet involvement (particularly for patients with mitral regurgitation), or when poor image quality on TTE limits image interpretation. The disadvantage compared with TTE is that it is invasive, requiring sedation and technical expertise distinct from TTE. TEE is not indicated until an initial assessment with TTE is made and findings suggest a need for additional information.

Cardiac magnetic resonance imaging or multidetector CT may provide information on left ventricular function, aortic dimensions, chamber sizes and volumes, and coronary anatomy. As with TEE, CMR imaging should not be performed until after an initial evaluation with TTE.

> **KEY POINT**
>
> - Transthoracic echocardiography is indicated for patients with systolic murmurs grade 3/6 or higher, late or holosystolic murmurs, diastolic or continuous murmurs, and murmurs with accompanying symptoms.

Bibliography

Premkumar P. Utility of echocardiogram in the evaluation of heart murmurs. Med Clin North Am. 2016;100:991-1001. [PMID: 27542419] doi:10.1016/j.mcna.2016.04.005

Item 111   Answer: D

Educational Objective: Evaluate tricuspid regurgitation with transthoracic echocardiography.

The most appropriate next step in management is transthoracic echocardiography. This patient has symptoms and signs consistent with tricuspid regurgitation. Severe tricuspid regurgitation may be well tolerated for a long period. Clinical signs of right-sided heart failure, such as elevated jugular venous pulse and peripheral edema, are an indication of severity. The murmur of tricuspid regurgitation is typically a holosystolic murmur heard along the left sternal border that increases during inspiration due to increased venous return. Causes of tricuspid regurgitation include rheumatic disease, radiation, endocarditis, myxomatous degeneration (prolapse), congenital abnormalities (Ebstein anomaly), carcinoid disease, and trauma (for example, chest wall impact or right ventricular biopsy). Placement of internal device leads for pacemakers and cardioverter-defibrillators is also a common cause of tricuspid regurgitation. In patients with suspected tricuspid regurgitation, transthoracic echocardiography is indicated to evaluate lesion severity, determine the cause, assess the size and function of the right-sided chambers, and estimate pulmonary artery pressures. Transesophageal echocardiography can also help demonstrate the relation of the device leads to tricuspid leaflets as a cause of tricuspid regurgitation.

Cardiovascular magnetic resonance (CMR) imaging may be helpful in the evaluation of tricuspid regurgitation if echocardiographic evaluation is suboptimal or inconclusive. In this patient, the pacemaker presents a contraindication to CMR imaging.

Answers and Critiques

Coronary angiography and right ventriculography are not useful in the diagnosis of tricuspid regurgitation. Unlike mitral regurgitation, ischemic coronary artery disease is not a common cause of tricuspid regurgitation. Evaluation of right heart pressures may be indicated following echocardiography, particularly if there is discordant information obtained by clinical and echocardiographic evaluation, but right heart catheterization is not necessary at this time.

> **KEY POINT**
>
> - In patients suspected of having tricuspid regurgitation, transthoracic echocardiography is indicated to evaluate lesion severity, determine the cause, assess the size and function of the right-sided chambers, and estimate pulmonary artery pressures.

Bibliography

Lin G, Nishimura RA, Connolly HM, Dearani JA, Sundt TM 3rd, Hayes DL. Severe symptomatic tricuspid valve regurgitation due to permanent pacemaker or implantable cardioverter-defibrillator leads. J Am Coll Cardiol. 2005;45:1672-5. [PMID: 15893186]

Item 112   Answer: A

Educational Objective: Manage drug-drug interactions in a patient with stable angina.

The most appropriate management is to decrease the dosage of ranolazine. This patient with stable angina is being transitioned from metoprolol, a β-blocker, to diltiazem, a calcium channel blocker. He is also currently taking several other antianginal therapies, notably ranolazine. Ranolazine decreases angina and modestly increases exercise times in patients with stable angina. Ranolazine inhibits the late sodium current, which in turn reduces sodium-dependent calcium currents, resulting in reduced wall tension and myocardial oxygen consumption. Ranolazine is primarily metabolized by cytochrome P450 3A4 (CYP3A4); therefore, caution should be exercised when prescribing ranolazine with CYP3A4 inhibitors, which will result in significantly increased plasma levels of ranolazine. Ranolazine should not be used with strong CYP3A4 inhibitors, such as keto-conazole, clarithromycin, and ritonavir. With moderate CYP3A4 inhibitors, including verapamil and diltiazem, the dosage should be decreased by 50% and should not exceed 500 mg twice daily. Ranolazine also has a modest QT-prolonging effect, but no proarrhythmic effect has been directly attributed to ranolazine.

The addition of diltiazem to this patient's medication regimen will not require increasing the dosage of atorvastatin. Diltiazem may in fact result in increased levels of atorvastatin, which is a CYP3A4 substrate.

There are no significant drug-drug interactions between lisinopril and diltiazem that would warrant switching to another ACE inhibitor.

Not adjusting this patient's medication regimen would result in excessive plasma levels of ranolazine and is not an acceptable option.

> **KEY POINT**
>
> - Ranolazine decreases symptoms of angina and modestly increases exercise times in patients with stable angina; it should not be used with strong CYP3A inhibitors, and dosage should be reduced when used in conjunction with moderate CYP3A inhibitors, such as diltiazem and verapamil.

Bibliography

Fihn SD, Gardin JM, Abrams J, Berra K, Blankenship JC, Dallas AP, et al; American College of Cardiology Foundation/American Heart Association Task Force. 2012 ACCF/AHA/ACP/AATS/PCNA/SCAI/STS guideline for the diagnosis and management of patients with stable ischemic heart disease: a report of the American College of Cardiology Foundation/American Heart Association task force on practice guidelines, and the American College of Physicians, American Association for Thoracic Surgery, Preventive Cardiovascular Nurses Association, Society for Cardiovascular Angiography and Interventions, and Society of Thoracic Surgeons. Circulation. 2012;126:e354-471. [PMID: 23166211] doi:10.1161/CIR.0b013e318277d6a0

Item 113   Answer: D

Educational Objective: Manage first-degree atrioventricular block accompanied by bifascicular block.

No further testing or intervention is required at this time. This asymptomatic patient has first-degree atrioventricular (AV) block (PR interval >200 ms), right bundle branch block, and left posterior fascicular block. Right bundle branch block is diagnosed by the findings of a widened QRS complex (>120 ms); an RSR′ pattern in lead V_1; and a wide negative S wave in leads I, V_5, and V_6. Blocks may also occur in the anterior or posterior divisions (fascicles) of the left bundle; these are termed fascicular blocks (or hemiblocks). Left anterior fascicular block is recognized by a positive QRS complex in lead I and a negative QRS complex in lead aVF. Left posterior fascicular block is recognized by a negative QRS complex in lead I and a positive QRS complex in lead aVF. Conduction disturbances involving the right bundle branch and one of the two fascicles (anterior or posterior) of the left bundle branch are commonly referred to as bifascicular block. The presence of first-degree AV block with bifascicular block is often called "trifascicular block"; however, the term is misleading because true trifascicular block would indicate complete AV block.

There is no need for extensive cardiac evaluation of patients with asymptomatic bifascicular block other than a careful history and physical examination to exclude the diagnosis of occult cardiac disease. Therefore, echocardiography and dobutamine echocardiography are not indicated because occult ischemic or structural heart disease is not suspected in this patient.

Pacemakers are indicated in patients with symptomatic bradycardia in the absence of a reversible cause, hence the importance of establishing symptoms when evaluating patients with bradycardia. Pacing is not indicated in asymptomatic patients with first-degree AV block accompanied by bifascicular block because the risk for progression to complete heart block is less than 2% to 3% per year. As such, pacemaker insertion is not needed in this patient.

- Asymptomatic first-degree atrioventricular block with bifascicular block does not require pacemaker implantation.

Bibliography

Da Costa D, Brady WJ, Edhouse J. Bradycardias and atrioventricular conduction block. BMJ. 2002;324:535-8. [PMID: 11872557]

Item 114   Answer: E

Educational Objective: Treat heart failure with reduced ejection fraction.

The most appropriate management of this patient with heart failure with reduced ejection fraction (HFrEF) is to continue the current medication regimen. Guideline-directed medical therapy for symptomatic heart failure includes treatment with an ACE inhibitor, β-blocker (specifically, metoprolol succinate, carvedilol, or bisoprolol), and an aldosterone antagonist. All of these agents reduce mortality in patients with HFrEF. This patient is already taking guideline-directed medical therapy at maximally tolerated doses, as evidenced by her symptomatic orthostatic hypotension; therefore, no changes need to be made to her medication regimen.

Ivabradine inhibits the I_f or "I-funny" channel of the sinoatrial node, resulting in a reduction in heart rate. In patients with HFrEF (left ventricular ejection fraction ≤35%) and New York Heart Association functional class II to IV symptoms who are in sinus rhythm with a heart rate of 70/min or higher and taking guideline-directed medical therapy, treatment with ivabradine has been associated with a reduction in heart failure hospitalizations. Before the resting heart rate is assessed for potential initiation of ivabradine, β-blockers should be titrated to maximally tolerated doses. Because this patient has a heart rate of 68/min and is already taking a maximally tolerated dose of carvedilol, she is not a candidate for ivabradine. It is important to note that ivabradine should be given in addition to β-blocker therapy, not in its place.

Valsartan-sacubitril is an angiotensin receptor–neprilysin inhibitor, a new drug class that combines an angiotensin receptor blocker with a neprilysin inhibitor. The neprilysin inhibitor prevents the breakdown of B-type natriuretic peptide, leading to enhanced diuresis, natriuresis, and myocardial relaxation. Compared with ACE inhibitor therapy, this drug combination has been shown to reduce the composite endpoint of cardiovascular death or heart failure hospitalization by 20% in symptomatic patients with HFrEF. However, in a clinical trial assessing response to valsartan-sacubitril, the major cause of withdrawal was hypotension. In this patient who is taking an ACE inhibitor and β-blocker and is experiencing symptomatic orthostatic hypotension, the addition of valsartan-sacubitril is not indicated. Adding valsartan-sacubitril to her current medication regimen, which includes lisinopril, would greatly increase her risk for angioedema and hypotension. ACE inhibitors should be discontinued at least 36 hours before initiating valsartan-sacubitril. If she did not have symptomatic hypotension, switching lisinopril to valsartan-sacubitril would be an appropriate option.

- Guideline-directed medical therapy for symptomatic heart failure with reduced ejection fraction includes an ACE inhibitor, β-blocker (specifically, metoprolol succinate, carvedilol, or bisoprolol), and aldosterone antagonist.

Bibliography

Yancy CW, Jessup M, Bozkurt B, Butler J, Casey DE Jr, Colvin MM, et al. 2016 ACC/AHA/HFSA focused update on new pharmacological therapy for heart failure: an update of the 2013 ACCF/AHA guideline for the management of heart failure: a report of the American College of Cardiology/American Heart Association Task Force on Clinical Practice Guidelines and the Heart Failure Society of America. J Am Coll Cardiol. 2016;68:1476-88. [PMID: 27216111] doi:10.1016/j.jacc.2016.05.011

Item 115   Answer: B

Educational Objective: Treat atrial septal defect.

Percutaneous atrial septal defect (ASD) device closure is the best management choice for this patient depending on favorability of anatomic features. Device closure is performed in the catheterization laboratory and is an option for patients with an isolated ostium secundum ASD. Indications for ASD device closure include right heart enlargement and symptoms. ASD closure is also reasonable for orthodeoxia-platypnea syndrome and before pacemaker placement because of the increased risk for systemic thromboembolism. An asymptomatic small ASD with no right heart enlargement can be monitored without closure. Surgical closure is indicated for nonsecundum ASDs, large secundum ASDs, anatomy unfavorable for device closure, and a secundum ASD in patients with coexistent cardiovascular disease requiring operative intervention, such as coronary artery disease or tricuspid regurgitation.

Cardiac magnetic resonance imaging can be used to detect a secundum ASD and can quantitate the effect of the defect by determining right ventricular volume; however, it is not indicated in this patient because the clinical assessment and echocardiogram are sufficient to guide the decision to close the ASD.

Endocarditis prophylaxis is recommended for patients with congenital heart disease characterized by unrepaired cyanotic disease, including palliative shunts and conduits; a congenital defect during the first 6 months after complete repair of the defect with prosthetic material or device; and repaired disease with residual defects. Patients with an uncomplicated ASD without a history of endocarditis do not require endocarditis prophylaxis.

Functional aerobic capacity measured by stress testing is not generally used to determine management in patients with ASDs.

- Right heart enlargement and symptomatic disease are indications for device closure of an ostium secundum atrial septal defect.

Bibliography

Warnes CA, Williams RG, Bashore TM, Child JS, Connolly HM, Dearani JA, et al; American College of Cardiology. ACC/AHA 2008 guidelines for the management of adults with congenital heart disease: a report of the American College of Cardiology/American Heart Association Task Force on Practice Guidelines (Writing Committee to Develop Guidelines on the Management of Adults With Congenital Heart Disease). Developed in Collaboration With the American Society of Echocardiography, Heart Rhythm Society, International Society for Adult Congenital Heart Disease, Society for Cardiovascular Angiography and Interventions, and Society of Thoracic Surgeons. J Am Coll Cardiol. 2008;52:e143-263. [PMID: 19038677] doi:10.1016/j.jacc.2008.10.001

Item 116   Answer: D

Educational Objective: Treat severe aortic stenosis with transcatheter aortic valve replacement in a patient with high surgical risk.

The most appropriate next step in management is transcatheter aortic valve replacement (TAVR). TAVR has emerged as a life-saving therapy for patients with severe aortic stenosis. In studies of patients with intermediate or high surgical risk, the outcomes of TAVR have been comparable or favorable to that of surgery, with similar rates of mortality and stroke. In the United States, TAVR is currently indicated for symptomatic patients with aortic stenosis and intermediate or high surgical risk, as assessed by a multidisciplinary heart team. Online tools, which are derived and regularly updated from national surgical databases, are available to assist with estimating surgical risk (for example, the Society of Thoracic Surgeons Adult Cardiac Surgery Risk Calculator [riskcalc.sts.org]). Although these calculators contain many data input fields, it is important to note that frailty as well as some other important patient and procedural characteristics are not part of the online assessment tools. Therefore, a comprehensive, holistic approach is required for determining patient surgical risk and candidacy for the various procedures to treat aortic stenosis. Frailty can be assessed with an examination of the patient's activities of daily living, independence in ambulation (for example, 6-minute walk distance), and various other geriatric tools.

Balloon aortic valvuloplasty may be considered as a bridge to transcatheter or surgical aortic valve replacement, but it has not been shown to improve the long-term prognosis of patients with aortic stenosis.

Medical therapy has not been found to be effective in slowing the disease progression in patients with aortic stenosis. Medical therapy would be pursued only if this patient declined aortic valve replacement or if he had morbidities that would preclude benefit from such surgery, such as a reduced life expectancy unrelated to valvular disease.

Surgical aortic valve replacement is not appropriate for this patient because his surgical risk was estimated to be high or prohibitive.

- Transcatheter aortic valve replacement has been found to be comparable to surgical intervention and is indicated for symptomatic patients with aortic stenosis and intermediate or high surgical risk, as assessed by a multidisciplinary heart team.

Bibliography

Smith CR, Leon MB, Mack MJ, Miller DC, Moses JW, Svensson LG, et al; PARTNER Trial Investigators. Transcatheter versus surgical aortic-valve replacement in high-risk patients. N Engl J Med. 2011;364:2187-98. [PMID: 21639811] doi:10.1056/NEJMoa1103510

Item 117   Answer: A

Educational Objective: Treat ST-elevation myocardial infarction complicated by heart failure.

The most appropriate treatment is eplerenone. This patient had an anterior ST-elevation myocardial infarction (STEMI) complicated by moderate left ventricular (LV) dysfunction and heart failure. Optimizing this patient's medical therapy is fundamental to preventing further impairment of LV function and promoting favorable LV remodeling. Although β-blockers and ACE inhibitors (or angiotensin receptor blockers [ARBs]) form the backbone of postinfarction medical therapy aimed at preserving LV function, it is important to recognize when additional agents may be indicated. The EPHESUS trial established the benefits of aldosterone antagonism with eplerenone in patients with acute myocardial infarction and concomitant LV dysfunction, and current guidelines recommend adding an aldosterone antagonist to ACE inhibitor and β-blocker therapy in STEMI patients with left ventricular ejection fraction of 40% or less and either heart failure symptoms or diabetes mellitus. Because of the potassium-sparing effect of eplerenone, serum potassium levels should be carefully monitored. Eplerenone should be used with caution in those with underlying kidney disease.

Long-acting nitrates, such as isosorbide mononitrate, have no role in the management of patients immediately after ST-elevation myocardial infarction. Nitrates may be used for future angina or may be coupled with hydralazine in those with persistent LV dysfunction despite maximally tolerated doses of a β-blocker and ACE inhibitor; however, administering isosorbide mononitrate is not the most appropriate next step in this patient's management.

Although an ARB such as valsartan may be useful as an alternative to ACE inhibitor therapy, adding an ARB to a medication regimen that already includes an ACE inhibitor and β-blocker has been associated with an excess of adverse events and is therefore not recommended.

Warfarin therapy is recommended to reduce the risk for systemic embolization in patients with LV apical clots following large anterior myocardial infarction, although this recommendation is not based on a large randomized dataset. In this patient, no clots were noted on the echocardiogram, and empiric anticoagulation is not indicated according to current guidelines.

KEY POINT

- In patients with ST-elevation myocardial infarction, left ventricular ejection fraction of 40% or less, and either heart failure symptoms or diabetes mellitus, an aldosterone antagonist is recommended in addition to ACE inhibitor and β-blocker therapy.

Bibliography

Pitt B, Remme W, Zannad F, Neaton J, Martinez F, Roniker B, et al; Eplerenone Post-Acute Myocardial Infarction Heart Failure Efficacy and Survival Study Investigators. Eplerenone, a selective aldosterone blocker, in patients with left ventricular dysfunction after myocardial infarction. N Engl J Med. 2003;348:1309-21. [PMID: 12668699]

Item 118   Answer: B

Educational Objective: Diagnose cardiac tamponade following catheter ablation of atrial fibrillation.

The catheter ablation–related complication that is most likely responsible for the patient's symptoms is cardiac tamponade. Although cardiac tamponade occurs in approximately 1% of patients who undergo catheter ablation procedures for atrial fibrillation, it is the most common serious complication and is likely to result in death if not recognized and treated urgently. Cardiac tamponade occurs within a mean of 10 days after the procedure, although it may occur within hours of the procedure or be delayed by weeks. Cardiac tamponade should be suspected when the patient has a compatible history, hypotension, elevated jugular venous pressure, narrow pulse pressure, and pulsus paradoxus. An enlarged cardiac silhouette may be seen on chest radiograph ("water-bottle heart"). The electrocardiogram typically demonstrates sinus tachycardia and electrical alternans. Echocardiography readily detects pericardial effusions and is the primary modality for diagnosing cardiac tamponade.

Patients who develop an atrioesophageal fistula most commonly present 1 to 4 weeks after the ablation procedure. Patients may exhibit a sudden onset of neurologic symptoms from esophageal air embolization. Patients may also present with fever, chest pain, seizures, transient ischemic attack after food intake, hematemesis, and endocarditis. MRI and CT are preferred as diagnostic studies.

Patients who develop dyspnea months to years after atrial fibrillation ablation may have pulmonary vein stenosis. Other symptoms may include cough, chest pain, and hemoptysis. Pulmonary vein stenosis occurs in approximately 1% to 3% of patients, but intervention to relieve symptoms is required in only 10% of these patients. Guidelines recommend CT or MRI as the preferred diagnostic test in symptomatic patients.

Vascular events, including hematomas, pseudoaneurysms at the arterial puncture site, and retroperitoneal hemorrhage from bleeding at the groin access site, are among the most common complications of catheter ablation. Symptoms include hypotension and ipsilateral flank pain. Symptom onset is typically within hours of the procedure. Diagnosis can be established with CT or ultrasonography.

Retroperitoneal hemorrhage cannot explain this patient's distant heart sounds, elevated central venous pressure, or pulsus paradoxus.

KEY POINT

- Cardiac tamponade occurs in approximately 1% of patients who undergo catheter ablation procedures for atrial fibrillation; it is the most common serious complication and is likely to result in death if not recognized and treated urgently.

Bibliography

Maan A, Shaikh AY, Mansour M, Ruskin JN, Heist EK. Complications from catheter ablation of atrial fibrillation: a systematic review. Crit Pathw Cardiol. 2011;10:76-83. [PMID: 21988947] doi:10.1097/HPC.0b013e318224b7bd

Item 119   Answer: D

Educational Objective: Treat heart failure with an implantable cardioverter-defibrillator and cardiac resynchronization therapy.

The most appropriate management is placement of an implantable cardioverter-defibrillator (ICD) with cardiac resynchronization therapy (CRT). This patient has symptomatic heart failure with reduced ejection fraction that is most likely secondary to cardiac sarcoidosis. Although sarcoidosis predominantly affects the lungs, cardiac sarcoidosis is found in up to 10% of patients with sarcoidosis at the time of autopsy, and the diagnosis should always be considered in patients with heart failure and concomitant pulmonary sarcoidosis. In patients with heart failure who have an ejection fraction less than 35%, continued symptoms despite maximally tolerated medical therapy, and expected survival of at least 1 year, ICD placement is indicated. When these criteria are accompanied by left bundle branch block with a QRS duration greater than or equal to 150 ms on electrocardiogram, as in this patient, CRT is also recommended. CRT improves left ventricular ejection fraction, functional capacity, and, most importantly, survival in symptomatic patients with an ejection fraction less than 35% and a wide QRS complex or left bundle branch block.

Diuretics, such as furosemide, are the principal therapy for volume overload in patients with heart failure. Patients should be treated with diuretics until they achieve a state of euvolemia. This patient does not have any evidence of volume overload and therefore does not require a diuretic.

β-Blockers, such as carvedilol, have a mortality benefit in patients with heart failure with reduced ejection fraction. It is generally reasonable to increase the β-blocker dosage every 2 to 4 weeks until the patient achieves a heart rate of approximately 60/min or has symptomatic hypotension. In this patient with a current heart rate below 60/min, increasing the β-blocker dosage is inappropriate.

Although cardiac sarcoidosis can be difficult to diagnose, endomyocardial biopsy is not indicated in suggestive cases. Cardiac sarcoidosis results in patchy myocardial involvement, and a negative biopsy result would not be reassuring that cardiac sarcoidosis is not present. The two imaging modalities that are most sensitive for diagnosing cardiac sarcoidosis are cardiac magnetic resonance imaging and PET.

When sarcoidosis is first diagnosed, treatment with glucocorticoids can improve ejection fraction and reduce arrhythmias. This patient has already been treated with prednisone for 6 months, and further therapy is unlikely to result in additional improvement. Therefore, she should receive an ICD with CRT.

KEY POINT

- Cardiac resynchronization therapy is indicated in patients with an ejection fraction less than or equal to 35%, New York Heart Association functional class II to IV heart failure symptoms despite guideline-directed medical therapy, sinus rhythm, and left bundle branch block with a QRS duration of 150 ms or greater.

Bibliography

Russo AM, Stainback RF, Bailey SR, Epstein AE, Heidenreich PA, Jessup M, et al. ACCF/HRS/AHA/ASE/HFSA/SCAI/SCCT/SCMR 2013 appropriate use criteria for implantable cardioverter-defibrillators and cardiac resynchronization therapy: a report of the American College of Cardiology Foundation appropriate use criteria task force, Heart Rhythm Society, American Heart Association, American Society of Echocardiography, Heart Failure Society of America, Society for Cardiovascular Angiography and Interventions, Society of Cardiovascular Computed Tomography, and Society for Cardiovascular Magnetic Resonance. J Am Coll Cardiol. 2013;61:1318-68. [PMID: 23453819] doi:10.1016/j.jacc.2012.12.017

Item 120   Answer: D

Educational Objective: Treat acute pericarditis.

High-dose aspirin and colchicine are indicated in this patient with acute pericarditis without high-risk features. Acute pericarditis is diagnosed in this patient by the presence of sharp chest pain of acute onset without evidence of myocardial necrosis, an electrocardiogram demonstrating widespread ST-segment elevation and PR-segment depression, and a small pericardial effusion. The elevated C-reactive protein level also supports acute pericarditis. Admission to the hospital is appropriate for patients with acute pericarditis who have at least one high-risk feature, including high fever (temperature >38 °C [100.4 °F]), subacute onset (gradual onset over several days), large pericardial effusion (>20 mm), oral anticoagulation therapy, or immunosuppression. First-line therapy includes aspirin (750-1000 mg) or ibuprofen (600 mg) every 8 hours for 1 to 2 weeks plus colchicine (0.5 mg/d) for 3 months. In this patient, initiation of anti-inflammatory therapy with early outpatient follow-up is appropriate.

Pericardiocentesis is reserved for treatment of patients with tamponade or for diagnosis in patients with pericardial effusion when there is a high clinical suspicion of a malignant, bacterial, or fungal cause.

Cardiac catheterization would be appropriate in the setting of an ST-elevation myocardial infarction to facilitate percutaneous coronary intervention. However, the widespread ST-segment elevation on this patient's electrocardiogram is atypical for ST-elevation myocardial infarction, which more commonly causes ST-segment elevation within a specific vascular distribution. Furthermore, the lack of biomarker evidence of myocardial necrosis after prolonged chest pain does not support a diagnosis of acute coronary syndrome.

Although this patient has risk factors for coronary artery disease, exercise treadmill stress testing has no role. Additionally, in the setting of acute pericarditis, exercise-associated ST-T–wave changes are not interpretable for ischemic coronary artery disease.

KEY POINT

- In patients with acute pericarditis, first-line treatment is high-dose aspirin or NSAIDs and adjuvant colchicine therapy.

Bibliography

Adler Y, Charron P, Imazio M, Badano L, Barón-Esquivias G, Bogaert J, et al; European Society of Cardiology (ESC). 2015 ESC guidelines for the diagnosis and management of pericardial diseases: the Task Force for the Diagnosis and Management of Pericardial Diseases of the European Society of Cardiology (ESC). Endorsed by the European Association for Cardio-Thoracic Surgery (EACTS). Eur Heart J. 2015;36:2921-64. [PMID: 26320112] doi:10.1093/eurheartj/ehv318

Index

Note: Page numbers followed by f and t denote figures and tables, respectively. Test questions are indicated by Q.